Principles and Practice of Veterinary Science

Principles and Practice of Veterinary Science

Edited by Gerardo Bailey

SYRAWOOD
PUBLISHING HOUSE

New York

Published by Syrawood Publishing House,
750 Third Avenue, 9th Floor,
New York, NY 10017, USA
www.syrawoodpublishinghouse.com

Principles and Practice of Veterinary Science
Edited by Gerardo Bailey

© 2017 Syrawood Publishing House

International Standard Book Number: 978-1-68286-476-0 (Hardback)

Cataloging-in-Publication Data

Principles and practice of veterinary science / edited by Gerardo Bailey.
  p. cm.
Includes bibliographical references and index.
ISBN 978-1-68286-476-0
1. Veterinary medicine. 2. Animals--Diseases. 3. Veterinary therapeutics. 4. Animal health. I. Bailey, Gerardo.
SF745 .P75 2017
636.089--dc23

Printed in the United States of America.

TABLE OF CONTENTS

PREFACE

Veterinary science is an extensive field of study. From theories to research to practical applications, case studies related to all contemporary topics of relevance in the field of veterinary science have been included in this book. Veterinary science deals with the diagnosis of diseases in animals along with its treatment and prevention. This book is a valuable compilation of topics, ranging from the basic to the most complex advancements in this discipline. For all readers who are interested in veterinary science, the case studies included in this book will serve as an excellent guide to develop a comprehensive understanding. It will help new researchers by foregrounding their knowledge in this branch. This book is an essential guide for both academicians and those who wish to pursue this discipline further.

Significant researches are present in this book. Intensive efforts have been employed by authors to make this book an outstanding discourse. This book contains the enlightening chapters which have been written on the basis of significant researches done by the experts.

Finally, I would also like to thank all the members involved in this book for being a team and meeting all the deadlines for the submission of their respective works. I would also like to thank my friends and family for being supportive in my efforts.

Editor

Prevalence of parasitic infection in captive wild animals in Bir Moti Bagh mini zoo (Deer Park), Patiala, Punjab

A. Q. Mir[1], K. Dua[1], L. D. Singla[2], S. Sharma[1] and M. P. Singh[3]

1. Department of Veterinary Medicine, Guru Angad Dev Veterinary and Animal Sciences University, Ludhiana - 141 004, Punjab, India; 2. Department of Veterinary Parasitology, Guru Angad Dev Veterinary and Animal Sciences University, Ludhiana - 141 004, Punjab, India; 3. Mahendra Choudhury Zoological Park, Chhatbir, Punjab, India.
Corresponding author: A. Q. Mir, e-mail: aqmirrp@gmail.com,
KD: kirtidua@yahoo.com, LDS: ldsingla@gmail.com, SS: drshukriti@yahoo.co.in, MPS: mps1032@rediffmail.com

Abstract

Aim: The study was conducted to know the prevalence of gastrointestinal parasites of captive wild animals at Bir Moti Bagh Mini Zoo (Deer Park), Patiala, Punjab.

Materials and Methods: A total of 31 fecal samples from eight species of captive animals including Civet cat (*Viverra zibetha*), Porcupine (*Hystrix indica*), Nilgai (*Boselaphus tragocamelus*), Spotted deer (*Axis axis*), Black buck (*Antelope cervicapra*), Sambar deer (*Cervus unicolor*), Hog deer (*Axis porcinus*), and Barking deer (*Muntiacus muntjak*) were screened using classical parasitological techniques including sedimentation and floatation technique.

Results: Out of 31 fecal samples examined, 20 were positive for parasitic ova/oocysts of different species indicating an overall prevalence of 68.0%. The six different types of parasites observed in the study included strongyle (67%), *Strongyloides* spp. (14%), coccidia (38%), *Trichuris* spp. (19%), ascarid (10%), and *Capillaria* spp. (10%). *Strongyles* were the most common parasites observed (67%) followed by coccidia (38%). Mixed helminth and protozoan infection were observed in 48% of animals. No cestode or trematodes were detected during the study.

Conclusion: The high prevalence of gastrointestinal parasites without overt clinical signs of disease or mortality as observed in this study is suggestive of subclinical infection. The findings will help in formulating the appropriate deworming protocol for parasitic control in these captive animals.

Keywords: captive wild animals, carnivores, parasitic infection, Punjab, rodent, ungulates.

Introduction

Zoos are an *ex-situ* form of conservation where animals are displayed in cages or enclosures for esthetic, educational or research, and conservation purposes [1]. Zoo populations are distinctive as they are maintained to educate the public regarding wildlife and their habitats and/or to preserve critically endangered species through captive breeding and reintroduction programs [2]. Parasites and infectious diseases have become a major concern in conservation of endangered species as they can lead to mortality, dramatic population declines, and even contribute to local extinction events [3-6]. Some studies have revealed that gastrointestinal parasites of wild animals in captivity include zoonotic species to humans and raise public health concerns [7-12].

Parasitic diseases often represent a major concern in zoo animals for the high environmental contamination due to the maintenance of animals in confined areas [13,14]. In wild conditions, animals have some natural resistance against parasitic diseases and there is a state of equilibrium between the parasite and the host and it seldom lead to harmful infection unless stressed [15]. In captivity wild animals may succumb to parasitic infections due to environmental stress such as change in the living conditions and space limitations [16,17]. The constant stress of captivity makes animals more susceptible to parasitic infection as the immune system of these captive animals becomes weak [14,18]. Studies on parasitic diseases of wildlife are still in infancy in India with only few systematic studies having been undertaken, and data are still on the base line [19].

To have a better understanding about the prevalence of the endoparasites affecting zoo animals, this study attempts to investigate the occurrence of helminth parasites of animals in Bir Moti Bagh Mini Zoo (Deer Park), Patiala, Punjab.

Materials and Methods

Ethical approval

The ethics committee for animal experiments from the Guru Angad Dev Veterinary and Animal Sciences University granted an approval (IAEC/2014/1) during XXXIII meeting of Institutional Animal Ethics Committee for the conduction of work.

Study site

The study was conducted at Bir Moti Bagh Mini Zoo (Deer Park) in the Patiala Wildlife Sanctuary located between 30°17'13.86"N latitude and 76°23'47.09"E longitude and at an altitude of 258 m (846 ft) during Jan-Feb, 2015. The sanctuary is located at a distance of 5 km from Patiala on Patiala-Dakala Road and is spread over 654 ha of state land. This mini zoo is home to nine species of mammals with 213 animals. The climate of the place is generally dry with rains during monsoon season. The average maximum and minimum temperature during January is 20.2°C and 7.1°C, respectively, while in June maximum temperature can go up to 44.4°C. The average annual rainfall in the district is 604.3 mm.

The zoo is separated into open enclosures for ungulates with different species having separate units except that of Black buck which is kept in two units. Civet cat and porcupines are housed in closed enclosures. The indoor and outdoor enclosures are cleaned on a routine basis with necessary prophylaxis. The prophylactic measures apart from regular deworming involved using the foot dips at the entrance of the zoo and also at each enclosure, tilling of enclosure area at regular intervals and adding some lime to destroy the larvae. The animals are fed black gram, cattle feed, and green fodder on daily basis with jaggery (gur) once a week. The zoo is a closed type having no introduction of any outside animal at least for past 5 years.

Animals sampled

A total of 31 fecal samples from eight species of animals belonging to ungulates, felines, and rodents were collected (Table-1). Among the eight species of captive animals surveyed in this study, 1 (3.2%) was felid, 2 (6.4%) were rodent, and 28 (90%) were ungulates. Fresh samples were collected in polythene bags from individual enclosures housing different species of animals. The properly labeled interlocked polythene bags containing the fecal samples were brought to the laboratory of the Department of Parasitology, Guru Angad Dev Veterinary and Animal Sciences University, for parasitological examination.

Sample processing

The fecal samples were subjected to detailed routine parasitological analysis for the presence of parasitic eggs/oocysts by direct smear examination, standard sedimentation, and floatation techniques [20].

Results and Discussion

This study revealed the presence of both helminth and protozoan parasites in Bir Moti Bagh Mini Zoo (Deer Park), Patiala, Punjab. Out of the total 31 fecal samples screened, 21 (68%) samples were positive for gastrointestinal parasitic infection as given in Table-1. Previously, different workers have reported the prevalence of similar parasitic infection in captive zoo animals from Nigeria, Italy, and Malaysia and among workers and inmates in a Nigerian zoo [10-12,21,22].

Table-1: Prevalence of parasitic infection in captive wild animals in Bir Moti Bagh mini zoo.

Animals	Total animals	Sample collected	Positive (%)	Parasite observed						Mixed infection
				Nematodes					Protozoa	
				Strongyle	Trichuris	Ascarid	Strongyloides	Capillaria	Coccidia	
Civet cat (V. zibetha)	01	01	01 (100)	01	-	01	-	-	-	01[a]
Porcupine (H. indica)	05	02	02 (100)	-	02	01	-	02	-	02[b,c]
Nilgai (B. tragocamelus)	09	04	04 (100)	02	01	-	01	-	04	03[d,e]
Spotted deer (A. axis)	62	08	04 (50)	03	01	-	-	-	01	01[f]
Black buck (A. cervicapra)	98	08	06 (75)	06	-	-	01	-	01	02[e,g]
Sambar (C. unicolor)	10	03	02 (66)	01	-	-	-	-	02	01[e]
Hog deer (A. porcinus)	26	04	01 (25)	01	-	-	-	-	-	-
Barking deer (M. muntjak)	02	01	01 (100)	-	-	-	01	-	-	-
Percent prevalence	213	31	21 (68)	14 (67%)	04 (19%)	02 (10%)	03 (14%)	02 (10%)	08 (38%)	10 (48%)

[a]Strongyle and Toxascaris leonine, [b]Trichuris, Capillaria and ascarid, [c]Trichuris and Capillaria, [d]Coccidia, Trichuris and Strongyloides, [e]Coccidia, Trichuris and Strongyle, [f]Trichuris and Coccidia, [g]Strongyle and Strongyloides. V. zibetha=Viverra zibetha, H. indica=Hystrix indica, B. tragocamelus=Boselaphus tragocamelus, A. axis=Axis axis, A. cervicapra=Antelope cervicapra, C. unicolor=Cervus unicolor, A. porcinus=Axis porcinus, M. muntjak=Muntiacus muntjak

However, the prevalence was higher than reported earlier by other authors [1,23,24]. The eggs/oocysts of six different types of parasites were observed in the study including strongyle (67%), *Strongyloides* spp. (14%), coccidia (38%), *Trichuris* spp. (19%), ascarid (10%), and *Capillaria* spp. (10%). *Strongyles* spp. were the most common parasites observed (67%) followed by coccidia (38%). Infections with trematodes and cestodes were not detected in this study. Helminth infection was more common than protozoal infection with nematode eggs observed in 19 (90%) affected animals while protozoans were observed in only 8 (38%) animals out of the total positive animals [21]. Similar findings were reported by Fagiolini *et al.* and Lim *et al.* [21,22], who also reported higher helminth than protozoal infection in Italian zoo. However, it is contrary to the studies of Levecke *et al.*, Cordon *et al.*, and Gomez *et al.* [7,18,25], who reported higher protozoal infection compared to helminthic infection. 48% of the parasitic infections were mixed infections comprising two or more helminth or protozoan parasites, whereas 52% of the infections comprised of only one parasite. Among the ungulates, the highest prevalence of mixed infection was observed in Nilgai (75%). *Toxascaris leonina* was observed in captive civet cat in this study, and earlier studies have also reported the parasite from captive felids [26].

The eggs/oocysts of six different types of parasites, *viz.*, strongyle, *Strongyloides* spp., coccidia, *Trichuris* spp., ascarid, and *Capillaria* spp. were observed in the study, and the majority of the animals examined in this study were infected with at least one intestinal parasite species. The gastrointestinal parasites species identified in this study have previously been recorded in captive animals in various zoos and zoological garden by other authors [27-29]. *Strongyles* were found to most prevalent parasites in this study which could be due to more conducive environment for the development of the pre-parasites stages in the hot and humid environmental conditions of this region [30,31].

The intensive husbandry of wild animals in zoos and zoological parks may be one of the reasons for the higher infection as high animal density in enclosures and their proximity to other species of animals provides opportunity for transmission of parasites [32]. Moreover, it has been observed that confinement of wild animals in zoo makes them more prone to different parasitic infections despite proper attention to feeding, water, and maintenance of hygiene in captivity [33]. The nematodes and some coccidian parasites have a direct life cycle, i.e., they do not involve any intermediate host and are transmitted by feco-oral route through contaminated feed, water, and soil and have the potential to accumulate in a captive environment [1]. Since all the parasites recorded in this study have direct life cycle and have the ability to survive in the environment, there is a high possibility of environmental contamination as the reason for their higher

prevalence [7,18,25]. Trematodes and cestodes were not detected in this study. This could be due to the fact that these parasites (mainly trematodes and some cestodes) require an intermediate host for their transmission and are less likely to accumulate in the captive environment [17]. Since the wild animals in zoos are maintained in closed enclosures giving no chance of accessibility to the intermediate hosts of trematodes and cestodes. The environmental contamination could be through contaminated water or fodder, and even zoo workers have also been reported to play a role in transmission by acting as vectors and transmitting parasites through their shoes, clothes, hands, food, or with working tools [8,34,35]. In the present zoo, there was no foot dip at the entrance of each cage/enclosure although the foot dip was present at the entrance of the zoo there is possibility that zoo workers cleaning the cages and enclosures could act as a vehicle (fomite) for the transmission of parasites as the pathogens may be present in the zoo environs.

Conclusion

As there was no reported mortality and clinical signs, and animal were apparently healthy during the period of examination, the high prevalence indicates subclinical infection which may flare up under stress conditions and can cause pathogenicity. Although overall management of zoo including nutrition, sanitation, and deworming practices was followed, the study identifies that there is scope for improvement in the management of the zoo by re-standardizing/re-investigating or re-scheduling anthelmintic program, regular examinations for parasitic infections and early season treatments to prevent infection.

Authors' Contributions

AQM performed the study and wrote the manuscript, KD and LDS helped in planning, execution of work, and edited the manuscript, SS helped in analysis, and MPS contributed for collection of samples from wild animals.

Acknowledgments

The authors are thankful to the Dean, Postgraduate Studies, Guru Angad Dev Veterinary and Animal Sciences University, Ludhiana and Chief Wildlife Warden, Punjab, for providing all available helps to undertake this investigation.

Competing Interests

The authors declare that they have no competing interest.

References

1. Thawait, V.K., Maiti, S.K. and Dixit, A.A. (2014) Prevalence of gastro-intestinal parasites in captive wild animals of Nandan Van Zoo, Raipur, Chhattisgarh. *Vet. World,* 7(7): 448-445.

2. Schulte-Hostedde, A.I. and Mastromonaco, G.F. (2015) Integrating evolution in the management of captive zoo populations. *Evol. Appl.,* 8(5): 413-422.

3.   Aguirre, A.A., Keefe, T.J., Reif, J.S., Kashinsky, L., Yochem, P.K., Saliki, J.T., Stott, J.L., Dubey, J.P., Goldstein, T., Braun, R. and Antonelis, G. (2007) Infectious disease monitoring of the endangered Hawaiian monk seal. *J. Wildl. Dis.*, 43: 229-241.

4.   Wisely, S.M., Howard, J., Williams, S.A., Bain, O., Santymire, R.M., Bardsley, K.D. and Williams, E.S. (2008) An unidentified filarial species and its impact on fitness in wild populations of the black-footed ferret (*Mustela nigripes*). *J. Wildl. Dis.*, 44: 53-64.

5.   Smith, K.F., Sax, D.F. and Lafferty, K.D. (2006) Evidence for the role of infectious disease in species extinction and endangerment. *Conserv. Biol.*, 20: 1349-1357.

6.   Smith, K.F., Acevedo-Whitehouse, K. and Pedersen, A.B. (2009) The role of infectious diseases in biological conservation. *Anim. Conserv.*, 12: 1-12.

7.   Levecke, B., Dorny, P., Geurden, T., Vercammen, F. and Vercruysse, J. (2007) Gastrointestinal protozoa in primates of four zoological gardens in Belgium. *Vet. Parasitol.*, 148: 236-246.

8.   Otegbade, A.C. and Morenikeji, O.A. (2014) Gastrointestinal parasites of birds in zoological gardens in south-west Nigeria. *Trop. Biomed.*, 31(1): 54-62.

9.   Adekunle, B.A. and Olayide, J.A. (2008) Preliminary investigation zooanthroposis in a Nigerian zoological garden. *Vet. Res.*, 2(3-4): 38-41.

10. Akinboye, D.O., Ogunfetimi, A.A., Fawole, O., Agbolade, O. and Ayinde, O.O. (2010) Control of parasitic infections among workers and inmates in a Nigerian Zoo. *Nig. J. Parasitol.*, 31: 35-38.

11. Opara, M.N., Osuji, C.T. and Opara, J.A. (2010) Gastrointestinal parasitism in captive animals at the zoological garden, Nekede Owerri, Southeast Nigeria. *Rep. Opin.*, 2(5): 21-28.

12. Ajibade, W.A., Adeyemo, O.K. and Agbede, S.A. (2010) Coprological survey and inventory of animals at Obafemi Awolowo University and University of Ibadan zoological gardens. *World J Zool.*, 5(4): 266-271.

13. Citino, S.B. (2003) Bovidae (except sheep and goat) and antilocapridae. In: Fowler, M.E. and Miller, R.E., editors. Zoo & Wild Animal Medicine. 5th ed. Saunders, W. B., Philadelphia, PA, p672.

14. Gracenea, M., Gomez, M.S., Torres, J., Carne, E. and Fernandez-Moran, J. (2002) Transmission dynamics of *Cryptosporidium* in primates and herbivores at the Barcelona Zoo: A long-term study. *Vet. Parasitol.*, 104: 19-26.

15. Gaur, S.N.S., Sethi, M.S., Tewari, H.C. and Prakash, O. (1979) A note on the prevalence of helminth parasites in wild and zoo animals in Uttar Pradesh. *Indian J. Anim. Sci.*, 46: 159-161.

16. Rana, M.A., Jabeen, F., Shabnam, M., Ahmad, I. and Hassan, M.M. (2015) Comparative study of endo-parasites in captive hog deer (*Axis porcinus*). *Int. J. Biosci.*, 6(1): 162-170.

17. Atanaskova, E. (2011) Endo-parasites in wild animals at the zoological garden in Skopje, Macedonia. *J. Threat. Taxa*, 3(7): 1955-1958.

18. Cordon, G.P., Prados, A.H., Romero, D., Moreno, S.M., Pontes, A., Osuna, A. and Rosales, M.J. (2008) Intestinal parasitism in the animals of the zoological garden "Pena Escrita" (Almunecar, Spain). *Vet. Parasitol.*, 156: 302-309.

19. Islam, S. (2006) Parasites and parasitic diseases of wildlife. Proceedings of XVII National Congress of Veterinary Parasitology and National Symposium on "Strengths, Challenges and Opportunities" in Veterinary Parasitology. p43-52.

20. Soulsby, E.J.L. (1982) Helminths, Arthropods and Protozoa of Domesticated Animals. 7th ed. Baillière Tindall, London.

21. Fagiolini, M., Riccardo, P.L., Piero, L., Paolo, C., Riccardo, M. and Stefania, P. (2010) Gastrointestinal parasites in mammals of two Italian zoological gardens. *J Zoo Wild. Med.*, 41(4): 662-670.

22. Lim, Y.A.L., Ngui, R., Shukri, J., Rohela, M. and Naim, H.R.M. (2008) Intestinal parasites in various animals at a zoo in Malaysia. *Vet. Parasitol.*, 157: 154-159.

23. Gurler, A.T., Beyhan, Y.E., Acici, M., Bolukbas, C.S. and Umur, S. (2010) Helminths of mammals and birds at the Samsun zoological garden, Turkey. *J. Zoo Wild. Med.*, 2: 218-223.

24. Adeniyi, I.C., Morenikeji, O.A. and Emikpe, B.O. (2015) The prevalence of gastro-intestinal parasites of carnivores in university zoological gardens in South West Nigeria. *J. Vet. Med. Anim. Health*, 7(4): 135-139.

25. Gomez, M.S., Torres, J., Gracenea, M., Montoliu, I., Feliu, C., Monleon, A., Fernadez, M.J. and Ensenanat, C. (1996) Intestinal parasitism protozoa and helminthes in primates at the Barcelona Zoo. *J Med. Prim.*, 25: 419-423.

26. Mamun, M.A., Shakif-Ul-Azam, M., Islam, N., Bari, T. and Khatun, M. (2014) Incidence of intestinal helminths in Asiatic lions (*Panthera leo persica*) at Dhaka Zoo, Bangladesh. *Zoo's Print*, 29(11): 22.

27. Arunachalam, K., Senthilvel, K. and Anbarasi, P. (2015) Endo parasitic infections in free living rhesus macaque (*Macaca mulatta*) of Namakkal, Tamil Nadu, India. *Zoo's Print*, 30(6): 20-21.

28. Singh, P., Gupta, M.P., Singla, L.D., Sharma, S., Sandhu, B.S. and Sharma, D.R. (2006) Parasitic infections in wild herbivores in the Mahendra Choudhury zoological park, Chhatbir, Punjab. *Zoo's Print. J.*, 21(11): 2459-2461.

29. Varadharajan, A., Ramesh, V. and Pythal, C. (2000) Does sex influence prevalence of parasitic infection among captive wild mammals? An observation at the zoological garden, Thiruvananthapuram, Kerala. *Zoo's Print. J.*, 15(7): 307-308.

30. Wadhawa, A., Tanwar, R.K., Singla, L.D., Eda, S., Kumar, N. and Kumar, Y. (2011) Prevalence of gastrointestinal helminths in cattle and buffaloes in Bikaner, Rajasthan, India. *Vet. World*, 4(9): 417-419.

31. Singla, L.D. (1995) A note on sub-clinical gastro-intestinal parasitism in sheep and goats in Ludhiana and Faridkot districts of Punjab. *Indian Vet. Med. J.*, 19: 61-62.

32. Moudgil, A.D. and Singla, L.D. (2013) Role of neglected wildlife disease ecology in emergence and resurgence of parasitic diseases. *Trends Parasitol. Res.*, 2(2): 18-23.

33. Kashid, K.P., Shrikhande, G.B. and Bhojne, G.R. (2002) Incidence of gastrointestinal helminths in captive wild animals at different locations. *Zoo's Print. J.*, 18(3): 1053-1054.

34. Dakshinkar, et al. (1983) Occurrence of *Trichuris* sp. in deer (Axis axis). *Veterinarian*, 7(11): 9.

35. Adetunji, V.E. (2014) Prevalence of gastro-intestinal parasites in primates and their keepers from two zoological gardens in Ibadan, Nigeria. *Sokoto J. Vet. Sci.*, 12(2): 25-30.

Assessment of immune response to a lyophilized peste-des-petits-ruminants virus vaccine in three different breeds of goats

S. S. Begum[1], G. Mahato[2], P. Sharma[3], M. Hussain[4] and A. Saleque[5]

1. Research Associate, ICAR-NRC on Yak, Dirang - 790 101, Arunachal Pradesh, India; 2. Department of Veterinary Epidemiology and Preventive Medicine, College of Veterinary Science, Assam Agricultural University, Khanapara Campus, Guwahati - 781 022, Assam, India; 3. Virologist, North East Regional Disease Diagnostic Laboratory, Khanapara, Guwahati - 781 022, Assam, India; 4. Senior Technical Officer, ICAR-NRC on Yak, Dirang - 790 101, Arunachal Pradesh, India; 5. Chief Scientist, Goat Research Station, Assam Agricultural University, Burnihat, Kamrup - 793 101, Assam, India.
Corresponding author: S. S. Begum, e-mail: dr.safeeda_begum@rediffmail.com,
GM: gaurangamahato@yahoo.com, PS: drparesh59@gmail.com, MH: hussainmokhtar61@gmail.com,
AS: saleque.abdus@yahoo.in

Abstract

Aim: Immune response to a lyophilized peste-des-petits-ruminants virus (PPRV) vaccine was evaluated in three different breeds of goats.

Materials and Methods: Three breeds of goats consisting six number of animals in three groups, i.e., Group A (local Assam hill goat), Group B (cross-bred), and Group C (Beetal goats) were randomly selected for evaluating the immune response to a lyophilized PPRV vaccine.

Results: A higher rise in the overall mean serum antibody titer was observed in Group A (40.50 ± 3.74) than in Group B (37.58 ± 37.58) and Group C (35.90 ± 3.29) during the study period.

Conclusion: Initially, a negative PPRV specific serum antibody titer was recorded in all the groups at 0th day of vaccination. Serum antibody titer in the vaccinated goats started rising gradually from the 14th day post vaccination. Later higher rise in the overall mean serum antibody titer in Group A (local Assam hill goat) lead to the conclusion that higher serum antibody titer in local non-descript breed might be due to their better adaptation to the environmental condition.

Keywords: goat, immune, peste-des-petits-ruminants, vaccine.

Introduction

Peste-des-petits-ruminants (PPR) is an important contagious viral disease of goats and sheep, often associated with high morbidity and mortality and was first reported in sheep and goats, in 1942, in Côte d'Ivoire, West Africa. It is emerging in new regions of the world, causing significant economic losses [1] and threatens the food security and sustainable livelihood of farmers across Africa, the Middle East, and Asia [2]. Although presence of PPR-like disease has been suspected earlier in a retrospective study [3], its presence was confirmed in India, in 1987, from Arasur village of Villupuram district of Tamil Nadu [4].

The disease causes more severe lesions in goats than sheep [5], and in India, the disease occurs round the year with the maximum outbreaks reported during the winter and rainy seasons. Therefore, vaccination just before the onset of rainy/winter season is considered as an appropriate step for the control of the disease. Of late, three groups of scientists have developed vero cell line based live attenuated PPR vaccines around the world using the different lineage of PPR virus (PPRV) of either goat or sheep origin for prophylaxis of disease [6-9]. Studies have been carried out to identify the sources of variation and also to unravel the genetic variance in the PPRV vaccine elicited immune response in goat kids [10]. Such studies have revealed significant variability for response to vaccination, which may be due to significant sources of variation such as environmental determinants, cohort, age at vaccination, and maternal environment. Study of comparative immunogenicity of two PPR vaccines in South Indian sheep and goats under field conditions gave no significant difference between the two strains, revealing that the two vaccine strains are equally efficacious [11].

Currently, PPR outbreaks are being reported regularly from different parts of the country [12-17], and there are very few reports on the prevalence of the disease in Assam. Furthermore, since vaccination is the mainstay for the control of PPR for goats in India, keeping these points in view, the present study was undertaken to assess the immune response of a lyophilized PPRV vaccine.

Materials and Methods

Ethical approval

Ethical approval for the study was obtained from Institutional Animal ethics Committee of College of Veterinary Science, Assam Agricultural University, Khanapara, Guwahati-781022, Assam.

Management profiles

The goats were maintained under semi-intensive system of management. The floors of the animal houses were either build with concrete cement or wooden planks and were cleaned regularly with broom and water by the concerned persons, and no bedding material was provided in any of the herd. Common feeding troughs were used for feed and water. Artificial insemination or natural breeding with selected bucks was done in the farm.

Selection of animal

Relevant data regarding age, sex, and previous history of infection were recorded for all the animals to ascertain the significance of these factors with positive cases of PPRV infection. During the study, apparently healthy goats were selected for vaccination. The status of parasitic infestation was evaluated on the basis of fecal examination and history of deworming whenever required, the animals were dewormed with Fentas plus @ 1 tablet per 10-30 kg body weight orally 10 days before vaccination.

Reference vaccine

The lyophilized PPRV vaccine was procured from Raksha-PPR, Indian Immunologicals (batch no.01PPR29/11).

Vaccination of animals

The vaccine was reconstituted with 100 ml of the diluent (provided with the vaccine) to prepare 100 doses, and then, it was administered subcutaneously at 1 ml per goat. The vaccinated goats were monitored for 48 h after primary vaccination, and no changes in the body temperature or any other clinical signs were observed.

Collection of serum samples

Serum samples from the vaccinated animals were collected at 0, 14, 30, 45, 60, and 90 days of post-vaccination for assay of PPRV specific antibody titer.

Assay of PPRV specific antibody titer was done using PPR c-ELISA kit for PPRV antibody detection that was obtained from Rinderpest Laboratory, Division of Virology, IVRI, Mukteswar.

Statistical analysis

Statistical analysis for assay of PPRV antibody was done using Statistical Package for Social Sciences, version 14.

Results and Discussion

Initially, a negative PPRV specific serum antibody titer was recorded in all the groups at 0th day of vaccination. Serum antibody titer in the vaccinated goats started rising gradually, and a higher rise in the overall mean serum antibody titer was observed in Group A (40.50 ± 3.74) than in Group B (37.58 ± 37.58) and Group C (35.90 ± 3.29) during the study period (Table-1).

From the present study, it was observed that higher serum antibody titer in local non-descript breed might be due to their relatively high resistance to disease and better adaptation to the environmental condition. The influence of stress factor in antibody production has also been observed, and it has been recorded that stress can inhibit the development of lymphocyte response to antigen, e.g. the response to a vaccine [18]. Exotic animals might have suffered from adaptability stress, and thereby, this may hamper insufficient production of antibody following immunization for which there was lower antibody titer in comparison to local non-descript and crossbred goats. Attenuated *Morbillivirus* vaccines also induce cell-mediated immunity [19], which may be important for protection. It is not clear which immune effectors (systemic neutralizing antibodies, cytotoxic T-cell, or mucosal immunity) can be correlated with protection following vaccination with the PPRV vaccine, but antibodies are most likely to be involved because the passive transfer of immunity via colostrum may provide protection [20,21].

The control group did not show any antibody titer to the vaccine throughout the study period, and statistical analysis showed a highly significant difference ($p<0.01$) of antibody titer between the groups, days of vaccination, and within the groups and days (Table-2).

Apart from the importation of animals from disease-free region, vaccination with the commercially available attenuated vaccine is one of the best measures for prevention of the disease. A number of attenuated vaccines in freeze-dried form, recombinant subunit vaccine, DNA vaccine, etc., are commercially

Table-1: Mean±SE of serum antibody titer of vaccinated and control group of goats.

GROUP no.	0 day	14 days	30 days	45 days	60 days	90 days	Overall mean
A (Local)	*	$27.07\pm8.56^{a}{}_{A}$	$51.27\pm0.13^{b}{}_{A}$	$52.68\pm0.12^{b}{}_{A}$	$54.78\pm0.41^{b}{}_{A}$	$57.20\pm0.78^{b}{}_{A}$	40.50 ± 3.74^{a}
B (Cross bred)	*	$40.55\pm0.27^{a}{}_{B}$	$42.29\pm0.62^{ab}{}_{B}$	$43.96\pm0.60^{ac}{}_{B}$	$48.04\pm1.38^{bc}{}_{A}$	$50.65\pm1.50^{c}{}_{AB}$	37.58 ± 37.58^{b}
C (Beetal)	*	$27.41\pm8.68^{a}{}_{A}$	$43.95\pm1.15^{b}{}_{B}$	$45.58\pm1.12^{b}{}_{A}$	$48.72\pm0.76^{b}{}_{A}$	$49.76\pm0.69^{b}{}_{B}$	35.90 ± 3.29^{b}
D (Control)	*	*	*	*	*	*	*
Overall mean	*	23.76 ± 4.19^{a}	34.38 ± 4.21^{b}	35.56 ± 4.34^{b}	37.89 ± 4.61^{bc}	39.40 ± 4.80^{c}	

*No antibody titer. Means bearing same subscript does not differ significantly in a row. Means bearing same superscript does not differ significantly in a column. SE=Standard error

Table-2: Analysis of variance for variate titer.

Source of variation	df	Sum of square	Mean sum of square	F value
Animal group	3	39366.28	13122.09	332.04**
Days	5	27024.44	5404.89	136.76**
Animal group×Day	15	10222.80	681.519	17.25**
Error	120	4742.34	39.52	

**p<0.01

available now-a-days for vaccinating the animals against PPR. Current vaccination schedules require the immunization of susceptible animal at least every 3 years [22,23], and vaccination in animals of 4-6 months age is recommended [24].

Animals vaccinated with an attenuated PPR vaccine are unable to transmit the challenge virus to animals with which they are in contact [25]. Furthermore, vaccinated animals produce high amount of neutralizing antibodies against the H, F, and F proteins similar to those recovered from a natural infection [26,27]. In a report, a single immunization with PPR vaccine conferred solid protection in sheep and goats for 3 years [28].

Conclusion

Based on the present study, we conclude that local breed of goats showed a higher immune response to Raksha-PPR vaccine (Indian immunological) than crossbred and Beetal breeds. Although live attenuated vaccines are able to induce both humoral and cell-mediated immune response and to keep long-term neutralizing antibodies against PPRVs at a high level, a potential possibility in the reversion of vaccine strains to virulence, albeit unreported so far, should not be neglected [29]. Availability of a marker vaccine (for differentiation of vaccinated animals and infected animals by use of an appropriate diagnostic tool) against PPR along with associated diagnostic tools may ease the PPR eradication program both in India and also at the global level [30].

Authors' Contributions

The present study was a part of SSB's original research work during Ph.D. thesis program. GM and PS had designed the plan of work. SSB and MH carried out the experiment in the farm, and SSB carried out the laboratory work. SSB, GM, PS, and AS analyzed the results. All the authors read and approved the final manuscript.

Acknowledgments

Thanks are due to Dr. D. Muthuchelvan, Senior Scientist, IVRI, Mukteshwar, for his support during this study. The authors are thankful to Director, North East Regional Disease Diagnostic Laboratory, Khanapara, Guwahati - 781 022, Assam and Dean, College of Veterinary Science, Assam Agricultural University, Khanapara, Guwahati - 781 022, Assam, for providing necessary facilities for the present study.

Competing Interests

The authors declare that they have no competing interests.

References

1.	Banyard, A.C., Wang, Z. and Parida, S. (2014) Peste des petits ruminants virus, Eastern Asia. *Emerg. Infect. Dis. J.*, 20: 2176-2177.

2.	Banyard, A.C., Parida, S., Batten, C., Oura, C., Kwiatek, O. and Libeau, G. (2010) Global distribution of peste des petits ruminants virus and prospects for improved diagnosis and control. *J. Gen. Virol.*, 91: 2885-2897.

3.	Taylor, W.P., Diallo, A., Gopalakrishna, S., Sreeramalu, P., Wilsmore, A.J., Nanda, Y.P., Libeau, G., Rajasekhar, M. and Mukhopadhyay, A.K. (2002) Peste des petits ruminants has been widely present in southern India since, if not before, the late 1980s. *Prev. Vet. Med.*, 52(3-4): 305-312.

4.	Shaila, M.S., Purashothaman, V., Bhavsar, D., Venugopal, K. and Venkatesan, R.A. (1989) Peste des petits ruminants of sheep in India. *Vet. Rec.*, 125:602.

5.	Muthuchelvan, D., Rajak, K.K., Ramakrishnan, M.M., Choudhary, D., Bhadouriya, S., Saravanan, P., Pandey, A.B. and Singh, R.K. (2015) Peste-des-petits-ruminants: An Indian perspective. *Adv. Anim. Vet. Sci.*, 3(8): 422-429.

6.	Diallo, A., Taylor, W.P., Lefevre, P.C. and Provosta, A. (1989) Attenuation of a virulent PPR strain potential homologous live vaccine. *Rev. Elevage Med. Vet. Des Pays Trop. (Paris).*, 42: 311-319.

7.	Singh, R.K., Balamurugan, V., Bhanuprakash, V., Sen, A., Saravanan, P. and Yadav, M.P. (2009) Possible control and eradication of peste des petits ruminants from India: Technical aspects. *Vet. Ital.*, 45(3): 449-462.

8.	Singh, R.P. (2011) Control strategies for peste des petits ruminants in small ruminants of India. *Rev. Sci. Tech.*, 30(3): 879-887.

9.	Singh, R.P., De, U.K. and Pandey, K.D. (2010) Virological and antigenic characterization of two peste des petits ruminants (PPR) vaccine viruses of Indian origin. *Comp. Immunol. Microbiol. Infect. Dis.*, 33(4): 343-353.

10.	Gowane, G.R., Akram, N., Misra, S.S., Prakash, V. and Kumar, A. (2016) Assessment of the antibody response to peste des petits ruminants (PPR) disease vaccination in a flock of Sirohi goat kids. *Small Rumin. Res.*, 138: 20-24.

11.	Santhosh, A.K., Gomes, A.R., Hegde, R., Rathnamma, D., Veeregowda, B.M., Byregowda, S.M., Renukaprasad, C., Bhanuprakash, V., Prabhudas, K., Hegde, N.R. and Isloor, S. (2013) Comparative immunogenicity of two peste des petitis ruminants (PPR) vaccines in South Indian sheep and goats under field conditions. *Indian J. Virol.*, 24(3): 373-379.

12.	Chauhan, H.C., Lambade, P.S., Sen, A., Dadawala, A.I., Ranaware, P.B., Chandel, B., Joshi, D.V., Patel, S.S., Pankaj, K., Shah, N.M. and Kher, H.N. (2011) The use of pathological and histopathological techniques in the diagnosis of peste des petits ruminants in India. *Vet. Ital.*, 47(1): 41-47.

13.	Kerur, N., Jhala, M.K. and Joshi, C.G. (2008) Genetic characterization of Indian peste des petits ruminants virus (PPRV) by sequencing and phylogenetic analysis of fusion protein and nucleoprotein gene segments. *Res. Vet. Sci.*, 85(1): 176-183.

14.	Muthuchelvan, D., De, A., Debnath, B., Choudhary, D., Venkatesan, G., Rajak, K.K., Sudhakar, S.B., Himadri, D., Pandey, A.B. and Parida, S. (2014) Molecular characterization of peste-des-petits ruminants virus (PPRV) isolated from an outbreak in the Indo-Bangladesh border of Tripura state of North-East India. *Vet. Microbiol.*, 174(3-4): 591-595.

15.	Nanda, Y.P., Chatterjee, A., Purohit, A.K., Diallo, A., Innui, K., Sharma, R.N., Libeau, G., Thevasagayam, J.A.,

Brüning, A., Kitching, R.P., Anderson, J., Barrett, T. and Taylor, W.P. (1996) The isolation of peste des petits ruminants virus from northern India. *Vet. Microbiol.*, 51(3-4): 207-216.

16. Raghavendra, A.G., Gajendragad, M.R., Sengupta, P.P., Patil, S.S., Tiwari, C.B., Balumahendiran, M., Sankri, V. and Prabhudas, K. (2008) Seroepidemiology of peste des petits ruminants in sheep and goats of southern peninsular India. *Rev. Sci. Tech. Int. Off. Epizoot.*, 27(3): 861-867.

17. Singh, R.P., Saravanan, P., Sreenivasa, B.P., Singh, R.K. and Bandyopadhyay, S.K. (2004) Prevalence and distribution of peste des petits ruminants virus infection in small ruminants in India. *Rev. Sci. Tech. Int. Off. Epiz.*, 23(3): 807-819.

18. Merlot, E. (2004) Conséquences du stress sur la function immunitaire chez les animaux d'élevage. *INRA Prod. Anim.*, 17(4): 255-264.

19. Lund, B.T., Tiwari, A., Galbraith, S., Baron, M.D., Morrison, W.I. and Barrett, T. (2000) Vaccination of cattle with attenuated rinderpest virus stimulates CD4 (+) T cell responses with broad viral antigen specificity. *J. Gen. Virol.*, 81: 2137-2146.

20. Gans, H.A. and Maldonado, Y.A. (2013) Loss of passively acquired maternal antibodies in highly vaccinated populations: An emerging need to define the ontogeny of infant immune responses. *J. Infect. Dis.*, 208: 1-3.

21. Ata, F.A., al Sumry, H.S., King, G.J., Ismaili, S.I. and Ata, A.A. (1989) Duration of maternal immunity to peste des petits ruminants. *Vet. Rec.*, 124: 590-591.

22. Diallo, A., Minet, C., Goff, C.l., Berhe, G., Albina, E., Libeau, G., Barrett, T. and le Goff, C. (2007) The threat of peste des petits ruminants: Progress in vaccine development for disease control. *Vaccine*, 25: 5591-5597.

23. Saravanan, P., Balamurugan, V., Sen, A., Sreenivasa, B.P., Singh, R.P., Bandyopadhyay, S.K. and Singh, R.K. (2010) Immune response of goats to a vero cell adapted live attenuated homologous PPR vaccine. *Indian Vet. J.*, 87: 1-3.

24. Balamurugan, V., Saravanan, P., Sen, A., Rajak, K.K., Venkatesan, G., Krishnamoorthy, P., Bhanuprakash, V. and Singh, R.K. (2012) Prevalence of peste des petits ruminants among sheep and goats in India. *J. Vet. Sci.*, 13: 279-285.

25. Kumar, N., Maherchandani, S., Kashyap, S.K., Singh, S.V., Sharma, S., Chaubey, K.K. and Ly, H. (2014) Peste des petits ruminants virus infection of small ruminants: A comprehensive review. *Viruses*, 6: 2287-2327.

26. Diallo, A., Barrett, T., Lefevre, P.C. and Taylor, W.P. (1987) Comparison of proteins induced in cells infected with rinderpest and peste des petits ruminants viruses. *J. Gen. Virol.*, 68: 2033-2038.

27. Sinnathamby, G., Naik, S., Renukaradhya, G.J., Rajasekhar, M., Nayak, R. and Shaila, M.S. (2001) Recombinant hemagglutinin protein of rinderpest virus expressed in insect cells induces humoral and cell mediated immune responses in cattle. *Vaccine*, 19: 3870-3876.

28. Zahur, A.B., Irshad, H., Ullah, A., Afzal, M., Latif, A., Ullah, R.W., Farooq, W., Samo, M.H., Jahangir, M., Ferrari, G., Hussain, M. and Ahmad, M.M. (2014) Peste des petits ruminants vaccine (Nigerian strain 75/1) confers protection for at least 3 years in sheep and goats. *J. Biosci. Med.*, 2: 27-33.

29. Liu, F., Wu, X., Liu, W., Li, L. and Wang, Z. (2014) Current prospectives on conventional and novel vaccines against peste des petits ruminants. *Vet. Res. Commun.*, 38: 307-322.

30. Singh, R.P. and Bandyopadhyay, S.K. (2015) Peste des petits ruminants vaccine and vaccination in India: Sharing experience with disease endemic countries. *Virus Dis.*, 26(4): 215-224.

3

Effect of dietary iodine on production of iodine enriched eggs

Shaikh Sumaiya[1], Sunil Nayak[1], R. P. S. Baghel[1], Anju Nayak[2], C. D. Malapure[1] and Rajesh Kumar[1]

1. Department of Animal Nutrition, College of Veterinary Science and Animal Husbandry, Jabalpur - 482 001, Madhya Pradesh, India; 2. Department of Veterinary Microbiology, College of Veterinary Science and Animal Husbandry, Jabalpur - 482 001, Madhya Pradesh, India.
Corresponding author: Sunil Nayak, e-mail: sunilnayak91@yahoo.com,
SS: drsumaiyakoul@gmail.com, RPSB: rameshbaghel@yahoo.co.in, AN: nayakanju@rediffmail.com,
CDM: cdmalapure@gmail.com, RK: rajeshkumarmahla46@gmail.com

Abstract

Aim: Objective of this study was to investigate the effect of different levels of iodine supplementation on iodine content of eggs in laying hens.

Materials and Methods: In the experiment, 135 laying hens (White Leghorn) of 55 weeks age were randomly distributed to 5 dietary treatments; each group contained 27 laying hens distributed in three replicates of 9 birds each. Diet T_1 was control basal layer diet without iodine enrichment in which iodine content (I_2) was as per NRC recommendation. Basal diets were supplemented with calcium iodate (Ca $(IO_3)_2$) at 5, 10, 15 and 20 mg/kg in T_2, T_3, T_4 and T_5 groups, respectively. The iodine content in the calcium iodate is 65.21%, therefore, the diets T_2, T_3, T_4 and T_5 contained 3.25, 6.50, 9.75 and 13.0 ppm iodine, respectively. The laying hens were fed the respective experimental diets *ad libitum* during the experimental period of 10-week. The iodine content of egg yolk and albumen was analyzed at the end of 5th and 10th week of the experiment. Economics of feeding for the production of iodine enriched egg was calculated at the end of the experiment.

Results: Increasing iodine levels in diet of hens from 0.45 to 13.0 ppm significantly increased egg iodine concentration, the highest concentration of egg iodine was observed in the group fed diet supplemented with 13.0 ppm iodine followed by those fed 9.75, 6.50, 3.25 and 0.45 ppm iodine in diet. There was no significant difference in the iodine levels of unboiled versus boiled eggs. Therefore, the consumers are ensured to receive the optimal levels of iodine from boiled iodine-enriched eggs. Among different diets, minimum and significantly lower feeding cost (Rs. per dozen or per kg eggs) was noticed in hens allotted T_3 diet (6.50 ppm I_2). However, feeding cost of hens receiving 3.25 and 9.25 ppm I_2 was statistically (p<0.05) similar to control group (T_1). Further, it was noticed that feeding cost (Rs. per dozen or per kg eggs) was significantly increased due to the inclusion of higher level of iodine (13.0 ppm).

Conclusion: It was concluded that supplementing iodine at 6.50 ppm in layers diet was economically better for the production of iodine enriched eggs followed by feed iodine supplementation at 3.25 ppm as compared to control and other treatment groups.

Keywords: eggs, iodine, layers, performance.

Introduction

Egg is considered as a complete food with the most of the nutrients required for well-being. In addition to the nutrients already available in the egg if we can alter or incorporate certain health beneficiary nutrients then these eggs will be the choice of food for health conscious people and can reduce the chances of occurrence of certain diseases. Enriched egg with trace minerals results in eggs with superior biological and nutritional value for human consumption [1]. Surveys carried out by Indian Council of Medical Research have shown that no state or union territory is free from the problem of iodine deficiency disorders (IDDs). Out of 586 districts in the country, 281 districts have been surveyed for IDD and 41 districts have been found to be endemic [2], therefore, an improvement of iodine supply is still a great challenge for nutritionists.

Iodine (I_2) is an essential micronutrient for humans and animals and its deficiency reduces the production of thyroid hormones, leads to the morphological and functional changes of the thyroid gland [3]. Fortification of various nutrients in egg is solely dependent on nutritional manipulation of the laying hen's ration [4]; therefore, iodine enrichment can be achieved by dietary manipulation of hen's diet. McDowell [5] pointed to a preferential interception of iodine in the hen ovary and an easy passage of iodine to oocytes. Experimental knowledge of factors participating in the relatively easy iodine passage to yolk makes it possible to increase iodine content in eggs.

The significance of this study is that the iodine supplementation in layer diets could increase the levels of iodine in hen eggs and can lead to prevention of iodine deficiency in humans.

The aim of this study was to investigate the effect of supplementation of iodine at different levels in layers diet on egg iodine content and economics of feeding.

Materials and Methods

Ethical approval

The experiment on animals including all procedures of this study was approved by Institutional Animal Ethics Committee.

Stock, diet and husbandry

In the experiment, 135 laying hens (White Leghorn) of 55 weeks age were randomly distributed to 5 dietary treatments; each group contained 27 laying hens distributed in three replicates of 9 birds each. T_1 was basal layer diet without iodine enrichment (control), in which iodine (I_2) content was as per NRC [6] recommendation (0.45 ppm). Basal diets were supplemented with calcium iodate ($Ca (IO_3)_2$) at 5, 10, 15 and 20 mg/kg in T_2, T_3, T_4 and T_5 groups, respectively. Therefore, dietary iodine (I_2) content in diets T_2, T_3, T_4 and T_5 was 3.25, 6.50, 9.75 and 13.00 ppm, respectively. All the diets were formulated as per NRC [6] recommendation using feed ingredients such as maize, soybean meal, and de-oiled rice polish. Ingredients and nutrient composition of all the diets are presented in Table-1. The experiment was for 10 weeks.

All the laying hens were shifted to experimental layer house. The system of rearing was cage system. The house was cleaned, white washed, fumigated, and sprayed with disinfectant before introducing the birds in it and was provided with a sufficient light source. Layer mash was offered *ad-libitum* to the hens in feeders. Care was taken that feeders are full of feed at all time and constant watch was kept to avoid feed wastage. An ample supply of clean and fresh drinking water was made available to the laying hens all the time through simple water channel type waterer. During the experiment, the eggs were collected thrice daily, i.e., at 9.00 am; 12.00 noon and at 3.00 pm replicate wise and where weighed at 4.00 pm daily.

Parameters studied

Total 60 eggs (12 eggs from each treatment) were collected randomly at the end of 5th and 10th week of the experiment for iodine estimation. The iodine concentration in the egg yolk and albumin was determined by a spectrophotometer method (440 nm) using alkaline ashing based on the Sandell-Kolthoff reaction [7]. The principle of the assessment was the reduction of Ce^{4+} to Ce^{3+} in the presence of As^{3+} and the catalytic effect of iodine. Mineralization took place in an alkaline medium at 600°C. In this method, organic sample fades away as the result of a high temperature and iodine released from the organic compound attaches to alcoholic group. The resulting product was not soluble in acid and thus the iodine content was determined chromatographically. In this method, iodine catalyzes a reductive oxidation reaction. In the same manner

Table-1: Ingredients and nutrient composition of layer diets (%).

Ingredients	Diets				
	T_1	T_2	T_3	T_4	T_5
Maize (kg)	53.00	53.00	53.00	53.00	53.00
DORP (kg)	16.80	16.80	16.80	16.80	16.80
SBM (kg)	19.00	19.00	19.00	19.00	19.00
DCP (kg)	0.400	0.400	0.400	0.400	0.400
LSP (kg)	03.00	03.00	03.00	03.00	03.00
Shell grit (kg)	07.00	07.00	07.00	07.00	07.00
Salt (kg)	0.360	0.360	0.360	0.360	0.360
$MnSO_4$ (kg)	0.054	0.054	0.054	0.054	0.054
$ZnSO_4$ (kg)	0.10	0.10	0.10	0.10	0.10
$CuSO_4$ (kg)	0.01	0.01	0.01	0.01	0.01
$FeSO_4$ (kg)	0.139	0.139	0.139	0.139	0.139
$Ca (IO_3)_2$ (kg)	0.004	0.032	0.065	0.097	0.13
Vitamin A, B_2, D_3, K (kg)*	0.025	0.025	0.025	0.025	0.025
Vitamin B complex (kg)*	0.005	0.005	0.005	0.005	0.005
Salinomycin (kg)	0.044	0.044	0.044	0.044	0.044
Total (kg)	100.00	100.00	100.00	100.00	100.00
Nutrient composition analyzed					
CP (%)	16.15	16.32	16.20	16.29	16.27
Ca (%)	03.47	03.56	03.38	03.65	03.73
Iodine (mg/kg)	0.45	03.25	06.50	09.75	13.00
Nutrient composition calculated					
ME (kcal/kg)	2602	2602	2602	2602	2602
Lysine (%)	0.66	0.66	0.66	0.66	0.66
Methionine (%)	0.26	0.26	0.26	0.26	0.26

*Vitamin premix provided (each 250 g contains): Vitamin A – 10,000,000 IU; Vitamin D_3 – 2,000,000 IU; Vitamin B_1 – 800 mg; Vitamin B_2 – 5 g; Vitamin B_6-1.6 g; Vitamin B_{12}- 20.5 g; Niacin - 12.0 g; Calcium D panthothenate - 8.0 g; Vitamin K_3- 1.0 g; Vitamin E - 8.0 g; Folic acid – 800 mg, DCP=Digestible crude protein, LSP=Left sacrum posterior, SBM=Soybean meal, DORP=De-oiled rice polish

the iodine content was also measured after boiling the eggs.

All the experimental diets were analyzed for proximate compositions as per AOAC [8]. The economics of feeding was calculated as the cost of feed consumed in rupees for production of one dozen eggs as well as for one kg egg mass.

Statistical analysis

The data obtained during the experiment were analyzed statistically using the methods described by Snedecor and Cochran [9]. Differences between the treatments were tested for significance by Duncan's new multiple range test using statistical software SPSS.

Results

Effects of dietary iodine on iodine composition of egg

The concentration of iodine in egg yolk and albumen (before and after boiling) of laying hens fed on various levels of iodine after 5th week of supplementation is presented in Table-2. The treatment means of the iodine concentration in eggs (before boiling) of laying hens fed on various levels of iodine after 5th week of supplementation indicated that the inclusion of different levels of iodine significantly (p<0.05) increased iodine content of egg yolk as well as albumen. Maximum and significantly (p<0.05) higher iodine content in egg yolk (1.17±0.025 µg/g) and egg albumin (0.12±0.001 µg/g) were recorded in layers assigned T_5 (13 ppm I_2) diet. Iodine content in egg yolk and albumen linearly decreased in layers assigned T_4 (9.7 ppm I_2), T_3 (6.50 ppm I_2), and T_2 (3.25 ppm I_2) diets, respectively. Minimum and significantly (p<0.05) lowest concentration of iodine content in egg yolk (0.19±0.005 µg/g) and egg albumin (0.02±0.002 µg/g) was found in layers assigned T_1 (control) diet. The treatment means of the iodine concentration in eggs (after boiling) indicated that the use of higher levels of iodine significantly (p<0.05) increased iodine content of egg yolk as well as albumen. Maximum and significantly (p<0.05) higher iodine content of egg (after boiling) was noted in layers assigned T_5 (13 ppm I_2) diet. Iodine content in boiled egg yolk and albumen linearly decreased in layers assigned T_4 (9.75 ppm I_2), T_3 (6.50 ppm I_2) and T_2 (3.25 ppm I_2) diets, respectively. It was observed that about 10-15% iodine was lost after boiling the eggs.

Iodine concentration in egg yolk and albumen (before and after boiling) of laying hens fed various levels of iodine after 10th week of supplementation (before and after boiling) is presented in the Table-3. The trend for iodine content in egg yolk and albumen was similar in the case of both boiled and unboiled eggs. The iodine content of eggs was significantly influenced due to the inclusion of different levels of iodine above recommended levels in the diet of laying hens. Among iodine supplemented groups, maximum

and significantly (p<0.05) higher iodine content of egg yolk and albumen was recorded in hens assigned T_5 (13 ppm I_2) diet. Iodine content in egg yolk and albumen linearly decreased in layers assigned T_4, T_3 and T_2 (9.75, 6.50 and 3.25 ppm I_2) diets, respectively. Significantly (p<0.05) lowest iodine concentration in egg yolk and albumin was found in layers assigned T_1 (control) diet. The treatment means of the iodine concentration indicated that, use of higher levels of iodine significantly (p<0.05) increased iodine content of egg yolk as well as albumen. Further, it was observed that about 10-15% iodine is lost on boiling the eggs.

Effect of iodine supplementation on economics of feeding

The economics of feeding for the production of iodine enriched eggs is presented in Table-4. The results of this study revealed that among iodine supplemented diets, significantly (p<0.05) lowest feeding cost (Rs. per dozen or per kg egg mass) was noticed in layers receiving 6.50 ppm iodine in their diet. However, feeding cost (Rs. per dozen or per kg egg mass) of layers receiving 3.25 and 9.75 ppm iodine in their diet was statistically similar (p>0.05) and comparable to control (0.45 ppm I_2). Further, inclusion of higher levels of iodine significantly (p<0.05) increased the feeding cost (Rs. per dozen or per kg eggs) in layers. Feed cost (Rs. per kg) was near about similar in all treatments since the price of iodine source was very low.

Discussion

Iodine content in eggs yolk and albumen, both after 5th week and 10th week of supplementation, linearly increased with the increasing iodine levels (0.45, 3.25, 6.50 and 13.0 ppm I_2) in their diets. This increment may be due to the higher iodine transfer from

Table-2: Concentration of iodine in eggs of laying hens fed on various levels of iodine after 5th week of supplementation (before and after boiling).

Treatments	Iodine level (ppm)	Yolk iodine (µg/g)		Albumen iodine (µg/g)	
		Before boiling	After boiling	Before boiling	After boiling
T_1	0.45	0.19^e±0.005	0.17^d±0.014	0.02^d±0.002	0.02^c±0.002
T_2	03.25	0.27^d±0.005	0.20^d±0.014	0.04^c±0.001	0.03^c±0.001
T_3	06.50	0.52^c±0.029	0.44^c±0.015	0.07^b±0.002	0.06^b±0.002
T_4	09.75	0.81^b±0.008	0.71^b±0.018	0.08^b±0.003	0.07^b±0.001
T_5	13.00	1.17^a±0.025	1.03^a±0.012	0.12^a±0.001	0.11^a±0.002

Mean values bearing different superscript differ significantly (p<0.05)

Table-3: Concentration of iodine in eggs of laying hens fed on various levels of iodine after 10th week of supplementation (before and after boiling).

Treatments	Iodine level (ppm)	Yolk iodine (µg/g)		Albumen iodine (µg/g)	
		Before boiling	After boiling	Before boiling	After boiling
T_1	0.45	0.20^e±0.014	0.18^e±0.017	0.02^e±0.001	0.02^e±0.001
T_2	03.25	0.28^d±0.014	0.23^d±0.020	0.05^d±0.001	0.04^d±0.002
T_3	06.50	0.60^c±0.014	0.51^c±0.014	0.07^c±0.001	0.06^c±0.002
T_4	09.75	0.84^b±0.023	0.72^b±0.020	0.09^b±0.002	0.08^b±0.002
T_5	13.00	1.20^a±0.021	1.03^a±0.002	0.12^a±0.002	0.11^a±0.002

Mean values bearing different superscript differ significantly (p<0.05)

Table-4: Economics of feeding for production of iodine enriched eggs.

Treatments	Iodine level (ppm)	Feed cost kg feed/dozen eggs (Rs.)	Feed cost kg feed/kg eggs (Rs.)
T_1	0.45	$32.56^b \pm 0.167$	$46.22^b \pm 0.763$
T_2	03.25	$32.43^b \pm 0.167$	$46.31^b \pm 0.480$
T_3	06.50	$32.06^c \pm 0.063$	$45.58^c \pm 0.184$
T_4	09.75	$32.81^b \pm 0.418$	$46.80^b \pm 0.663$
T_5	13.00	$34.07^a \pm 0.126$	$50.47^a \pm 0.223$

Mean values bearing different superscript differ significantly ($p < 0.05$)

feed to egg. The results of iodine concentration are consistent with the findings of Kaufmann et al. [10], who found a significant linear correlation (r=0.93) between iodine content in feed mixture up to 5 mg/kg and iodine content in yolk. Yang et al. [11] indicated that laying hens might be a good carrier for transporting iodine, from diet to egg. Ramune et al. [12] found that in eggs from laying hens receiving feed containing 1 and 4 ppm iodine, egg iodine content was 24% and 196 % more than control group. Moreover, Songserm et al. [13] revealed that 4000 mg supplemental iodine/ton diet in two forms potassium iodide or potassium iodate increased the iodine concentration of eggs. In support to the results of this study introduction of iodine supplement from 1 to 5 mg/kg into the diet of hens enabled the significant enrichment of the egg iodine content [14]. Saki et al. [15] indicated that increased albumen and yolk iodine is proportional to level of supplementary iodine in diet ($p < 0.05$). Similarly, Gjorgovska and Kiril [16] stated that when laying hen feed enriched with 5 mg iodine/kg diet, the yolk from eggs of such hens is better source of iodine and can fulfill 11-15% of daily requirements for adult people if they consume one egg per day. Travnicek et al. [17] found that when iodine content in feed mixtures was raised from 0.22 to 1.18 mg/kg dietary dry matter, iodine content in egg yolk was increased significantly. Malak et al. [18] in their experiment also observed that increasing iodine levels from 0.3 to 9.6 ppm in hens diet significantly increased egg iodine concentration and the highest concentration of egg iodine was observed for the hens fed diet supplemented with 9.6 ppm followed by those fed 4.8 ppm iodine, while these high levels of iodine negatively affected the egg production. They concluded that supplementation of laying hen diet with 2.4 mg iodine/kg diet gave iodine enriched egg which can fulfill 44% of daily requirements of iodine for children of 1-10 years. The results of this study regarding egg iodine concentration are also in concurrent with the findings of Rottger et al. [19] who recorded linear correlation between iodine content in feed and egg yolk.

In this study, the reduction in the iodine content of eggs after boiling ranged between 10% and 15%. In concurrent to this lower iodine recovery in the case of egg boiled for 30 min was also reported by Lipiec

et al. [20]. While, Songserm et al. [13] studied iodine stabilization of iodine-enriched eggs before boiling followed by two methods of boiling, i.e. short time (soft boiled egg) and long time (hardboiled egg) and reported no any significant ($p > 0.05$) difference in the iodine levels of boiled and unboiled eggs.

Among iodine supplemented diets, minimum and significantly ($p < 0.05$) lowest feeding cost (Rs per dozen or per kg egg mass) was noticed in layers receiving 6.50 mg/kg iodine in their diet. Further, the inclusion of higher levels of iodine significantly ($p < 0.05$) increased the feeding cost in layers. In support to our results, Malak et al. [18] also reported improved economic efficiency of laying hens fed 0.6, 1.2, 2.4 and 4.8 ppm iodine in their diet as compared to control.

Conclusion

From the results of the present experiment, it was concluded that iodine at 6.50 ppm in layers diet was economically better for the production of iodine enriched eggs followed by feed iodine supplementation at 3.25 ppm as compared to control and other treatment groups.

Authors' Contributions

SN and RPSB have designed the plan of work. SS carried out the laboratory work and analyzed the results. AN and CDM drafted and RK revised the manuscript. All the authors read and approved the final manuscript.

Acknowledgments

The authors are thankful to The Dean, Collage of Veterinary Science and Animal Husbandry, Jabalpur for providing support and necessary laboratory facilities to carry out this research.

Competing Interests

The authors declare that they have no competing interests.

References

1. Al-Massad, M., Al-Shdefat, R. and Khashroum, A. (2011) The effects of microbial phytase and dietary calcium level on the performance and eggshell quality in laying hens fed marginal phosphorus diets. *Asian J. Anim. Sci.*, 5: 118-126.

2. ACC/SCN. (2004) Fifth Report on the World Nutrition Situation: Nutrition for Improved Development Outcomes. ACC/SCN, Geneva.

3. Krzepiłko, A., Zych-Wężyk, I. and Molas, J. (2015) Alternative ways of enriching the human diet with iodine. *J. Pre-Clin. Clin. Res.*, 9(2): 167-171.

4. Nimalaratne, C. and Wu, J. (2015) Hen egg as an antioxidant food commodity: A review. *Nutrients*, 7: 8274-8293.

5. McDowell, L.R. (1992) Minerals in Animal and Human Nutrition. Academic Press Inc., Harcourt Brace Jovanovich, USA. p524.

6. NRC. (1994) Nutrient Requirements of Poultry. 9th ed. National Academy of Sciences, USA. p19-34.

7. Trokhimenko, O.M. and Zaitsev, V.N. (2004) Kinetic determination of iodide by the sandell-kolthoff reaction using diphenylamine-4-sulfonic acid. *J. Anal. Chem.*, 59: 491-494.

8. AOAC. (2000) Official Methods of Analysis. 17th ed. Association of Official Analytical Chemists, Washington, DC.

9. Snedecor, G.W. and Cochran, W.G. (2004) Statistical Methods. 9th ed. The Iowa State University Press, Ames, Iowa, USA.

10. Kaufmann, S., Wolfram, G., Delange, F. and Rambeck, W.A. (1998) Iodine supplementation of laying hen feed: A supplementary measure to eliminate iodine deficiency in humans. *Z. Ernahrungswiss*, 37(3): 288-293.

11. Yang, L.I.E., Coa, S., Cheng, M., Chen, L. and Chen, K. (2004) Effects of iron, zinc, iodine and selenium levels in rations on activities of metabolic enzymes of layers and egg quality. *J. Huazhong Agric. Univ.* China, 51: 352-413.

12. Ramune, C., Bobiniene, R., Vytautassirvydis, D., Gudaviciute, M. and Inga, K. (2008) Effect of stable iodine preparation on the quality of poultry products. *Vet. Zootech-Lith.*, 42(64): 1392-2130.

13. Songserm, O., Chewprecha, W., Sinawat, S., Chotvichien, S. and Suakam, P. (2006) Iodine supplementation in layer diets for commercial production of iodine-enriched eggs. The Proceedings of 44th Kasetsart University Annual Conference Animals, Veterinary Medicine. p257-264.

14. Słupczynska, M., Jamroz, D., Orda, J. and Wiliczkiewicz, A. (2014) Effect of various sources and levels of iodine, as well as the kind of diet, on the performance of young laying hens, iodine accumulation in eggs, egg characteristics, and morphotic and biochemical indices in blood. *Poult. Sci.*, 93(10): 2536-2547.

15. Saki, A.A., Farisar, M.A., Aliarabi, H., Zamani, P. and Abbasinezhad, M. (2012) Iodine enriched egg production in response to dietary iodine in laying hens. *J. Agric. Technol.*, 8(4): 1255-1267.

16. Gjorgovska, N. and Kiril, F. (2010) Enriching table eggs with iodine. *Lucrări Ştiinţifice*, 53(15): 332-335.

17. Travnicek, J., Korupova, V., Herzig, I. and Kursa, J. (2006) Iodine content in consumer hen eggs. *Vet. Med.*, 51: 93-100.

18. Malak, N.Y.A., Osman, S.M.H., Bahakaim, A.S.A., Omar, A.S. and Ramadan, N.A. (2012) Effect of using different levels of iodine in layer's diets on egg iodine enrichment. *Egypt. Poult. Sci.*, 32: 851-864.

19. Rottger, A.S., Halle, I., Wagner, H., Breves, G., Danicke, S. and Flachowsky, G. (2012) The effects of iodine level and source on iodine carry-over in eggs and body tissues of laying hens. *Arch. Anim. Nutr.*, 66(5): 385-401.

20. Lipiec, E., Warowicka, O., Ruzik, L., Zhou, Y., Jarosz, M. and Połec-Pawlak, K. (2012) Investigation of iodine bioavailability from chicken eggs versus iodized kitchen salt with *in vitro* method. *Eur. Food Res. Technol.*, 234: 913-919.

4

Effectiveness of a recombinant human follicle stimulating hormone on the ovarian follicles, peripheral progesterone, estradiol-17β, and pregnancy rate of dairy cows

Mohamed Ali and Moustafa M. Zeitoun

Department of Animal Production and Breeding, Qassim University, College of Agriculture and Veterinary Medicine, Buraidah 6622, Saudi Arabia.
Corresponding author: Mohamed Ali, e-mail: mohamed0_9@yahoo.com,
MMZ: mmzeitoun@yahoo.com

Abstract

Aims: This study aimed at elucidating the effects of recombinant human follicle stimulating hormone (r-hFSH) on the ovarian follicular dynamics, progesterone, estradiol-17β profiles, and pregnancy of dairy cows.

Materials and Methods: Three groups (G, n=5 cows) of multiparous dairy cows were used. G1 (C) control cows were given controlled internal drug release (CIDR) and prostaglandin F2α; G2 (L) cows were given low dose (525 IU and G3 (H) cows were given high dose (1800 IU) of r-hFSH on twice daily basis at the last 3 days before CIDR removal. All cows were ultrasonically scanned for follicular growth and dynamics, and blood samples were collected every other day for two consecutive estrus cycles for the determination of estradiol-17β and progesterone.

Results: Estrus was observed in all C and L but not in H cows. Dominant follicle was bigger in L compared to C and H cows. Dominant follicle in C (16.00 ± 2.5 mm) and L cows (17.40 ± 2.3 mm) disappeared at 72 h after CIDR removal. However, in H cows, no ovulation has occurred during 7 days post-CIDR removal. Progesterone was not different (p>0.10) among groups, whereas estradiol-17β revealed significant (p<0.01) reduction in H (15.96 ± 2.5 pg/ml) cows compared to C (112.26 ± 26.1 pg/ml) and L (97.49 ± 15.9 pg/ml) cows. Pregnancy rate was higher in L cows (60%) compared with C cows (20%). However, H cows were not artificially inseminated due to non-ovulation. Only a cow of C group has calved one calf, however, 2 of the L cows gave birth of twins and a cow gave single calf.

Conclusion: Administration of a low dose (525 IU) of r-hFSH resulted in an optimal size of dominant follicle, normal values of progesterone and estradiol-17β, and 40% twinning rate, howeverusing 1800 IU of r-hFSH, have adverse effects on ovarian follicular dynamics and hormonal profiles with non-pregnancy of dairy cows raised under hot climate.

Keywords: dairy cows, estradiol-17β, follicles, progesterone, recombinant human follicle stimulating hormone.

Introduction

Superovulation of superior cows has been an approach targeting the need for large number of good quality embryos to be transferred [1]. Although much has been done to improve the result of the superovulatory treatment, there are still obstacles facing the purity of hormone, and consequently, the good quality embryos collected from a donor.

Due to the long acting half-life of equine chorionic gonadotrophin (eCG) in the blood of the stimulated females, adverse effects occur on the embryo quality to be eligible for transfer [2]. On the other hand, follicle stimulating hormone (FSH) was found to be more efficient to produce better quality embryos, though it requires to be administered in a series of injections due to its short acting half-life of about 5 h [3]. The preparation of FSH differs from batch to another and also its potency varies according to the species source [4]. Several experiments of superovulation in cattle have been conducted last decades using porcine, bovine, and ovine FSH [1,2].

The preparations to induce superovulation include; eCG derived from pregnant mares (i.e., previously named; pregnant mare's serum gonadotrophin), extracts of domestic animal pituitaries, particularly those of the pig, ovine, and horse of various degree of purity and FSH to luteinizing hormone (LH) ratios, recombinant bovine somatotrophin combined with FSH; and gonadotrophin of pituitary origin extracted from human postmenopausal urine (human menopausal gonadotrophin).

In this study, we focused on using a new preparation of FSH in cattle, that is, a recombinant human follicle stimulating hormone (r-hFSH) produced in Chinese hamster ovarian cells by recombinant DNA technology [5]. The therapeutic indications for r-hFSH in women are anovulation [including polycystic ovarian syndrome (PCOS)], stimulation of multifollicular development, and severe LH and FSH deficiency. It also causes stimulation of spermatogenesis in men who have congenital or acquired hypogonadotropic hypogonadism with concomitant human chorionic gonadotrophin therapy. Therefore, this study aimed to determine the effect of a low versus high dose of r-hFSH on the follicular dynamics, progesterone, and estradiol-17β profiles, and pregnancy rates in dairy cows raised under hot climate.

Materials and Methods

Ethical approval

This study has been approved by the animal rights and ethical use committee of Qassim University.

Animal's management and location

This study was conducted at the Experimental Agriculture and Veterinary Research Station, Qassim University, Saudi Arabia, during August 2014-March 2015. 15 Friesian and crossbred multiparous cows (~3-4 years) were selected for the study. These cows were healthy, cycling normally, and non-pregnant as confirmed by transrectal ultrasound palpation. The ovaries were also palpated for the presence of either follicles or an active corpus luteum (CL). Cows were supplemented with commercial concentrates (16% crude protein) at a rate of 8 kg/cow/day. Freshwater and mineral blocks were available *ad libitum*.

Experimental outline

All cows were inserted with controlled internal drug release device (CIDR® device; inter-Ag, New Zealand) for 7 days. This device is readily coated with 1.38 g of progestagen in a silicon rubber elastomer. Cows were randomly and equally divided into three groups (control [C], low dose [L], and high dose [H]). Control cows were inserted with CIDR for 7 days and given cloprostenol (500 μg i.m., Estrumate®, Schering-Plough Animal Health, USA) at CIDR removal. Low dose cows (L) were inserted with CIDR as control and given r-hFSH (i.m., GONAL-f, MERK, SERONO, Switzerland) in descending pattern on twice daily basis on day 5, 6, and 7 at doses of 300, 150, and 75 IU (i.e., total dose of 525 U), respectively. High dose cows (H) were also inserted with CIDR for 7 days and received FSH (i.m.) on twice daily basis on day 5, 6, and 7 at doses of 900, 600, and 300 IU (i.e., total dose of 1800 U), respectively. All cows in L and H groups were given (i.m.) 500 μg estrumate at the fifth dose of FSH. Figure-1 shows the experimental outline of the experiment.

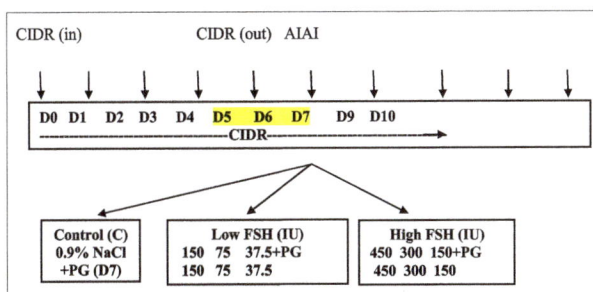

Figure-1: Diagrammatic outline of the experimental design.

Estrus exhibition and insemination

24 h after the conclusion of the treatment, estrus signs were visually observed in all cows in the C and L groups. However, none of the cows of H group exhibited estrus within 7 days post super-ovulatory treatment. Artificial insemination was performed immediately after estrus exhibition and repeated twice at 12 h interval in all estrus cows. Straws (0.5 ml) of fertile tested bull containing 20 X 10^6 live sperm were used for inseminating the estrus cows.

Ultrasound examination

The ovaries were examined by an ultrasound scanner (Pie-medical, Netherlands) with a 5 MHz transrectal probe to determine the time of ovulation and follicular populations. Ovulation occurrence was considered at the day preceding the sudden disappearance of the dominant follicle during examination. For confirmation that ovulation had occurred, the cow was reexamined 24 h later and continuously examined to determine the sizes of follicles on once a week during the subsequent 30 days. Pregnancy was also determined in C and L cows by the ultrasound examination after 30 days of insemination. Cows in H group were scanned for ovulation and follicular dynamics.

Blood sampling and sera processing

Tail venipuncture blood samples were collected in plain vacutainer® tubes for hormone assay once daily beginning at day of CIDR removal for 3 consecutive days. Thereafter, blood samples were collected once a week during the next 30 days. Blood samples were cooled at 5°C for 2 h and centrifuged (3000 rpm/5°C), sera were harvested and stored deep frozen (- 20°C) until analysis.

Progesterone (P4) and estradiol 17-β (E2) determinations

EIA Commercial kits (Human, Germany) were used for the determinations of P4 and E2. The sensitivity of progesterone ranges between 0.03 and 0.07 ng/ml. The intra- and inter-assay coefficient of variations for progesterone values were 3.7% and 5.1%, respectively [6]. The sensitivity of estradiol 17-β was 3.6 pg/ml. The intra- and inter-assay coefficient of variations were 3.2% and 5.6%, respectively [7].

Statistical analysis

Data were analyzed using SPSS statistical software release. Number of cows displayed estrus, inseminated and became pregnant was expressed as a percentage of the total number within a group. Due to the non-normally distributed nature of the data, Kruskal–Wallis one-way ANOVA (non-parametric statistical test) was used to test for the presence of statistically significant difference among three groups. Data for hormones were analyzed by the least square analysis of variance by repeated measures [8]. Proportional data (pregnancy rate and estrus expression) were analyzed by Chi-square.

Results

Estrus, conception, and calving

Table-1 shows that percent of the estrus presentation was higher in L (100%) compared with C (60%) cows. Contrariwise, none of the H cows exhibited estrus signs during the 7 days subsequent to CIDR removal, which resulted in non-pregnancy in this group. Administration of a low dose of r-hFSH accelerated (p<0.01) the occurrence of estrus in dairy cows by 22.2 h earlier than that found in control cows. Furthermore, pregnancy rate was 3-folds (60%) in the

L cows compared with C (20%) cows. Moreover, two of the pregnant L cows calved twins (one cow calved 2 males and another cow calved a male and female) and the third cow calved a single female. Contrariwise, the only pregnant control cow calved a single male. Mean birth weight for the calf born with twins was 38 kg, however, single calf weighed 42 kg at birth.

Ovarian follicular dynamics

Figure-2a illustrates number of medium follicles in different treatment groups. The size of medium

Table-1: Effect of administration of r-hFSH on the estrus exhibition and pregnancy rate in dairy cows.

Treatment	Number of animals	Number of cows exhibiting estrus (%)	Mean time from CIDR removal to estrus (hours)	Pregnancy rate (%)	Number of calves born
Control (C)	5	3 (60)	75.00±4.0[a]	20 (1)	1
Low FSH (L)	5	5 (100)	52.80±2.9[b]	60 (3)	5
High FSH (H)	5	0 (0)	ND*	0	0

[ab]Means in the same column with different superscripts are significantly different (p<0.01). *ND=Not detected, r-hFSH=Recombinant human follicle stimulating hormone, CIDR=Controlled internal drug release

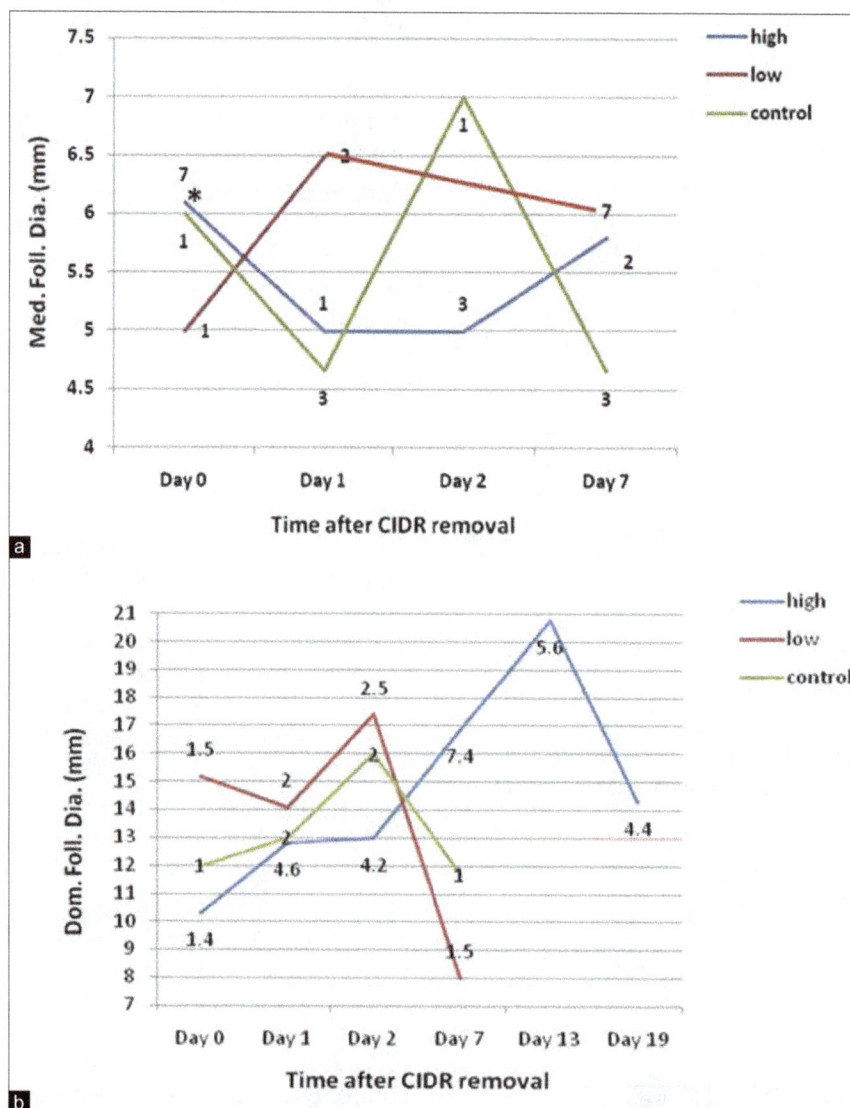

Figure-2: Number of medium (a) and large (b) follicles during days post controlled internal drug release removal in control, low and high-recombinant human follicle stimulating hormone -treated dairy cows.

follicles at CIDR removal was 6.00±0.0, 5.00±0.0, and 6.14±0.4 mm in C, L, and H cows, respectively, with no statistically significant difference. However, seven medium follicles were found in three cows in H group, only one medium follicle was found in each cow in C and L cows. At 24 h post-CIDR removal, mean size of medium follicles in C cows was 4.66±0.33 mm (i.e. total of three follicles in two cows), while size of medium follicles was slightly bigger (6.5±0.5 mm) in two cows of L group. In H cows, only one medium follicle with diameter of 5 mm in one cow was observed.

After 48 h of CIDR withdrawal, no medium follicles were found in L cows, whereas there found one follicle (7 mm) and three follicles (5 mm) per cow in C and H cows, respectively. At day 7 post-CIDR removal, mean number of medium follicles were 1.5, 1, and 3.5 in C, L, and H cows, respectively. Likewise, mean size of medium follicles was 4.66±0.2, 5.66±0.6, and 5.85±0.4 in C, L, and H cows, respectively.

Figure-2b exhibits the population of large follicles throughout the experiment. At day of CIDR removal, number of large follicles was 1, 1.5, and 1.4 in C, L, and H cows, respectively, however, this number was 2, 2, and 4.5 follicles at day 1 and 2, 2.5, and 4.2 follicles at 2 post-CIDR removal in C, L, and H cows, respectively. At day 7, number of large follicles was 1, 1.5, and 7.4 in C, L, and H cows, respectively. Beyond day 7, only H cows were scanned at days 13 and 19 post-CIDR removal and contained decreased large follicles (i.e., 5.6 and 4.4 at day 13 and 19, respectively).

Diameter of large follicles reveals different trends among treatments. The largest follicles at CIDR removal was observed in L cows (15.25±2.6 mm) compared with C (12.0±1.1 mm) and H (10.3±2.2 mm) cows with none significant difference. Near time of ovulation (i.e., around day 2 post-CIDR removal), diameter of largest follicle was 16, 17.4, and 13 mm in C, L, and H cows, respectively, being higher (p<0.05) in C and L than H cows. The ultrasound diagnosis revealed that ovulation has occurred at 90 and 65 h in C and L cows, respectively, post-CIDR removal, however, none of the H cows presented estrus or ovulation during 14 days post-CIDR removal. At day 7, the diameter of largest follicle was larger (p<0.05) in H (16.9±1.8 mm) cows compared with C (11.75±2.1 mm) and L (8.0±0.01 mm) cows. In H cows, the largest follicle approached 20.8 mm at day 13 and regressed to 14.3 mm at day 19. These H cows were subsequently recycled with gonadotropin-releasing hormone for regular cycling which obviously done after about 50 days of CIDR removal.

Blood progesterone and estradiol-17β

Progesterone in blood circulation revealed mean values of 10, 10.79, and 9.56 ng/ml (Figure-3) being none significant (p>0.10) among treatments. On the other hand, estradiol-17β (Figure-4) revealed a significant (p<0.05) decline in H cows (15.96 pg/ml)

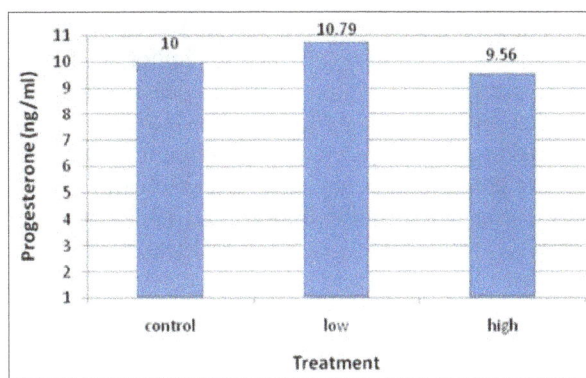

Figure-3: Blood progesterone level in control, low and high-recombinant human follicle stimulating hormone-treated cows.

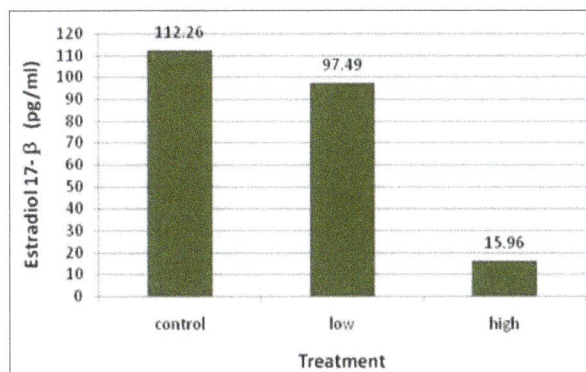

Figure-4: Blood estradiol 17-β level in control, low and high-recombinant human follicle stimulating hormone-treated cows.

compared with C (112.26 pg/ml) cows, which was not different than L (97.49 pg/ml) cows.

Discussion

Since FSH has shown good superovulatory responses accompanied with better number of good quality transferable embryos compared with eCG in gilts [9], deer [10], beef cows [2], goats [11], and dairy cows [12]. Administration of descending dose of FSH has shown acceptable superovulation in dairy cows. The use of bovine, porcine, and ovine FSH has been a common practice in the superovulation regimes in dairy cattle [13]. However, implementing hFSH in the superovulatory programs of dairy cows has not been attempted before. Therefore, the current study focused to examine the use of r-hFSH. It has been found that hFSH is capable of promoting the activation of primordial follicles and maintaining the ultrastructural integrity of caprine preantral follicles cultured *in vitro* for 7 days [14].

The homology of the α-subunit of the hFSH and bovine FSH molecule was found to be 75% [15]. Positions of cysteine residues are highly conserved among species, implying that the disulfide bridges within the α-subunit are identical among α-subunits of different species. Furthermore, it has been reported that the nature of the carbohydrate residues that distinguish the α-subunits of the various gonado-trophins within a species is of great importance [16]. Moreover, as the β-subunit determines the biological specificity of the gonadotrophin [15], it is often referred to as the hormone-specific subunit. For example, the bovine hormones were found to contain very little sulfated (S) and sialylated (N) (0-2% of total oligosaccharides) linkages, whereas human and ovine hormones have relatively large amounts of S-N (10% of ovine FSH and 23% of human LH oligosaccharides are of the S-N type). However, bovine, ovine, and human pituitary glycoprotein hormones display a very similar spectrum of sulfated oligosaccharides [17].

The species-specific differences in the molecular structure of gonadotrophin are well known, even though there is still certain percent of homology among species [18]. It is well known that granulosa cells in female ovaries and sertoli cells in male testicles are the target cells for FSH expressing its specific receptors [19].

Application of recombinant technology has allowed the engineering of a variety of analogs with distinct biological features and therapeutic potential [18]. Several researchers confirmed the interspecies FSH interaction to stimulate folliculogenesis and steroidogenesis [20].

The administration of an excess dose of FSH (1800 IU equivalent to 132 µg) in the current study not only resulted in the disappearance of estrus signs but also impeded the rupture of large follicles (anovulatory response) leading to a PCOS. Apparently, this high dose compromised the hypothalamo-pituitary-ovarian axis leading to a sharp decline in estradiol-17β secretion. The existence of PCOS in H cows might be attributed to the hormonal imbalance occurred in cows [21]. Kanitz *et al.* [22] found that using excessive dosages of FSH can disturb the ovulation process at two levels; at the level of pituitary and the ovarian level. This means that these high doses of FSH might suppress or decrease the LH surge leading to a decreased and/or impediment of the ovulation of large follicles. Another cause for the reduced ovulation rate, in this case, might be attributed to the down regulation of follicular FSH receptors by high doses of homologous ligand. Therefore, each FSH product has an optimal dose range [21].

Various pharmaceutical products with gonad-otrophin activity and even various batches within a product can differ in their bioactivity and/or immuno-activity [23]. The differences in the bioactivity of various species-derived FSH were mainly ascribed to the degree of glycosylation of the molecule and to the occurrence of isoforms [24].

The sharp decrease in estradiol-17β levels accompanying the high FSH was previously reported *in vitro* [25] and *in vivo* [26]. The decreased E2 in H cows are most likely a result to the negative feedback of the excess FSH on the hypothalamo-pituitary-ovarian axis [27]. Concurrently, the P4 level in H cows

revealed similar value to C and L cows. The cystic follicles in H cows were ultrasonically diagnosed as luteinized follicles, leading to compensation of the inefficiency of the original CL. The presence of luteinized follicles might interpret the lack of E2 secretion by granulosa cells, which are replaced by lutein cells [18]. Contrariwise, administration of a low dose of r-hFSH (525 IU=38.5 µg) resulted in higher than control response of estrus exhibition (100% vs. 60%) and pregnancy rate (60% vs. 20%). Cows given low FSH delivered two sets of healthy twins with an average birth weight of 38 kg/calf.

Conclusion

Using r-hFSH in stimulating dairy cows during the hot climate was as efficient as using other FSH products derived from bovine, ovine, and porcine pituitaries. The use of a low dosage (525 IU equivalent to 38.5 µg) of r-hFSH in dairy cows would be considered a practical regime to stimulate the inactivity of the ovaries of dairy cows during hot summer months. Moreover, this low dosage of r-hFSH resulted in an increased outcome of born calves (twinning). Much interest must be further paid to the best timing during ovarian follicular dynamics for the FSH to be administered.

Authors' Contributions

MA has managed the cows, applied treatments, observed estrus, scanned ovarian structures, neonatal care, and weighing and analyzed data. MMZ has accomplished hormonal analyses, helped in the ultrasound measurements, tabulated the data, and wrote and edited the manuscript. Both authors read and approved the final manuscript.

Acknowledgments

The authors acknowledge the support of the College of Agriculture and Veterinary Medicine, Qassim University, KSA for providing animals. We wish to express our sincere thanks to Mr. Mansour Al-Towajeri, for his assistance to control cows and blood sampling.

Competing Interest

The authors declare that they have no competing interests.

References

1. Mapletoft, R.J. and Bo, G.A. (2013) Innovative strategies for superovulation in cattle. *Anim. Reprod.*, 10: 174-179.
2. Mattos, M.C.C., Bastos, M.R., Guardieiro, M.M., Carvalho, J.O., Francoc, M.M., Mourão, G.B., Barros, C.M. and Sartori, R. (2011) Improvement of embryo production by the replacement of the last two doses of porcine follicle-stimulating hormone with equine chorionic gonadotropin in Sindhi donors. *Anim. Reprod. Sci.*, 125: 119-123.
3. Gabriel, A., Reuben, B. and Mapletoft, J. (2014) Historical perspectives and recent research on superovulation in cattle. *Theriogenology*, 81: 38-48.
4. Gervais, A., Hammel, Y.A. and Pelloux, S. (2003) Glycosylation of human gonatrophins: Characterization and batch-to-batch consistency. *Glycobiology*, 13: 179-189.

5. Kim, D.J., Seok, S.H., Baek, M.W., Lee, H.Y., Juhn, J.H., Lee, S., Yun, M. and Park, J.H. (2010) Highly expressed recombinant human follicle stimulating hormone from Chinese hamster ovary cells grown in serum-free medium and its effect on induction of folliculogenesis and ovulation. *Fertil. Steril.*, 93: 2652-2660.

6. Radwanska, E., Frankenberg, J. and Allen, E. (1978) Plasma progesterone levels in normal and early pregnancy. *Fertil. Steril.*, 30: 398-402.

7. Goldstein, D., Zuckerman, H., Harpaz, S., Barkai, J., Gev, A., Gordon, S., Shalev, E. and Schwartz, M. (1982) Correlation between estradiol and progesterone in cycles with luteal phase deficiency. *Fertil. Steril.*, 37: 348-354.

8. SPSS. (2007) Statistical Package for the Social Sciences. Version 16 for Windows. SPSS, Chicago, USA.

9. Hu, J., Bao, G., Ma, X., Li, W., Lei, A., Yang, C., Gao, Z. and Wang, H. (2010) FSH is superior to ECG for promoting ovarian response in Chinese Bamei gilts. *Anim. Reprod. Sci.*, 122: 313-316.

10. Zanetti, E.S., Munerato, M.S., Cursino, M.S. and Duarte, J.M.B. (2014) Comparing two different superovulation protocols on ovarian activity and fecal glucocorticoid levels in the brown brocket deer (*Mazama gouazoubira*). *Reprod. Biol. Endocrinol.*, 12: 24-32.

11. Rahman, M.R., Rahman, M.M., Wan Khadijah, W.E. and Abdullah, R.B. (2014) Follicle Stimulating Hormone (FSH) dosage based on body weight enhances ovulatory responses and subsequent embryo production in goats. *Asian-Aust. J. Anim. Sci.*, 27: 1270-1274.

12. Son, H.N., Hanh, N.V., Huu, Q.X. and Chau, L.T. (2013) Effect of bovine ovarian status on superovulation. *Tạp Chí Sinh Học*, 35: 243-247.

13. Mapletoft, R.J. (2006) Bovine embryo transfer. In: I.V.I.S, editor. IVIS Reviews in Veterinary Medicine. Ithaca, NY: International Veterinary Information Service, R0104.1106. Available from: http://www.ivis.org. Accessed on 05-01-2016.

14. da Costa, S.L., da Costa, E.P., Pereira, E.C.M., Benjamin, L.A., Verde, I.B.L., Celestino, J.L.H. and de Figueiredo, J.R. (2015) The human follicle stimulating hormone (HFSH) keeps the normal ultrastructure of caprine preantral follicles cultured *in vitro*. *Semina: Ciências Agrárias, Londrina*, 36(3), S1: 1965-1978.

15. Mullen, M.P., Cooke, D.J. and Crow, M.A. (2013) Structural and functional roles of FSH and LH as glycoproteins regulating reproduction in *Mammalian species*. In: Vizcarra, J., editor. Gonadotropin. Ch. 8InTech,International Publisher p155-180.

16. Bousfield, G.R. and Dias, J.A. (2011) Synthesis and secretion of gonadotropins including structure-function correlates. *Rev. Endocr. Metabol. Disord.,* 12: 289-302.

17. Green, E.D. and Baenziger, J.U. (1988) Asparagine-linked oligosaccharides on lutropin, follitropin, and thyrotropin. I. Structural elucidation of the sulfated and sialylated oligosaccharides on bovine, ovine, and human pituitary glycoprotein hormones. *J. Bio. Chem.*, 263: 25-35.

18. Ulloa-Aguirre, A. and Timossi, C. (1998) Structure-function relationship of follicle-stimulating hormone and its receptor. *Hum. Reprod. Update*, 4: 260-283.

19. George, J.W., Dille, E.A. and Heckert, L.L. (2011) Current concepts of follicle-stimulating hormone receptor gene regulation. *Biol. Reprod.*, 84: 7-17.

20. Okamoto, T. and Nishimoto, I. (1992) Detection of G protein-activator regions in M4 subtype muscarinic cholinergic and tc2-adrenergic receptors based upon characteristics in primary structure. *J. Biol. Chem.*, 267: 8342-8346.

21. Butler, S.T., Pelton, S.H. and Butler, W.R. (2004) Insulin increases 17β-estradiol production by the dominant follicle of the first postpartum follicle wave in dairy cows. *Reproduction*, 127: 537-545.

22. Kanitz, W., Becker, F., Schneider, F., Kanitz, E., Leiding, C., Nohner, H.P. and Pöhland, R. (2002) Superovulation in cattle: Practical aspects of gonadotropin treatment and insemination. *Reprod. Nutr. Dev.*, 42: 587-599.

23. Braileanu, G.T., Albanese, C., Card, C. and Chedrese, P.J. (1998) FSH bioactivity in commercial preparations of gonadotropins. *Theriogenology*, 49: 1031-1037.

24. Stanton, P.G., Pozvek, G., Burgon, P.G., Robertson, D.M. and Hearn, M.T. (1993) Isolation and characterization of human LH isoforms. *J. Endocrinol.*, 138: 529-543.

25. Tamilmani, G., Varshney, V.P., Dubey, P.K., Pathak, M.C. and Sharma, G.T. (2013) Influence of FSH on in vitro growth, steroidogenesis and DNA synthesis of buffalo (*Bubalus bubalis)* ovarian preantral follicles. *Anim. Reprod.*, 10: 32-40.

26. Burns, D.S., Jimenez-Krassel, F., Ireland, J.L., Knight, P.G. and Ireland, J.J. (2005) Numbers of antral follicles during follicular waves in cattle: Evidence for high variation among animals, very high repeatability in individuals, and an inverse association with serum follicle-stimulating hormone concentrations. *Biol. Reprod.*, 73: 54-62.

27. Singh, J., Dominguez, M., Jaiswal, R. and Adams, G.P. (2004) A simple ultrasound test to predict the superstimulatory response in cattle. *Theriogenology*, 62: 227-243.

5

Prevalence and burden of gastrointestinal parasites of Djallonke sheep in Ayeduase, Kumasi, Ghana

Moses Owusu[1], Jemima Owusu Sekyere[2] and Frederick Adzitey[3]

1. Department of Pathobiology, School of Veterinary Medicine, College of Health Sciences, Kwame Nkrumah University of Science and Technology, Kumasi, Ghana; 2. Department of Nursing, Signature Healthcare of Madison, Madison, Tennessee, United States of America; 3. Department of Animal Science, Faculty of Agriculture, University for Development Studies, Tamale, Ghana.
Corresponding author: Moses Owusu, e-mail: owusu.moses@ymail.com,
JOS: jemi.sekyere@yahoo.com, FA: adzitey@yahoo.co.uk

Abstract

Aim: This study was conducted to determine the prevalence and burden of gastrointestinal (GIT) parasites of Djallonke sheep in Ayeduase, Kumasi from January 2015 to July 2015.

Materials and Methods: The presence of nematodal eggs and coccidial oocysts in fecal samples were analyzed using the saturated sodium chloride floatation technique. Identification of eggs or oocysts was done on the basis of morphology and size of the eggs or oocysts.

Results: Out of 110 fecal samples of sheep examined, 108 were infected with GIT parasites, representing a prevalence rate of 98.2%. The total infection rate of GIT nematodes and coccidia oocysts were 94.5% and 51.8%, respectively. Strongyle nematode (94.5%) was the most prevalent GIT nematode detected, followed by strongyloides (27.3%). The average nematodal burden in g/feces was significantly higher ($p<0.001$) in young rams under 1 year (3482.0) than gimmers (1539.0), lamb (825.0), ewes (420.7), and rams over 1 year (313.3). Nematodal burden in gimmers was significantly higher ($p<0.001$) than that of lambs, ewes, and rams over 1 year. Nematodal counts of lambs, ewes, and rams did not differ significantly ($p>0.05$) from each other. The average coccidia oocysts count in g/feces was significantly higher ($p<0.001$) in lambs (2475.0) than rams under 1 year (286.0), gimmers (263.6), ewes (158.6), and rams over 1 year (150.0). There was no significant difference ($p>0.05$) in the coccidia oocysts count of rams under 1 year, gimmers, ewes, and rams over 1 year. From the studied animals, 40%, 6.36%, 48.18%, and 5.45% had heavy, moderate, light, and no infestation, respectively, with GIT nematodes.

Conclusion: Djallonke sheep in Ayeduase, Kumasi, were infested with varying amounts of GIT parasites. The infestation of Djallonke sheep by GIT parasites also varies among different age groups and sexes.

Keywords: burden, Djallonke sheep, gastrointestinal parasites, prevalence.

Introduction

The rich potential from the small ruminant sector is not efficiently exploited due to several constraints including malnutrition, inefficient management, and diseases [1,2]. In this regard, diseases due to parasites take the lion's share in limiting the productivity of these animals all over the world. This is especially true in many tropical and subtropical regions. Small ruminants under intensive and extensive production systems are extremely susceptible to the effects of a wide range of helminths [2]. The prevalence of gastrointestinal (GIT) helminths is related to the agro-climatic conditions such as quantity and quality of pasture, temperature, humidity, and grazing behavior of the host [3].

GIT parasite infections are a world-wide problem for both small- and large-scale farmers, but the impact in general is greater in Sub-Saharan Africa [2]. Among the parasitic diseases, endoparasites are of greatest importance in sheep and goats. Common parasites of sheep and goats include coccidia, roundworms, tapeworms, and liver flukes [4]. Strongyle nematodes are the main cause of parasitic gastro-enteritis in sheep and goats in Ghana [5]. Young animals and those with weakened immune systems due to other diseases are most affected by internal parasites [6].

Economic losses are caused by GIT parasites in a variety of ways: They cause losses through lowered fertility, reduced work capacity, involuntary culling, a reduction in food intake and lower weight gains, lower milk production, treatment costs, and mortality in heavily parasitized animals [7]. A combination of treatment and management is necessary to control parasites so that they will not cause economic loss to the producer [6]. Internal parasites get out of control and cause damage when their numbers grow beyond what the animal can tolerate.

It is, therefore, necessary to carry out a study to determine the prevalence and burden of GIT parasites in sheep. This will determine whether there is the need to develop preventive and treatment measures to curb production losses. The objective of this work was to determine the prevalence and burden of GIT parasites in Djallonke sheep in Ayeduase.

Materials and Methods

Ethical approval

The research was conducted after approval of research committee and institutional ethics committee.

Study area

The study was conducted in Ayeduase in the Kumasi Metropolis. The metropolis is located in the north-eastern part of the Ashanti Region of the Republic of Ghana between latitude 6°35" and 6°40" N and longitude 1°30" and 1°35" E [8]. During the study period, Ayeduase received an average annual rainfall of 1100-1600 mm and a mean monthly temperature of 33.33-34.0°C [8]. The vegetation of the metropolis falls within the moist semi-deciduous section of the South-East Ecological zone [8].

Collection and examination of fecal samples

A total of 110 rectal fecal samples from apparently healthy sheep were collected from 12 different flocks in Ayeduase. Fecal samples were placed in screw-capped plastic bottles, labeled and immediately transported under 4°C to the Ashanti Regional Veterinary Diagnostic Laboratory in Kumasi for analyzes. The category of sheep and the number of samples examined are presented in Table-1. The numbers examined varied because the number and ages of sheep in a farmer's flock vary.

The presence of nematodal eggs and coccidial oocysts in all fecal samples was analyzed using the saturated sodium chloride floatation technique [9-11].

Table-1: Category of sheep and number of samples examined in Ayeduase.

Category of sheep	Number of samples analyzed
Rams above 1 year	15
Rams below 1 year	25
Ewes	29
Gimmers	33
Lambs	8
Total	110

Identification of eggs or oocysts was done on the basis of morphology and size of the eggs or oocysts [10]. In this study, the authors wished to determine species, but financial constraints and lack of some equipment/instruments in our laboratory did not permit that. Fecal egg counts per gram were determined for each sample following the McMaster egg counting technique, and the degree of infection was categorized based on Hansen and Perry [10]. Animals with egg counts from 50-799, 800-1200, and above 1200 were categorized as lightly, moderately, and heavily infected, respectively [9-11].

Data analysis

Data obtained was analyzed using analysis of variance of the Genstat Edition four.

Results and Discussion

The results for the prevalence of GIT parasites in sheep are presented in Table-2. Microscopic examination of the 110 sheep fecal samples revealed that 98.2% (108) of sheep were infested with one or more GIT parasites. Emiru et al. [12], Admasu and Nurlign [13], and Gadahi et al. [14] also found that 84.3%, 58.7%, and 53.3% of sheep fecal samples, respectively, were infested with one or more GIT parasites. The total infestation rate of GIT nematodes was 94.5% (104) while that of coccidia was 51.8% (57). Similarly, to this study Aragaw and Gebreegziabher [15] reported an overall prevalence rate of nematodes in sheep to be 93.1%. Wang et al. [16] found an overall prevalence of coccidial infection in sheep to be 92.9% (287/309) which is higher than what was found in this study. Out of 104 samples that were infested with nematodes 51.1% (53/104) of them were also infested with coccidia.

The nematodes detected were the strongyle type (104/110) and Strongyloides spp. (30/110); and thus, the strongyle type nematodes were the most prevalent GIT nematodes detected. Furthermore, all the samples infested with strongyloides were also infested with strongyle. Nematode parasites (54.1%), Eimeria (14.6%), and Moniezia (13.4%) were also found to infest small ruminants [12].

The prevalence of nematodes in sheep was highest in gimmers (100%) and rams below 1 year (100%), followed by ewes (93.1%), rams over 1 year (86.7%), and lambs (75%). This means that more

Table-2: Prevalence of gastrointestinal parasites of sheep in Ayeduase.

Category Sheep	Number of samples examined	Number of samples infected with one or more GIT parasites (%)	Number of samples infected with nematodes (%)	Number of samples infected with coccidia oocysts (%)
Rams over 1 year	15	15 (100)	13 (86.7)	9 (60)
Rams below 1 year	25	25 (100)	25 (100)	14 (56)
Ewes	29	28 (96.6)	27 (93.1)	13 (44.8)
Gimmers	33	33 (100)	33 (100)	14 (42.4)
Lambs	8	7 (87.5)	6 (75)	7 (87.5)
Total	110	108 (98.2)	104 (94.5)	57 (51.8)

GIT=Gastrointestinal

gimmers and rams below 1 year were infested with GIT nematodes, followed by ewes, rams over 1 year and lambs. The low prevalence of nematodes in lambs could be because, in some flocks, sampled lambs had just started nibbling and may not have ingested contaminated feed that leads to GIT parasites infestation. Quantitative analyzes of sheep fecal samples showed that the nematodal burden of rams under 1 year was significantly higher (p<0.001) than gimmers, lambs, ewes, and rams over 1 year (Table-3). Quantitatively, the number of gimmers infested with nematodes was also significantly higher (p<0.001) than that of lambs, ewes, and rams over 1 year. Thus, the total number of nematodes isolated from rams under 1 year was the highest, followed by those isolated from gimmers, lambs, ewes, and rams over 1 year.

The prevalence of coccidia oocysts in sheep was highest in lambs (87.5%), followed by rams over 1 year (60%), rams below 1 year (56%), ewes (44.82%), and gimmers (42.4%) (Table-2). Quantitative analyzes of sheep fecal samples showed that the coccidial burden in lambs was significantly higher (p<0.001) than rams under 1 year, gimmers, ewes, and rams over 1 year. Contrarily, to the results obtained for nematodal burden, lambs were most infested with coccidia oocysts both qualitatively and quantitatively. In agreement with this study Emiru et al. [12] found significant differences (p<0.05) in the prevalence of GIT parasites between the different age groups. Young, unhealthy, and malnourished sheep will be more susceptible to nematode and coccidia parasites. Sheep are infested with nematode and coccidia parasites when they eat feed or drink water contaminated with the eggs of these parasites.

The intensity of infestation of GIT nematodes in sheep in Ayeduase is shown in Table-4. Out of the total sheep fecal samples (110) examined, 40% (44), 6.4% (7), and 48.2% (53) had heavy, moderate, and light infestations, respectively, with GIT nematodes, while no GIT nematode ova was detected in fecal samples from 5.5% (6) of the study population. Admasu and Nurlign [13] reported that 91 (58.7%), 34 (21.9%), and 30 (19.4%) of sheep were lightly, moderately, and highly infested by GIT parasites.

The prevalence of GIT parasites by sex is shown in Table-5. Female sheep (98.6%) and male sheep (97.6%) were infested with one or more GIT parasites. More female sheep 66 (95.7%) were infested with nematodes than male sheep 38 (92.7%). With regards to coccidia oocysts, more male sheep 23 (57.5%) were infested than female sheep 34 (49.3%). Admasu and Nurlign [13] found no significant differences (p>0.05) in the prevalence of GIT parasites between sex, while Emiru et al. [12] found significant differences (p<0.05) in the prevalence of GIT parasites between sex.

Conclusion

Djallonke sheep in Ayeduase are infested with nematodal and coccidial parasites. The prevalence rate of these GIT parasites varies among different age groups and sexes. The intensity of infestation by GIT nematodes also varies from no to heavy infestation. There is the need for farmers in Ayeduase to improve on their biosecurity and feeding habits to prevent GIT

Table-3: Prevalence and burden of nematodes ova and coccidia oocysts of sheep in Ayeduase.

Parasite type	Sheep type						
	Ewes	Lambs	Gimmers	Ram+	Ram−	LSD*	p value
Nematodes eggs/g of feces	420.7[a]	825[a]	1539.4[b]	313.3[a]	3482[c]	810.8	<0.001
Coccidia oocysts/g of feces	158.6[a]	2475[b]	263.6[a]	150[a]	286[a]	747.4	<0.001

Ram+=Rams over 1 year, Ram−=Rams under 1 year, LSD=Least significant difference, p value=Probability value, means in the same row with different superscript are significantly different (p<0.05)

Table-4: Intensity of gastrointestinal nematodes infestation of sheep in Ayeduase.

Category sheep	Heavy (%)	Moderate (%)	Light (%)	No infestation (%)
Rams over 1 year	-	-	13 (86.7)	2 (13.3)
Rams below 1 year	25 (100)	-	-	-
Ewes		2 (6.9)	25 (86.2)	2 (6.9)
Gimmers	19 (57.6)	5 (15.2)	9 (27.3)	-
Lambs	-	-	6 (75)	2 (25)
Infestation intensity (%)	44 (40)	7 (6.4)	53 (48.2)	6 (5.5)

Table-5: Prevalence of gastrointestinal parasites by sex.

Sex	Number of samples examined	Number of samples infected with one or more GIT parasites (%)	Number of samples infected with nematodes (%)	Number of samples infected with coccidia oocysts (%)
Male	41	40 (97.6)	38 (92.7)	23 (57.5)
Female	69	68 (98.6)	66 (95.7)	34 (49.3)
Total	110	108 (98.2)	104 (94.5)	57 (51.8)

GIT=Gastrointestinal

parasite infestations in their flocks. Sheep should be dewormed during the dry season (December to March) to reduce the shedding of ova and larvae and pasture contamination during the subsequent rains. They should be dewormed again during the peak rainy season (June-July) to prevent massive pasture contamination with ova and larvae from young adults developed from infections picked up during the early part of the rains.

Authors' Contributions

FA supervised the overall research work. MO and JOS went to the field to collect the data and carried out the research. MO and FA wrote the first draft before being revised by all the authors. All authors also read and approved the final manuscript.

Acknowledgments

We are grateful to the School of Veterinary Medicine, Kwame Nkrumah University of Science and Technology, Kumasi for providing us with equipment to carry out this research.

Competing Interests

The authors declare that they have no competing interests.

References

1. Adzitey, F. (2013) Animal and meat production in Ghana - An overview. *J. World's Poult. Res.,* 3: 1-4.
2. Ibrahim, N., Tefera, M., Bekele, M. and Alemu, S. (2014) Prevalence of gastrointestinal parasites of small ruminants in and around Jimma Town Western Ethiopia. *Acta Parasitol.,* 5: 26-32.
3. Pal, R.A. and Qayyum, M. (1993) Prevalence of gastrointestinal nematodes of sheep and goats in upper Punjab, Pakistan. *Pak. Vet. J.,* 13: 138-141.
4. Bagley, C.V. (1997) Internal Parasites. Utah State University Extension, Logan UT. 84322-5600. Available from: http://www.tvsp.org/pdf/sheep/internal-parasites.pdf. Accessed on 10-10-2015.
5. Blackie, S. (2014) A review of the epidemiology of gastrointestinal nematode infections in sheep and goats in Ghana.

J. Agric. Sci., 6: 109-118.
6. Scarfe, A.D. (1993) Approaches to managing gastro-intestinal nematode parasites in small ruminants. Available from: http://www.clemson.edu/agronomy/goats/handbook/nematode.html. Accessed on 10-10-2015.
7. Fikru, R., Teshale, S., Reta, D. and Yosef, K. (2006) Epidemiology of gastrointestinal parasites of ruminants in Western Oromia, Ethiopia. *J. Appl. Res. Vet. Med.,* 4(1): 51-57.
8. MOFA. (2009) Agricultural Potentials/Opportunities. Available from: http://www.mofa.gov.gh/site/?page_id=859. Accessed on 12-08-2015.
9. Soulsby, E.J.L. (1986) Helminthes, Arthropods and Protozoa of Domesticated Animals. 7th ed. Bailliere, Tindall, London, UK. Available from: http://www.abebooks.com/Helminths-Arthropods-Protozoa-Domesticated-Animals-Soulsby/14412228721/bd. Accessed on 10-10-2015.
10. Hansen, J. and Perry, B. (1994) The Epidemiology, Diagnosis and Control of Helminth Parasites of Ruminants. A Hand Book. 2nd ed. ILRAD (International Laboratory for Research on Animal Diseases), Nairobi, Kenya. p171. Available from: https://www.cgspace.cgiar.org/bitstream/handle/10568/2735/ILRAD93.pdf?sequence=1. Accessed on 10-10-2015.
11. Urquhart, G., Aremour, J., Dunchan, J.L., Dunn, A.M. and Jeninis, F.W. (1996) Veterinary Parasitology. 2nd ed. The University of Glasgow, Black Well Sciences, Scotland. Available from: http://www.abebooks.com/Helminths-Arthropods-Protozoa-Domesticated-Animals-Soulsby/14412228721/bd. Accessed on 10-10-2015.
12. Emiru, B., Ahmed, Y., Tigre, W., Feyera, T. and Deressa, B. (2013) Epidemiology of gastrointestinal parasites of small ruminants in Gechi District, Southwest Ethiopia. *Adv. Biomed. Res.,* 7: 169-174.
13. Admasu, P. and Nurlign, L. (2014) Prevalence of gastrointestinal parasites of small ruminants in Kuarit District, North West Ethiopia. *Afr. J. Bas. Appl. Sci.,* 6: 125-130.
14. Gadahi, J.A., Arshed, M.J., Ali, Q., Javaid, S.B. and Shah, S.I. (2009) Prevalence of gastrointestinal parasites of sheep and goats in and around Rawalpindi and Islamabad, Pakistan. *Vet. World,* 2: 51-53.
15. Aragaw, K. and Gebreegziabher, G. (2014) Small intestinal helminth parasites in slaughtered sheep and goats in Hawassa, Southern Ethiopia. *Afr. J. Bas. Appl. Sci.,* 6: 25-29.
16. Wang, C.R., Xiao, J.Y., Chen, A.H., Chen, J., Wang, Y., Gao, J.F. and Zhu, X.Q. (2010) Prevalence of coccidial infection in sheep and goats in Northeastern China. *Vet. Parasitol.,* 174: 213-217.

6

Peperomia pellucida leaf extract as immunostimulator in controlling motile aeromonad septicemia due to *Aeromonas hydrophila* in red hybrid tilapia, *Oreochromis* spp. farming

S. W. Lee[1], K. Y. Sim[1], W. Wendy[2] and A. K. Zulhisyam[1]

1. Faculty of Agro Based Industry, Universiti Malaysia Kelantan Jeli Campus, 17600, Jeli, Kelantan, Malaysia;
2. School of Fisheries and Aquaculture Sciences, Universiti Malaysia Terengganu, Kuala Terengganu, 21030, Terengganu, Malaysia.
Corresponding author: S. W. Lee, e-mail: leeseongwei@yahoo.com,
KYS: sk.yuen@umk.edu.my, WW: wendy@umt.edu.my, AKZ: zulhisyam.a@umk.edu.my

Abstract

Aim: This study was revealed the potential of *Peperomia pellucida* leaf extract as an immunostimulator agent in controlling motile aeromonad septicemia due to *Aeromonas hydrophila* in red hybrid tilapia, *Oreochromis* sp.

Materials and Methods: In the present study, minimum inhibitory concentration (MIC) of *P. pellucida* leaf extract against *A. hydrophila* was determined through two-fold microbroth dilution method. The plant extract was screening for its active compound using a gas chromatograph mass spectrometer, and the effectiveness of *P. pellucida* leaf extract as an immunostimulator agent was evaluated. The experimental fish were fed with medicated feed at three different concentrations (25 mg/kg, PP-25; 50 mg/kg, PP-50; and 100 mg/kg, PP-100) of *P. pellucida* leaf extract for 1 week before they were intraperitoneally exposed to *A. hydrophila*. Enzyme-linked immunosorbent assay was carried out to determine the value of antibody response to *A. hydrophila* in fish from a group of fish that received medicated feed, and the percentage of total cumulative mortality of the experimental fish were observed at the end of the experiment.

Results: The results showed that the major bioactive compound is phytol (40%), and the MIC value was 31.5 mg/L. The value of antibody response to *A. hydrophila* in fish from a group of fish which received medicated feed (PP-25, 0.128±0.014 optical density [OD]; PP-50, 0.132±0.003 OD; and PP-100, 0.171±0.02 OD) was found significantly higher (p<0.05) compared to fish did not receive medicated feed (0.00 OD). Whereas, percentage cumulative mortality of fish from all groups of fish received medicated feed (PP-25, 18.0±3.2%; PP-50, 18.2±2.8%; and PP-100, 17.7±1.8%) were found significantly lower (p<0.05) compared to a group of fish did not receive medicated feed (83.2±1.4%).

Conclusion: The findings of the present study indicated the huge potential of *P. pellucida* leaf extract as natural immunostimulator agent for aquaculture uses.

Keywords: *Aeromonas hydrophila*, immunostimulator, motile aeromonad septicemia, red hybrid tilapia.

Introduction

Recently, aquaculture activities are expanding rapidly to generate more aquaculture production in fulfilling demand from the market. The expansion of aquaculture industry is due to the declining of fishery production and overexploitation of fishery product from the open sea. Subsequently, aquaculture is gearing toward intensification with the expectation to produce more fish. However, bacterial disease is recognized as a major constraint to the development of aquaculture industry. One of the bacterial diseases known as motile aeromonad septicemia (MAS) due to

Aeromonas hydrophila was reported to cause devastation to tilapia fish farms.

A. hydrophila was reported found in many aquatic animals. For instance, Lee *et al.* [1] claimed that *A. hydrophila* was found in diseased Malaysian giant prawn, *Macrobrachium rosenbergii*. Other study was also reported that this bacterium was responsible to the mass mortality of ornamental fish in the aquarium shop. Based on the literature survey, *A. hydrophila* was found in Mantis Shrimp, *Squilla* sp., African catfish, *Clarias gariepinus*, American bullfrog, *Rana catesbeiana* [2], Asian seabass, *Lates calcarifer* [3], golden pompano, *Trachinotus blochii* [4], silver catfish, *Pangasius sutchi*, and red hybrid tilapia, *Oreochromis* sp. [5].

Traditionally, commercial antibiotic was used in fish health management. However, cases of antibiotic resistance have been alarming the industry due to the misuse and over use of the commercial antibiotics in aquaculture. Therefore, this study was performed to reveal the potential of *Peperomia pellucida* leaf extract as an alternative antimicrobial agent for aquaculture uses.

Materials and Methods

Ethical approval

The study was conducted following approved guidelines of the Institutional Animal Ethics Committee.

Bacterial isolate

A. hydrophila isolated from diseased red hybrid tilapia, *Oreochromis* sp., at commercial farms in Kelantan, Malaysia was used in the experiment. The bacterial isolate was cultured using brain heart infusion broth (Oxoid, England) for 18 h at room temperature. The bacterial pellet was harvested by centrifugation at 13,500 rpm for 10 min. The harvested bacterial pellet was washed twice using physiological saline, and the concentration of the bacterial isolate was adjusted to 10^9 colony forming unit/mL for challenged by intraperitoneal injection of 100 µl of each inoculum, at a dose causing 50% mortality (LD_{50}).

Plant extraction

P. pellucida leaf extract was prepared immediately after bought from the local market. The plants were clean using tap water and subjected to oven dried for 24 h at 40°C. *P. pellucida* leaf was extracted according to Lee *et al.* [6]. The extract was then stored at −20°C for further use.

Minimum inhibitory concentration (MIC) values determination

MIC values were determined using two-fold micro broth dilution method in 96-wells microtiter plate format. The bacterial suspension was prepared as described above. Bacterial suspensions were inoculated into wells of a microtiter plate in the presence of the plant extract with concentration start from 0.15 to 31.5 mg/L and kanamycin as the positive control [7]. The growth of tested bacterial, *A. hydrophila*, was checked after 24 h (s) incubation via enzyme-linked immunosorbent assay (ELISA) reader (Bio-Rad, USA) at 540 nm. MIC value is determined as the lowest concentration of antimicrobial agent inhibits the visible growth of the inoculated bacteria [8].

Determination of plant extracts chemical composition

The chemical composition of the plant extract was carried out as described by Lee and Wendy [9]. The chromatographic procedure was performed using a gas chromatograph mass spectrometer QP2010-GC-MS (Shimadzu, Japan) with autosampler. The sample was diluted 25 times with acetone and 1 µl of sample was injected into a column. A fused silica capillary column HP5-MS (30 m × 0.32 mm, film thickness 0.25 µm) was used. Helium was the carrier gas, and a split ratio of 1/100 was used. The oven temperature used was maintained at 60°C for 8 min. The temperature was then gradually raised at a rate of 3°C per min to 180°C and maintained at 180°C for 5 min. The

temperature at the injection port was 250°C. The components of the test solution were identified by comparing the spectra with those of known compounds stored in the internal library.

Medicated feed

The fish pellets (Cargill, Malaysia) were purchased commercially before they were mixed with crude extract of *P. pellucida* leaf. Medicated feed was prepared in three different concentrations of *P. pellucida* leaf extract at 25 mg/kg, PP-25; 50 mg/kg, PP-50; and 100 mg/kg, PP-100. In the preliminary toxicity test, crude extract of *P. pellucida* showed adverse effect on the fish when given at concentrations of 150 mg/kg and above. The extract was coated onto fish pellet at a desired concentration and oven dried at 30°C for 24 h. The prepared fish pellet was then kept at −20°C for further use.

Efficacy of medicated feed experiment

The antimicrobial agent efficacy test was carried out to determine the effectiveness of *P. pellucida* leaf extract in preventing and controlling MAS in red hybrid tilapia due to *A. hydrophila*. A total of 15 groups of fish, where each group contains 10-15 fish were maintained in 20 L aquaria. Six groups of fish were used as control, where each three groups served as negative and positive control, respectively. Nine groups of fish were used in the treatment using three different concentration of *P. pellucida* leaf extract (25 mg/kg, PP-25; 50 mg/kg, PP-50; and 100 mg/kg, PP-100), with triplicates for each treatment. The experimental fish were given medicated fish pellet at 2% body weight of fish a day for 1 week before the fish were exposed to *A. hydrophila* by intraperitoneal injection. The mortality of the infected fish was observed and recorded for 4 weeks. Simultaneously, the medicated and unmedicated fish pellet was continuously given to the fish for 4 weeks. Fish from each treatment was randomly sampled for weekly ELISA. The calculation of the fish mortality as shown below:

$$\frac{\text{Total cumulative died fish} \times 100\%}{\text{Total experimental fish in aquaria}}$$

Indirect ELISA

ELISA was carried out as described by Shelby *et al.* [10] with some modification. Briefly, fish were bled from the caudal vein and the blood was collected into a micro-centrifuge tube. The blood was then allowed to clot for 1 h at 25°C. The fish serum was harvested through centrifugation at 300 g and stored at −80°C for further use. The MAS antigen was prepared by a whole cell dilution of *A. hydrophila* with carbonate buffer to 500 µg/mL. A 100 µL of MAS antigen was added to each well of the microtiter plate for 1 h at 25°C. The wells were then blocked with 3% bovine serum albumin (Sigma, USA) for 1 h at 25°C. After the incubation period, the wells were washed 5 times with phosphate-buffered saline (PBS) plus teewn-20

(PBS-T). A volume of 100 µL of a serum sample (1 µL of serum diluted in 999 µL of PBS-T) were added to three replicate wells of the plate followed by 30 min incubation at 25°C. The wells were then washed 3 times with PBS-T. After washing, 100 µL of goat anti-tilapia immunoglobulin serum (diluted 1: 5000 in PBS-T) was added to the wells followed by 30 min incubation at 25°C. Again, after 3 times washing with PBS-T, 100 µL of rabbit anti-goat peroxidase conjugate (diluted 1: 5000 PBS-T) was added into the wells. Finally, the wells were washed again with PBS-T followed by the addition of 100 µL of *o*-phenylenediamine in urea-peroxide buffer into each well. The ELISA reaction was stopped at 15 min by adding 50 µl of 3 M H_2SO_4. The optical densities (OD) of the reactions were read with the microplate reader (Bio-Rad, USA) at 490 nm. Negative controls consisted of wells coated with antigen and no sample serum and wells with no antigen and a serum sample. The control reactions gave an optical density reading at 0.04 or less.

Statistical analysis

Statistical differences between mortality and ELISA values were analyzed with one-way analysis of variance using Tukey *post-hoc* multiple comparison tests at 5% of a significant level.

Results and Discussion

The results showed that the major bioactive compound is phytol (40%), and the MIC value was 31.5 mg/L. The value of antibody response to *A. hydrophila* in fish from a group of fish which received medicated feed (PP-25, 0.128±0.014 OD; PP-50, 0.132±0.003 OD; and PP-100, 0.171±0.02 OD) was found significantly higher ($p < 0.05$) compared to fish did not receive medicated feed (0.00 OD). Whereas, percentage of cumulative mortality in fish from all groups of fish received medicated feed (PP-25, 18.0±3.2%; PP-50, 18.2±2.8%; and PP-100, 17.7±1.8%) was found significantly lower ($p < 0.05$) compared to a group of fish did not receive medicated feed (83.2±1.4%) (Table-1).

In the present study, the major compound of *P. pellucida* leaf extract was phytol (39.12%) followed by 2-naphthalenol, decahydro- (27.10%), hexadecanoic acid, methyl ester (16.12%) and 9,12-octadecadienoic acid (Z,Z)-, methyl ester (17.66) (Table-2). However, none of the identified compounds in the present study were reported by Bayma *et al.* and Xu *et al.* [11,12], which may due to a different approach in characterizing chemical compounds in the plant extract. Previous studies have revealed the antimicrobial activity of *P. pellucida* leaf extract against various types of bacteria. For instance, Lee *et al.* [7] showed that the major compound of *P. pellucida* leaf extract is phytol which claimed to be responsible to the antimicrobial and antioxidant activity of the plant. This statement is supported by the study of Kumar *et al.* [13], where the study claimed that phytol is an important

Table-1: Cumulative mortality (%) of fish of the present study.

Treatment	Cumulative mortality (%)
Control	83.2±1.4
PP-25	18.0±3.2
PP-50	18.2±2.8
PP-100	17.7±1.8

Table-2: Compound composition of *P. pellucida* leaf extract.

Compound	Composition (%)
Phytol	39.12
2-Naphthalenol, decahydro-	27.10
Hexadecanoic acid, methyl ester	16.12
9,12-Octadecadienoic acid (Z, Z)-, methyl ester	17.66
Total	100

P. pellucida = *Peperomia pellucida*

diterpene and possessed both antimicrobial and anticancer activities. In the literature, many studies were exploring the benefits of *P. pellucida* leaf extract. Nwokocha *et al.* [14] reported that *P. pellucida* was used as an anti-hypertensive remedy. However, none of the study revealed the potential of *P. pellucida* leaf extract as immunostimulator agent for aquaculture uses. Hence, this is the first report on the potential of *P. pellucida* leaf extract as an alternative of commercial antibiotic in fish health management.

Many studies have reported antimicrobial activity of plant against pathogenic bacteria from aquaculture sites. For example, *Allium sativum* extract [8], *Cymbopogon nardus* essential oil [9], *Andrographis paniculata* leaf extract [15], *Michelia champaca* seed and flower extracts [16], *Syzygium aromaticum* flower bud [17], *Citrus microcarpa* [18], *Murdannia bracteata* leaf extract [6], and many more. However, the mentioned studies were focus only on the *in vitro* antimicrobial activity of the plants. On the other hand, this study highlighted the mechanism and mode of action of the *P. pellucida* leaf extract in stimulating the immune system of the fish against infection of MAS due to *A. hydrophila*. In the near future, more immunological assays should be carried out to support the findings of the present study. For instance, immunological assays such as phagocytosis assay and chemiluminescence assay where these assays may give information on humoral and specific immune systems of fish and the response of the fish to pathogens [19].

Conclusion

Based on the finding of the present study showed the huge potential of *P. pellucida* leaf extract as immunostimulator in controlling motile septicemia motile (MAS) due to *A. hydrophila* infected in red hybrid tilapia, *Oreochromis* sp. Hence, we proposed that this plant extract can be incorporated in the fish feed to manage fish health. However, further study should be carried out in the near future before we can come to a conclusion.

Peperomia pellucida leaf extract as immunostimulator in controlling motile aeromonad septicemia due...

27

Authors' Contributions

SWL and KYS designed and supervised the study. SWL, WW, and AKZ conducted a study and analyzed the data. All authors contributed in the draft, revision, and approval of the final manuscript.

Acknowledgments

This project was funded by Minister of Education Malaysia under Niche Research Grant Scheme (vot no: R/NRGS/A0.700/00387A/006/2014/00152.

Competing Interests

The authors declare that they have no competing interests.

References

1. Lee, S.W., Najiah, M., Wendy, W., Zarol, A. and Nadirah, M. (2009) Multiple antibiotic resistance and heavy metal resistance profile of bacteria isolated from giant freshwater prawn (*Macrobrachium rosenbergii*) hatchery. *Agric. Sci. China*, 8(6): 740-745.

2. Lee, S.W., Najiah, M., Wendy, W., Nadirah, M. and Faizah, S.H. (2009) Occurrence of heavy metals and antibiotic resistance in bacteria from organs of American bullfrog (*Rana catesbeiana*) cultured in Malaysia. *J. Ven. Anim. Toxins. Incl. Trop. Dis.*, 15(2): 353-358.

3. Lee, S.W., Najiah, M. and Wendy, W. (2010) Bacterial flora from a healthy freshwater Asian sea bass (*Lates calcarifer*) fingerling hatchery with emphasis on their antimicrobial and heavy metal resistance pattern. *Vet. Arch.*, 80(3): 411-420.

4. Lee, S.W., Najiah, M. and Wendy, W. (2010) Bacteria associated with golden pompano (*Trachinotus blochii*) broodstock from commercial hatchery in Malaysia with emphasis on their antibiotic and heavy metal resistances. *Front. Agric. China*, 4(2): 332-336.

5. Lee, S.W., Najiah, M., Wendy, W. and Nadirah, M. (2010) Antibiogram and heavy metal resistance of pathogenic bacteria isolated from moribund cage cultured silver catfish (*Pangasius sutchi*) and red hybrid tilapia (*Tilapia* sp.). *Front. Agric. China*, 4(1): 116-120.

6. Lee, S.W., Wendy, W., Julius, Y.F.S., Desy, F.S. and Ahmad, A.I. (2010) Characterization of antioxidant, antimicrobial, anticancer property and chemical composition of *Murdannia bracteata* leaf extract. *Pharmacol. Online*, 3: 930-936.

7. Lee, S.W., Wendy, W., Julius, Y.F.S. and Desy, F.S. (2011) Characterization of anticancer, antimicrobial, antioxidant property and chemical composition of *Peperomia pellucida* leaf extract. *Acta Med. Iran.*, 49(10): 670-674.

8. Lee, S.W. and Najiah, M. (2008) Inhibition of *Edwardsiella tarda* and other fish pathogens by *Allium sativum* L. (Alliaceae) extract. *Am. Eurasian J. Agric. Environ. Sci.*, 3(5): 692-696.

9. Lee, S.W. and Wendy, W. (2013) Chemical composition and antimicrobial activity of *Cymbopogon nardus* citronella essential oil against systemic bacteria of aquatic animals. *Iran. J. Microbiol.*, 5(2): 147-152.

10. Shelby, R.A., Klesius, P.H., Shoemaker, C.A. and Evans, J.J. (2002) Passive immunization of tilapia, *Oreochromis niloticus* (L.), with anti *Streptococcus iniae* whole sera. *J. Fish Dis.*, 25: 1-6.

11. Bayma, J.D., Arruda, M.S., Muller, A.H., Arruda, A.C. and Canto, W.C. (2000) A dimeric ArC compound from *Peperomia pellucida*. *Phytochemistry*, 55: 779-782.

12. Xu, S., Li, N., Ning, M.M., Zhou, C.H., Yang, Q.R. and Wang, M.W. (2006) Bioactive compounds from *Peperomia pellucida*. *J. Nat. Prod.*, 69(2): 247-250.

13. Kumar, P.P., Kumaravel, S. and Lalitha, C. (2010) Screening of antioxidant activity, total phenolics and GC-MS study of *Vitex negundo*. *Afr. J. Biochem. Res.*, 4(7): 191-195.

14. Nwokocha, C.R., Owu, D.U., Kinlocke, K., Murray, J. and Delgoda, R. (2012) Possible Mechanism of action of the hypotensive effect of *Peperomia pellucida* and Interactions between human cytochrome P450 enzymes. *Med. Aromat. Plants*, 1: 105.

15. Lee, S.W., Wendy, W., Julius, Y.F.S. and Desy, F.S. (2011) Characterization of antimicrobial, antioxidant, anticancer properties and chemical composition of Malaysian *Andrographis paniculata* leaf extract. *Pharmacol. Online*, 2: 996-1002.

16. Lee, S.W., Wendy, W., Julius, Y.F.S. and Desy, F.S. (2011) Characterization of antimicrobial, antioxidant, anticancer property and chemical composition of *Michelia champaca* seed and flower extracts. *S. J. Pharm. Sci.*, 4(1): 19-24.

17. Lee, S.W., Najiah, M., Wendy, W. and Nadirah, M. (2009) Chemical composite on and antimicrobial activity of the essential oil of *Syzygium aromaticum* flower bud (Clove) against fish systemic bacteria isolated from aquaculture sites. *Front. Agric. China*, 3(3): 332-336.

18. Lee, S.W. and Najiah, M. (2009) Antimicrobial property of 2-hydroxypropane-1,2,3-tricarboxylic acid isolated from *Citrus microcarpa* extract. *Agric. Sci. China*, 8(6): 740-745.

19. Stewart, A., Vaughn, O., Scott, L., Steve, H., Carolyn, F. and James, W. (2008) Measurement of the Innate Cellular Immune Response of Hybrid Striped Bass and Rainbow Trout. Bulletin for the Western Regional Aquaculture Center (WRAC) Publication, Washington, DC.

7

Loop mediated isothermal amplification: An innovative gene amplification technique for animal diseases

Pravas Ranjan Sahoo[1], Kamadev Sethy[2], Swagat Mohapatra[3] and Debasis Panda[3]

1. Department of Veterinary Biochemistry, Odisha University of Agriculture & Technology, Bhubaneswar, Odisha, India; 2. Department of Animal Nutrition, Odisha University of Agriculture & Technology, Bhubaneswar, Odisha, India; 3. Department of Veterinary Physiology, Odisha University of Agriculture & Technology, Bhubaneswar, Odisha, India.
Corresponding author: Pravas Ranjan Sahoo, e-mail: pravasvet86@gmail.com,
KS: babuivri@gmail.com, SM: swagat.physiology@gmail.com, DP: bapu8280@mail.com

Abstract

India being a developing country mainly depends on livestock sector for its economy. However, nowadays, there is emergence and reemergence of more transboundary animal diseases. The existing diagnostic techniques are not so quick and with less specificity. To reduce the economy loss, there should be a development of rapid, reliable, robust diagnostic technique, which can work with high degree of sensitivity and specificity. Loop mediated isothermal amplification assay is a rapid gene amplification technique that amplifies nucleic acid under an isothermal condition with a set of designed primers spanning eight distinct sequences of the target. This assay can be used as an emerging powerful, innovative gene amplification diagnostic tool against various pathogens of livestock diseases. This review is to highlight the basic concept and methodology of this assay in livestock disease.

Keywords: designed primers, loop-mediated isothermal amplification assay, transboundary animal diseases.

Introduction

India is a developing country, which economy is mainly contributed by the livestock sector. As there is more emerging of transboundary diseases, high molecular level research is being going on in India for devastating the economy loss [1]. For this purpose, nucleic acid amplification is one of the most valuable tools not only for the diagnosis of infectious diseases but also used in advanced gene level research. Traditional polymerase chain reaction (PCR) of its apparent high simplicity and reliability is mostly widely used as a standard approach in all biotechnological and medical diagnostic laboratories but due to its requirement for a high precision thermal cycler, it prevents this powerful method from being widely used such as in private clinics as a routine diagnostic tool. Other different modified amplification methods such as nucleic acid sequence based amplification, self-sustained sequence replication and strand displacement amplification (SDA) work efficiently with elimination some heat denaturation step without need of thermal cycler. First, two techniques have some compromise in sensitivity, which has to overcome and SDA overcomes this problem dueto the use of four primers and isothermal conditions for amplification but still has some disadvantage such as increased backgrounds due to digestion of irrelevant DNA contained in the sample and the necessity of costly modified nucleotides as substrate [2]. So, to overcome these above problems, another single-tube amplification technique should be developed that can amplify a few copies of DNA to 10^9 in less than an hour under isothermal conditions with greater specificity. The loop-mediated isothermal amplification (LAMP) assay may fulfill all the above parameters for which it can be used as low-cost alternative for detection of different transboundary animal disease. This technique has the potential to revolutionize molecular biology because it allows DNA amplification under isothermal conditions and is highly compatible with point of care analysis [3]. So, this review may help the understanding of the basic principle, methodology and advances of LAMP assay in the livestock sector.

Principle

LAMP is an isothermal nucleic acid amplification technique, in which amplification is carried out at a constant temperature without the need of thermal cycler. It is a powerful and novel nucleic acid amplification method, which detects the DNA at a very low level compared to other methods. This method amplifies very few copies of target DNA with high specificity, efficiency, and rapidity under isothermal conditions using a set of four specially designed primers and a DNA polymerase with strand displacement activity [4]. It has two steps of LAMP amplification comprising non cyclic and cyclic steps. In this process, two or three sets of primers are used specific to the target sequence which is amplified at a constant temperature of 60-65°C by a polymerase having high strand displacement activity. For identification of 6 distinct regions on the target gene, usually, 4 different primers are used which increases the specificity. Further use of "loop primers" cause increase rate the acceleration rate of the reaction for which the amplification is obtained within 30 min. The amount of DNA produced in this assay is considerably higher than traditional PCR based amplification due to the specific nature of these primers. Amplification and detection of gene are completed in a single step by incubating the gene sample, DNA polymerase, and substrates at constant temperature. In case of reverse transcription loop LAMP (RT-LAMP) assay, the process is initiated by reverse transcriptase from the backward internal primer (BIP), by binding to a target sequence on the 3' end of the RNA template and synthesizing a copy DNA strand. Simultaneously, a new cDNA strand is created with the help of DNA polymerase by binding of the B3 primer to this side of the template strand while displacing the previously made copy. The single stranded copy now loops at the 3' end as it binds to itself. The forward internal primer (FIP) binds to the 5' end of this single strand and accompanied by DNA polymerase and synthesizes a complementary strand. The F3 primer, with DNA polymerase, binds to this end and generates a new double-stranded DNA molecule while displacing the previously made single strand. This new single strand that has been released, will act as the starting point for the LAMP cycling amplification. The DNA has a dumbbell like structure as the ends fold in and self anneal. This structure becomes a stem loop when the FIP or BIP primer once again initiates DNA synthesis at one of the target sequence locations. This cycle can be started from either the forward or backward side of the strand using the appropriate primer. Once this cycle has begun, the strand undergoes self-primed DNA synthesis during the elongation stage of the amplification process. This amplification takes place in only an hour, under isothermal conditions between 60°C and 65°C.

Methodology

The whole procedure of this assay is very simple and rapid by incubating mixture of gene sample and six proper designed specific primers in a single tube with reverse transcriptase and Bst DNA polymerase at 63°C. The LAMP amplification includes a set of six primers comprising two outers, two internal and two loop primers that recognize eight distinct regions on the target sequence [5]. The primers are designed as two outer primers, such as forward outer primer (F3) and backward outer primer (B3), having strand displacement activity during the non-cyclic step only and also two internal primers, such as FIP and BIP, having both sense and antisense sequence which helps in loop formation. Further, two loop primers, i.e.,forward loop primer and backward loop primer are designed to amplify the additional sites that are not accessed by internal primers. The amplified product is detected by agarose gel electrophoresis as well as by real time monitoring, which is based on photometry for turbidity. The turbidity is due to magnesium pyrophosphate precipitate which is being increasing in quantity as a byproduct of amplification. So, one can detect the amplification product by the naked eye whether it is of larger or smaller reaction volumes. The detection procedure can be done in real time either by measuring the turbidity or by fluorescence using intercalating dyes such as SYTO 9 [6]. A visible color change can be seen with naked eyes using dyes such as SYBR green. The dye molecules intercalate or directly label the DNA, which can be correlated with the number of copies making the LAMP be quantitative. Manganese loaded calcein can be used for detection of DNA amplification in the tube during *in vitro* DNA synthesis [2]. A small amount of low molecular weight polyethyleneimine is added to the LAMP reaction solution to detect LAMP products in a sequence-specific manner [7].

Sensitivity and Specificity of LAMP

LAMP assay is found to be 10-100 fold more sensitive than PCR with a detection limit of 0.01-10 pfu of virus [8].

LAMP in Diagnosis of Animal Diseases

Due to its simplicity, ruggedness, and low cost, LAMP has the potential to be used as a simple screening assay in the field or at the point of care by veterinarian [9]. This assay without the use of expensive thermocyclers is being used for diagnosis infectious disease in developing countries [10]. In the medical field, LAMP is widely being studied for detecting infectious diseases such as tuberculosis [11], malaria [12] and sleeping sickness [13]. LAMP has been successfully applied for rapid and real time detection of both DNA and RNA viruses. A one step single tube real time accelerated RT-LAMP assay has been developed for rapid detection of each of several recently emerged human viral pathogens i.e., Dengue, Japanese encephalitis, Chikungunya, West Nile, SARS, highly pathogenic avian influenza H5N1, and Norwalk viruses [14-18]. Amplification of DNA viruses, such as human papillomavirus type 6, 11, 16, and 18, was done by LAMP due to its high sensitivity, specificity, rapidity, and simplicity [19]. Although this assay has been started in the veterinary field, it needs to be concerned. LAMP assays that have been developed for the detection of 18 viruses deemed notifiable of ruminants, swine, and poultry by the World Organization for Animal Health [20]. Among the animal viruses, a one-step, RT-LAMP assay has been developed for detection of foot and mouth disease virus in less than 1 h in a single tube without thermal cycling [21].This assay is done by amplifying a fragment of the 3D RNA polymerase gene at 65°C in the presence of primer mixture, reverse transcriptase, and Bst polymerase. Similarly, a single step RT-LAMP was developed against G-protein sequence for detection of viral hemorrhagic septicemia virus [22]. A set of primers designed against on canine parvovirus in fecal sample, a LAMP has been reported by Cho *et al* [23]. A new of LAMP assay coupled with lateral flow dipstick for the detection of classical swine fever virus has been developed by Chowdry *et al* [24]. This assay was developed against *Coxiella burnetii* targeting the *com1* gene as an actual alternative to conventional PCR [25]. LAMP test targeting the *p40* gene of *Mycoplasma agalactiae*, for the diagnosis of classical contagious agalactia was developed by Rekha *et al* [26]. This test for detection of *Mycoplasma synoviae* strains in poultry using specifically designed primers targeting *hemagglutin A* (vlh) gene was developed by Kursa *et al* [27]. This assay for specific and rapid detection of *Brucella abortus* was developed from clinical samples of cattle [28]. This assay was found to be useful in the detection of Marek's disease in feathers and internal organs of infected chickens [29]. One step RT-LAMP method for rapid detection of the hemagglutinin and neuraminidase genes of H7N9 virus was developed Zhang *et al* [30]. A LAMP assay with 6 primers targeting a highly conserved region of the GRA1 gene was developed to diagnose *Toxoplasma gondii* [31]. It has been emerged as a novel nucleic acid amplification method for diagnosis of visceral leishmaniasis [32]. The assay with the best performance was targeted to the egl gene, which shows high analytical specificity for diverse strains of the beta proteo bacterium *Ralstonia solanacearum* [33]. This assay is currently used as standalone diagnostic test for *Clostridium difficile* infection [34]. In addition to above developments, LAMP assay can be extensively applied in the field of molecular diagnosis of cancer, identification of genetically modified organisms, detection of food adulteration, eutrophication, food allergens, pesticides, identification of medicinal plants, drug resistance, and DNA methylation studies [35].

Advantages of LAMP

Due to its ability to amplify nucleic acid under isothermal conditions in the range of 65°C, it only needs simple and low cost effective equipment. LAMP stands out to be a good and effective diagnostic test for empowering in developing countries as it does not require sophisticated equipment and skilled personnel and proves to be cost effective [36]. Its specificity is extremely high because it can amplify a specific gene by discriminating a single nucleotide difference [37]. Its amplification efficiency of LAMP is very high because there is no time loss of thermal change. The enzyme inhibition reaction at the later stage of amplification is less likely to occur because this assay is being undergoing at optimum temperature of the enzyme. The nucleic acid amplified by the LAMP method is detected through the naked eye by observing the turbidity derived from the precipitate. It can be visually detected through fluorescence by utilizing calcein in loop amp fluorescent detection reagent [2]. The fluorescence is generated by binding of pyrophosphate ions, i.e., the by-product of the amplification, to the manganese ions from calcein. The fluorescence is further intensified as calcein combines with magnesium ions. It involves both amplification and detection of the gene in a single step, by incubating the mixture of gene sample, primers, DNA polymerase with strand displacement activity and substrates at a constant temperature. Due to its high amplification efficiency, DNA can be amplified 10^9-10^{10} times in 15-60 min. There is no need denaturation step i.e., conversion of double-stranded DNA into a single stranded form, so it requires less time. LAMP assay has the great advantage of monitoring amplification by SYBR Green I dye mediated naked eye visualization and by real-time monitoring using an inexpensive turbid meter according to the situation [38].

Disadvantages of LAMP

Although LAMP has above advantages, it has some following disadvantages. Kikuchi *et al.* stated that it is more sensitive and specific than PCR as [39], but it seems to be less sensitive than PCR to inhibitor in case of complex samples such as blood, likely due to the use of a *Bst* DNA polymerase rather than *Taq* polymerase as in PCR [40]. It is less versatile than PCR. LAMP is useful primarily as a diagnostic or detection technique but not useful for cloning purposes. Proper designing of primer is a major constraint in this assay [41]. Multiplexing approaches for LAMP are less developed than for PCR. The larger number of primers per target in LAMP increases the primer-primer interactions. The product of LAMP is a series of concatemers of the target region, giving rise to a characteristic "ladder" or banding pattern on a gel, rather than a single band as with PCR.

Conclusion

LAMP is an innovative, new generation, gene amplification technique that can amplify the target sequence with a high degree of sensitivity and specificity under isothermal condition. The invention of this method a decade ago has given new impetus toward the development of point of care diagnostic tests based on amplification of pathogen DNA, a technology that has been the precinct of well developed laboratories [42]. Due to its easy detection procedure, i.e., on real-time nucleic acid amplification, this assay can be used as pen side point of care diagnostic tool for infectious animal disease. Thus, it will provide a great platform for quick and accurate identification of different pathogens in medical as well as veterinary field.

Authors' Contributions

Each and every author has contributed the relevant literature in preparation of this work of review. PRS carried out his investigations and experimentations on the mentioned topic. KS searched various related topics for better reference purpose. SM corrected the grammatical errors exists in the manuscript and DP designed the proper format of the manusript. All authors read and approved the final manuscript.

Acknowledgments

The authors are thankful to the Dean, College of Veterinary Science & A.H and to Hon'ble Vice Chancellor, Odisha University of Agriculture & Technology, Bhubaneswar, India. The authors are thankful to the Head, Department of Veterinary Biochemistry, for providing facilities and fund for the study.

Competing Interests

The authors declare that nobody has a conflict of interest in relation to this manuscript.

References

1. Belak, S., Thoren, P., Leblanc, N. and Viljoen, G. (2009) Advances in viral disease diagnosis and molecular epidemiological technologies. *Exp. Rev. Mol. Diagn.,* 9: 367-381.
2. Tomita, N., Mori, Y., Kanda, H. and Notomi, T. (2008) Loop-mediated isothermal amplification (LAMP) of gene sequences and simple visual detection of products. *Nat. Protoc.,* 3(5): 877-882.
3. Zhang, X, Lowe, S.B. and Gooding, J.J. (2014) Brief review of monitoring methods for loop-mediated isothermal amplification (LAMP). *Biosens. Bioelectron.,* 61: 491-499.
4. Saharan, P., Dhingolia, S., Khatri, P., Duhan, J.S. and Gahlawat, S.K. (2014) Loop-mediated isothermal amplification (LAMP) based detection of bacteria: A review. *Afr. J. Biotechnol.,* 13(19): 1920-1928.
5. Parida, M., Sannarangaiah, S., Dash, P.K., Rao, P.V.L. and Morita, K. (2008) Loop mediated isothermal amplification (LAMP): A new generation of innovative gene amplification technique; perspectives in clinical diagnosis of infectious diseases. *Rev. Med. Virol.,* 18: 407-421.
6. Njiru, Z.K., Mikosza, A.S., Armstrong, T., Enyaru, J.C., Ndung'u, J.M. and Thompson, A.R. (2008) Loop mediated isothermal amplification (LAMP) method for rapid detection of *Trypanosoma brucei* rhodesiense. *PLoS Negl. Trop. Dis.,* 2(1): e147.
7. Mori, Y., Hirano, T. and Notomi, T. (2006) Sequence specific visual detection of LAMP reactions by addition of cationic polymers. *BMC Biotechnol.,* 6: 3.
8. Parida, M.M., Horioke, K., Ishida, H., Dash, P.K., Saxena, P., Jana, A.M., Islam, M.A., Inoue, S., Hosaka, N. and Morita, K. (2005) Rapid detection and differentiation of dengue virus serotypes by a real-time reverse transcription-loop-mediated isothermal assay. *J. Clin. Microbiol.,* 43: 2895-2903.
9. Sen, K. and Ashbolt, N.J. (2011) Environmental Microbiology: Current Technology and Water Application. Caister Academic Press, Norfolk, UK.
10. Macarthur, G. (2009) Global Health Diagnostics: Research, Development and Regulation. Academy of Medical Sciences Workshop Report (PDF). Academy of Medical Sciences, Great Britain.
11. Dhanasekaran, S., Chandran, S.P. and Kenneth, J. (2011) Efficacy of loop mediated isothermal amplification (LAMP) assay for the laboratory identification of *Mycobacterium tuberculosis* isolates in a resource limited setting. *J. Microbiol. Methods.,* 84(1): 71-73.
12. Poon, L.L., Wong, B.W., Ma, E.H., Chan, K.H., Chow, L.M., Abeyewickreme, W., Tangpukdee, N., Yuen, K.Y., Guan, Y., Looareesuwan, S. and Peiris, J.S. (2006) Sensitive and inexpensive molecular test for falciparum malaria: Detecting *Plasmodium falciparum* DNA directly from heat-treated blood by loop-mediated isothermal amplification. *Clin. Chem.,* 52(2): 303-306.
13. Njiru, Z.K., Mikosza, A.S., Matovu, E., Enyaru, J.C., Ouma, J.O., Kibona, S.N., Thompson, R.C. and Ndung'u, J.M. (2008) African trypanosomiasis: Sensitive and rapid detection of the sub-genus *Trypanozoon* by loop-mediated isothermal amplification (LAMP) of parasite DNA. *Int. J. Parasitol.,* 38(5): 589-599.
14. Toriniwa, H. and Komiya, T. (2006) Rapid detection and quantification of Japanese encephalitis virus by real-time reverse transcription loop-mediated isothermal amplification. *Microbiol. Immunol.,* 50(5): 379-387.
15. Parida, M.M., Santhosh, S.R., Dash, P.K., Tripathi, N.K., Saxena, P., Srivastav, A. and Sahni, A.K. (2007) Development and evaluation of reverse transcription loop-mediated isothermal amplification assay for rapid and real-time detection of Japanese encephalitis virus. *J. Clin. Microbiol.,* 44(11): 4172-4178.
16. Parida, M.M., Santhosh, S.R., Dash, P.K., Tripathi, N.K., Lakshmi, V., Mamidi, N., Shrivastva, A., Gupta, N., Saxena, P., Pradeep Babu, J., Lakshmana Rao, P.V. and Morita, K. (2007) Rapid and real-time detection of chikungunya virus by reverse transcription loop mediated isothermal amplification assay. *J. Clin. Microbiol.,* 45(2): 351-357.
17. Imai, M., Ninomiya, A. and Minekawa, H. (2006) Rapid diagnosis of H5N1 avian influenza virus infection by newly developed influenza H5 hemagglutinin gene-specific loop-mediated isothermal amplification method. *Vaccine.,* 24(44-46): 6679-6682.
18. Fukuda, S., Takao, S., Kuwayama, M., Shimazu, Y. and Miyazaki, K. (2006) Rapid detection of norovirus from fecal specimens by real-time reverse transcription-loop-mediated isothermal amplification assay. *J. Clin. Microbiol.,* 44(4):1376-1381.
19. Hagiwara, M., Sasaki, H., Matsuo, K., Honda, M., Kawase, M. and Nakagawa, H. (2007) Loop mediated isothermal amplification method for detection of human papilloma virus type 6, 11, 16, and 18. *J. Med. Virol.,* 79(5): 605-615.
20. Mansour, S.M., Ali, H., Chase, C.C. and Cepica, A. (2015) Loop-mediated isothermal amplification for diagnosis of 18 World Organization for Animal Health (OIE) notifiable viral diseases of ruminants, swine and poultry. *Anim. Health Res. Rev.,* 22: 1-18.
21. Dukes, J.P., King, D.P. and Alexandersen, S. (2006) Novel reverse transcription loop-mediated isothermal amplification for rapid detection of foot-and-mouth disease virus. *Arch. Virol.,* 151(6): 1093-1106.
22. Soliman, H. and El-Matbouli, M. (2006) Reverse transcription loop-mediated isothermal amplification (RT-LAMP) for rapid detection of viral hemorrhagic septicaemia virus (VHS). *Vet. Microbiol.,* 114(3-4): 205-213.
23. Cho, H.S., Kang, J.I. and Park, N.Y. (2006) Detection of canine parvovirus in fecal samples using loop mediated isothermal amplification. *J. Vet. Diagn. Invest.,* 18(1): 81-84.
24. Chowdry, V.K., Luo, Y., Widén, F., Qiub, H.J., Shan, H., Belák, S. and Liu, L. (2014) Development of a loop-mediated isothermal amplification assay combined with a lateral flow dipstick for rapid and simple detection of classical swine fever virus in the field. *J. Virol. Methods.,* 197: 14-18.
25. Raele, D.A., Garofolo, G., Galante, D. and Cafiero, M.A. (2015) Molecular detection of *Coxiella burnetii* using an alternative loop-mediated isothermal amplification assay (LAMP). *Vet. Ital.,* 51(1): 73-78.
26. Rekha, V., Rana, R., Thomas, P., Viswas, K.N., Singh, V.P., Agarwal, R.K., Arun, T.R., Karthik, K. and Sophia, I. (2015) Development of loop-mediated isothermal amplification test for the diagnosis of contagious agalactia in goats. *Trop. Anim. Health Prod.,* 47(3): 581-587.
27. Kursa, O., Woźniakowski, G., Tomczyk, G., Sawicka, A. and Minta, Z. (2015) Rapid detection of mycoplasma

synoviae by loop-mediated isothermal amplification. *Arch. Microbiol.*, 197(2): 319-325.

28. Karthik, K., Rathore, R., Thomas, P., Arun, T.R., Viswas, K.N., Agarwal, R.K., Manjunathachar, H.V. and Dhama, K. (2014) Loop mediated isothermal amplification (LAMP) test for specific and rapid detection of *Brucella abortus* in cattle. *Vet. Q.,* 34(4): 174-179.

29. Woźniakowski, G. and Samorek-Salamonowicz, E. (2014) Direct detection of Marek's disease virus in poultry dust by loop-mediated isothermal amplification. *Arch. Virol.,* 159(11): 3083-3087.

30. Zhang, J., Feng, Y., Hu, D., Lv, H., Zhu, J., Cao, M., Zheng, F., Zhu, J., Gong, X., Hao, L., Srinivas, S., Ren, H., Qi, Z., Li, B. and Wang, C. (2013) Rapid and sensitive detection of H7N9 avian influenza virus by use of reverse transcription loop mediated isothermal amplification. *J. Clin. Microbiol.,* 51(11): 3760-3764.

31. Cao, L., Cheng, R., Yao, L., Yuan, S. and Yao, X. (2014) Establishment and application of a loop-mediated isothermal amplification method for simple, specific, sensitive and rapid detection of *Toxoplasma gondii. J. Vet. Med. Sci.,* 76(1): 9-14.

32. Khan, M.G., Bhaskar, K.R., Salam, M.A., Akther, T., Pluschke, G. and Mondal, D. (2012) Diagnostic accuracy of loop-mediated isothermal amplification (LAMP) for detection of *Leishmania* DNA in buffy coat from visceral leishmaniasis patients. *Parasit. Vectors,* 35: 280.

33. Lenarčič, R., Morisset, D., Pirc, M., Llop, P., Ravnikar, M. and Dreo, T. (2014) Loop-mediated isothermal amplification of specific endo glucanase gene sequence for detection of the bacterial wilt Pathogen *R. solanacearum. PLoS One,* 9(4):e96027.

34. Lloyd, A., Pasupuleti, V., Thota, P., Pant, C., Rolston, D.D., Hernandez, A.V., Benites-Zapata, V.A., Fraser, T.G., Donskey, C.J. and Deshpande, A. (2015) Accuracy of loop-mediated isothermal amplification for the diagnosis of *Clostridium difficile* infection: A systematic review. *Diagn. Microbiol. Infect. Dis.,* 82(1): 4-10.

35. Kundapur, R.R. and Nema, V. (2016) Loop-mediated isothermal amplification: Beyond microbial identification. *Cogent Biol.*, 2(1): 1137110.

36. Dhama, K., Karthik, K., Chakraborty, S., Tiwari, R., Kapoor, S., Kumar, A. and Thomas, P. (2014) Loop-mediated isothermal amplification of DNA (LAMP): A new diagnostic tool lights the world of diagnosis of animal and human pathogens: A review. *Pak. J. Biol. Sci.,* 17(2): 151-166.

37. Tavares, R.G., Staggemeier, R., Borges, A.L.P., Rodrigues, M.T., Castelan, L.A., Vasconcelos, J., Anschau, M.E. and Spalding, S.M. (2011) Molecular techniques for the study and diagnosis of parasite infection. *J.Venom. Anim.Toxins Incl.Trop. Dis.,* 17(3): 239-248.

38. Nakamura, N., Ito, K., Takahashi, M., Hashimoto, K., Kawamoto, M.,Yamanaka, M.,Taniguchi, A., Kamatani, N. and Gemma, N. (2007) Detection of six single-nucleotide polymorphisms associated with rheumatoid arthritis by a loop-mediated isothermal amplification method and an electrochemical DNA chip. *Anal. Chem.,*79(24): 9484-9493.

39. Aikawa, T., Horino, S. and Ichihara, Y. (2015) A novel and rapid diagnostic method for discriminating between feces of Sika deer and Japanese serow by loop-mediated isothermal amplification. *Mamm Genome.*, 26: 355-363.

40. Kermekchiev, M.B., Kirilova, L.I., Vail, E.E. and Barnes, W.M. (2009) Mutants of Taq DNA polymerase resistant to PCR inhibitors allows DNA amplification from whole blood and crude soil samples. *Nucleic. Acids Res.,* 37(5): e40.

41. Torres, C., Vitalis, E.A., Baker, B.R., Gardner, S.N., Torres, M.W. and Dzenitis, J.M. (2011) LAVA: An open-source approach to designing LAMP (loop-mediated isothermal amplification) DNA signatures. *BMC Biochem.,*12: 240.

42. Njiru, Z.K. (2012) Loop-mediated isothermal amplification technology: Toward point of care diagnostics. *PLoS Negl. Trop. Dis.* 6(6): e1572.

8

The efficacy of Na-butyrate encapsulated in palm fat on performance of broilers infected with necrotic enteritis with gene expression analysis

M. G. Eshak[1], M. A. Elmenawey[2], A. Atta[2], H. B. Gharib[2], B. Shalaby[3] and M. H. H. Awaad[4]

1. Department of Cell Biology, National Research Centre, Dokki, Cairo, Egypt; 2. Department of Animal Production, Faculty of Agriculture, Cairo University, Cairo, Egypt; 3. Department of Bacteriology, Animal Health Research Institute, Dokki, Cairo, Egypt; 4. Department of Poultry Diseases, Faculty of Veterinary Medicine, Cairo University, Cairo, Egypt.
Corresponding author: M. H. H. Awaad, e-mail: awaad3@gmail.com,
MGE: mgergis@yahoo.com, MAE: elmenawey7@yahoo.com, AA: abdomatta@hotmail.com,
HBG: hassangharib2001@gmail.com, BS: basmashalaby300@hotmail.com

Abstract

Aim: To study the efficacy of Na-butyrate encapsulated in palm fat on performance of broiler chickens experimentally infected with necrotic enteritis (NE) with the determination of its protective effect against the changes in the gene expression profiles and deoxyribonucleic acid (DNA) fragmentation.

Materials and Methods: A total of 800 one-day-old male Arbor Acres Plus broiler chickens were randomly allocated into four groups for 5 weeks. Na-butyrate was supplemented at dosages of 1 kg/ton for starter diet, 0.5 kg/ton for grower diet, and 0.25 kg/ton for finisher diet (presence or absence). Birds of groups 1 and 2 were inoculated by crop gavages with 4×10^8 CFU/ml/bird of *Clostridium perfringens* in phosphate buffered saline for 4 successive days, from 14 to 17 days of age to produce NE.

Results: Addition of Na-butyrate, encapsulated in palm fat, to ration of experimentally infected broilers with NE resulted in increased final body weight, at 35 days of age, reduced total feed consumption, improved feed conversion ratio, reduced cumulative mortality, and increased production number. There were increased intestinal diameter, intestinal length, and significantly increased the weight of bursa of Fabricius(BF) with higher hemagglutination inhibition titers against Newcastle disease (ND) vaccination versus untreated infected and untreated negative control birds. The results showed increased expression levels of alpha-toxin and glyceraldehyde-3-phosphate dehydrogenase in the bursa tissues of broilers infected with *C. perfringens*. However, the expression levels of these genes in broilers treated with Na-butyrate were similar to the non-infected control group. Supplementation of broilers with Na-butyrate increased the expression level of insulin-like growth factor-1 (IGF-1) and decreased the DNA fragmentation induced by *C. perfringens*.

Conclusion: Na-butyrate significantly improved chicken broiler body weights, increased relative weights of BF, increased antibody titers against ND vaccination, numerically lowered mortality due to *C. perfringens* infection, increased the expression level of IGF-1, and decreased the DNA fragmentation induced by *C. perfringens*. Obtained results point out the effectiveness of Na-butyrate encapsulated in palm fat in improving the production performance variables, immune response, and intestinal morphology in experimentally induced NE as well as in non-infected chicken broilers.

Keywords: chickens, deoxyribonucleic acid fragmentation, gene expression analysis, Na-butyrate, necrotic enteritis.

Introduction

It is already established that chicken gastrointestinal tract (GIT) provides a means by which the body derives nutrition, furnishes protective mechanisms to safeguard the host, and serves as an environment for other living organisms [1]. *Clostridium perfringens* belongs to the resident microbiota [2]; however, this microorganism along with predisposing factors such as mucosal damage is prerequisites for developing of necrotic enteritis (NE) [3]. Many recent studies of NE have focused on finding different ways to control this disease [4].

Butyrate is of special interest due to its numerous positive effects on the health of gut and extraintestinal tissues. Butyrate is the most important energy source of the colonocytes [5]. It regulates the proliferation and differentiation of the gastrointestinal epithelium [6] and induces apoptosis in genetically disordered cells [7]. As a consequence, butyrate has a protective effect against colorectal cancer, which was reported in some *in vitro* [8] and also *in vivo* animal studies [9]. Due to its selective antimicrobial action on most enteric pathogens [10], butyrate improves the balance of the intestinal microflora which can influence the health of the host animal or the human host [11].

Accordingly, this study was dedicated to determine the effect of using Na-butyrate encapsulated in palm fat (which is a protected acidifier encapsulated in a vegetable fat matrix, resulting in a slow release of the acids during transport through the intestinal tract) on the productive performance variables of experimentally induced NE in chicken broilers with determination of its protective effect against the changes in the gene expression profiles and deoxyribonucleic acid (DNA) fragmentation.

Materials and Methods

Ethical approval

The experiment was carried out according to the National regulations on animal welfare and approved by the Institutional Animal Ethical Committee. This study was carried out at the Poultry Research Center, Department of Animal Production, Faculty of Agriculture, Cairo University, Giza, Egypt.

Experimental birds

One-day-old male Arbor Acres Plus broiler chickens (n=800) were assigned at random to four equal experimental groups (1-4) of 200 birds assigned into 10 replicates of deep litter pens (2*1 m) with 20 birds per replicate. The brooding temperature was set at 32°C on the first day, gradually reduced to 24°C by the end of the third week, and kept at that level until the end of the experiment. The lighting pattern was 23 h L:1 h D. All chicks were vaccinated against ND at the 7th and 21st day of age using live Hitchner B1 and La Sota strain vaccines, respectively. Live infectious bursal disease vaccine (IBD 228-E vaccine) was administered at the 14th day of age. Drinking water method was used as a route of administration of the live vaccines. On the 10th day of age, 0.5 ml inactivated avian influenza vaccine (H5N1) was injected subcutaneously in the back of neck [12]. Broilers were housed in the semi-closed house. The composition of the diets and their calculated analysis are shown in Table-1. The diets used were formulated to meet

Table-1: Composition of the broilers 3-phase diets (g/kg as fed) and their calculated chemical composition.

Corn gluten meal 60%	70	70	66.5
Soya oil	30	43.8	40
Di-calcium phosphate	18	18	18
Lime stone	13	13	13
D.L. Methionine	2.2	2.1	2.3
Lysine hydrochloride	2.9	2.8	3.6
Sodium chloride	4	4	4
Premix*	3	3	3
Calculated analysis			
Crude protein %	23.0	21.0	19.0
Metabolizable energy (kcal/kg)	3000	3100	3200

*Each 3 g of premix contained: Vitamin A (trans-retinyl acetate), 9,000 IU; Vitamin D3 (cholecalciferol), 2,600 IU; Vitamin E (dl-á-tocopheryl acetate), 16 mg; Vitamin B1, 1.6 mg; Vitamin B2, 6.5 mg; Vitamin B6, 2.2 mg; Vitamin B12 (cyanocobalamin), 0.015 mg; Vitamin K3, 2.5 mg; choline (choline chloride), 300 mg; nicotinic acid, 30 mg; pantothenic acid (d-calcium pantothenate), 10 mg; folic acid, 0.6 mg; d-biotin, 0.07 mg; manganese (MnO), 70 mg; zinc (ZnO), 60 mg; iron (FeSO H O), 40 mg; copper (CuSO 5H O), 7 mg; iodine [Ca(IO)], mg; selenium (NaSeO), 0.3 mg

the nutrient requirements of the broiler chicks during starter, grower, and finisher periods according to the National Research Council [13]. Semduramicin was added to all rations at a concentration of 25 ppm as a coccidiostat. No antibiotics were administrated in water or feed, for the whole experimental period (35 days). Birds had free access to feed and water.

Experimental design

Birds of groups 1 and 3 received Na-butyrate in palm fat (which is fat coated sodium of alimentary fatty acid). Its ingredient is n-Butyric acid sodium salt 30±2%. Na-butyrate supplementation in ration was given at a dosages according to the manufacturer's recommendations (starter diet: 1 kg/ton, grower diet: 0.5 kg/ton, and finisher diet: 0.25 kg/ton). Birds of groups 2 and 4 received control ration without treatment. Birds of groups 1 and 2 were inoculated by crop gavages with 4×10^8 CFU/ml/bird of *C. perfringensin* phosphate buffered saline (PBS) for 4 successive days, from 14 to 17 days of age [14]. The used strain of *C. perfringens* was type A B2 NET B, isolated from cases of chicken NE. Broilers of groups 3 and 4 were kept without infection.

Measured parameters
Productive performance

Chicken performance response variables were determined according to North [15]; weekly individual body weight (wt.) was measured on all birds. Weekly feed consumption (g/d/bird), feed conversion ratio (FCR) (g feed/g live body wt. gain), and mortality rate were measured for each replicate. Dead birds were weighed to include their weights in the feed conversion estimates. An index of productivity is the so-called production number, which equals (Kilograms of growth per day * (100-mortality%)/ Feed conversion ratio)*100 [16] was estimated for each replicate, at the end of the experimental period.

Intestinal length and diameter

Intestinal length (duodenum + jejunum + ileum) and diameter (in the middle of ileum) were measured on three birds from each replicate (chosen at random), on the 35th day of age.

Relative weights of spleen, thymus, and BF

At 35 days of age, determination of the relative spleen, thymus, and BF weights, as a percent of the fasting live body weights, was performed on the chosen 3 birds from each replicate.

Humoral anti-ND vaccine antibody titers

For determination of the effect of NE infection and feed supplementation with Na-butyrate on humoral immunity, blood samples were collected from wing veins of 30 randomly selected birds from each replicate, at 2, 3, 4, and 5 weeks of age. Serum samples were subjected to HI test for determining antibody titers against ND vaccination as described by Swayne *et al.* [17].

The present study was also aimed to: (1) Investigate the role the immune proteins encoding genes (alpha-toxin and glyceraldehyde-3-phosphate dehydrogenase [GPD]) in bursa tissues of broilers treated with *C. perfringens*, (2) Examine the alteration in insulin-like growth factor-1 (IGF-1) gene expression due to *C. perfringens* exposure in liver tissues, (3) Study the effect of *C. perfringens* on the DNA fragmentation in the intestinal tissues of treated broilers, and (4) Evaluate the protective effect of Na-butyrate against the changes in the gene expression and DNA fragmentation induced by *C. perfringens* in broiler organs.

DNA fragmentation in intestine using gel electrophoresis laddering assay

Apoptotic DNA fragmentation of 10 birds from each treatment (one from each replicate), at 5 weeks of age, was qualitatively analyzed by detecting the laddering pattern of nuclear DNA according to Gibb *et al.* [18]. Briefly, intestinal tissues were homogenized, washed in PBS, and lysed in 0.5 ml of DNA extraction buffer (50 mM Tris–HCl, 10 mM EDTA. 0.5% Triton, and 100 µg/ml proteinase K, pH 8.0) for overnight at 37°C. The lysate was then incubated with 100 µg/ml, DNase-free, RNase for 2 h at 37°C, followed by three extractions of an equal volume of phenol/chloroform (1:1 v/v) and a subsequent re-extraction with chloroform by centrifuging at 15,000 rpm for 5 min at 4°C. The extracted DNA was precipitated in two volumes of ice-cold 100% ethanol with 1/10 volume of 3 M sodium acetate, pH 5.2 at −20°C for 1 h, followed by centrifuging at 15,000 rpm for 15 min at 4°C. After washing with 70% ethanol, the DNA pellet was air-dried and dissolved in 10 mM Tris–HCl/1 mM EDTA, pH 8.0. The DNA was then electrophoresed on 1.5% agarose gel and stained with ethidium bromide in Tris/acetate/EDTA (TAE) buffer (pH 8.5, 2 mM EDTA, and 40 mM Tris–acetate). A 100-bp DNA ladder (Invitrogen, USA) was included as a molecular size marker, and DNA fragments were visualized and photographed by exposing the gels to ultraviolet trans illumination.

Gene expression analysis

Extraction of total RNA: The bursa and liver tissues of 10 birds from each treatment (one from each replicate), at 5 weeks of age, were used individually to extract total RNA using TRIzol® Reagent (Invitrogen, Germany). Total RNA of each tissue was treated individually with 1 U of RQ1, RNAse-free, DNAse (Invitrogen, Germany) to digest DNA residues, re-suspended in DEPC-treated water, and photospectrometrically quantified at A260. The purity of total RNA was assessed by the 260/280 nm ratio (between 1.8 and 2.1). In addition, integrity was assured with ethidium bromide-stain analysis of 28S and 18S bands by formaldehyde-containing agarose gel electrophoresis. Aliquots were used immediately for reverse transcription (RT), otherwise stored at −80°C.

Synthesis of the cDNA using RT reaction

The complete Poly (A)⁺ RNA isolated from birds tissues was reverse transcribed into cDNA in a total volume of 20 µl using Revert Aid™ First Strand cDNA Synthesis Kit (MBI Fermentas, Germany). An amount of total RNA (5µg) was used as a reaction mixture, termed as master mix (MM). The MM was consisted of 50 mM $MgCl_2$,5× RT buffer (50 mM KCl; 10 mM Tris-HCl; pH 8.3), 10 mM of each dNTP, 50 µM oligo-dT primer, 20 U ribonuclease inhibitor (50 kDa recombinant enzyme to inhibit RNase activity), and 50 U M-MuLV reverse transcriptase. The mixture of each sample was centrifuged for 30 s at 1000 g and transferred to the thermocycler (Biometra GmbH, Göttingen, Germany). The RT reaction was carried out at 25°C for 10 min followed by 1 h at 42°C and finished with a denaturation step at 99°C for 5 min [19,20]. Afterward, the reaction tubes containing RT preparations were flash-cooled in an ice chamber until being used for DNA amplification through semi-quantitative real time-polymerase chain reaction (sqRT-PCR).

sqRT-PCR

PCR reactions were set up in 25 µL reaction mixtures containing 12.5 µL 1× SYBR® Premix Ex TaqTM (TaKaRa, Biotech. Co. Ltd.), 0.5 µL 0.2 µM sense primer, 0.5 µL 0.2 µM antisense primer, 6.5 µL distilled water, and 5 µL of cDNA template. The reaction program was allocated to 3 steps. The first step was at 95.0°C for 3 min. The second step consisted of 40 cycles in which each cycle divided into 3 steps: (a) At 95.0°C for 15 s; (b) at 55.0°C for 30 s; (c) at 72.0°C for 30 s. The third step consisted of 71 cycles which started at 60.0°C and then increased about 0.5°C every 10 s up to 95.0°C. At the end of each sqRT-PCR, a melting curve analysis was performed at 95.0°C to check the quality of the used primers. Each experiment included a distilled water control. The quantitative values of RT-PCR of Alpha-toxin (Forward: CCG CTC GAG TTG GGA TGG AAA AAT TGA T; Reverse: CCG GAA TTC TTT ATA TTA TAA GTT GAA TTT [21], GPD (Forward: CCG CTC GAG GGT AAA AGT AGC TAT TAA CGG; Reverse: CCG GGT ACC TTA GAA ACT AAG CAT TTT AAA [21] and IGF-1 (Forward: GCT GTT TCC TGT CTA CAG TG; Reverse: GTA CTC TGC AGA TGG CAC AT, GenBank accession no. M32791) genes were normalized on the bases of β-actin (β-actin-F): 5′- TGT GAT GGT GGG AAT GGG TCA G -3′, B-actin-R: 5′- TTT GAT GTCACG CAC GAT TTC C -3′, expression [22]. At the end of each sqRT-PCR, a melting curve analysis was performed at 95.0°C to check the quality of the used primers.

Calculation of gene expression

The amplification efficiency (Ef) was calculated from the slope of the standard curve using the following formula [23]: $Ef=10^{-1/slope}$ Efficiency (%) = (Ef−1) × 100. The relative quantification of the target to the reference was determined using the ΔC_T method if E for the target (Alpha-toxin, GPD, and IGF-1), and the reference primers (β-Actin) are the same [24]. Ratio$_{(reference/target\ gene)}$ $= Ef_T^{C\ (reference)-C(target)}$ Gene expression data are expressed as means±standard error of mean.

Statistical analyzes

One-way analysis of variance has been adopted using SAS software general linear models procedure [25]. Percentage data were subjected to arcsine transformation before analysis. Mean values were compared using Duncan's multiple range test [26] when significant differences existed. Significance was set at p<0.05.

Results

Production performance

The results revealed that NE infected birds consumed the basal diet had significantly the lowest body weights, at 35 days of age versus the other three groups. However, non-infected birds consumed diet with Na-butyrate had significantly the heaviest body weights. The other two treatment groups (control birds and infected birds consumed Na-butyrate) body weights were intermediate with no significant differences between them. Data of feed consumption and FCR indicated that there were no significant effects due to either *C. perfringens* infection or Na-butyrate supplementation (Table-2). Numerical higher

mortality rate was present in infected consumed basal diet group as compared with the other three groups. Supplementation of Na-butyrate to non-infected birds decreased the total mortality percentage. Our data indicated that the other two experimental groups had intermediate mortalities with no significant differences between them (Table-2).

NE infection resulted in a significant decrease in the production number as compared to non-infected birds that consumed Na-butyrate diet (Table-3). However, there were no significant differences between these two groups and the other groups. However, the lowest production number was that of the infected group while the highest production number was that of the non-infected Na-butyrate-treated group.

Intestinal length and diameter

The birds infected with NE had significantly shorter intestine as compared to the non-infected ones that consumed Na-butyrate diet and the control group. However, there were no significant differences between infected birds that consumed Na-butyrate diet and control group. There were no significant effects of either NE infection or Na-butyrate supplementation on the intestinal diameter (Table-4).

Relative weights of spleen, thymus, and bursa of Fabricius

There were no significant effects of either NE infection or Na-butyrate supplementation on the

Table-2: Effect of Na-butyrate feed supplementation on performance and mortality of CPI and non-infected broilers.

Body weight (g)	1 d	1 weeks	2 weeks	3 weeks	4 weeks	5 weeks
Na-butyrate+CPI	45.3±0.1	173.4±0.7	486.3±2.1^{ab}**	960.7±6.4^a	1427±7.2^b	1852±8.8^b
CPI	45.1±0.2	174.0±0.6	482.1±3.6^b	938.1±6.5^b	1398±7.6^c	1822±9.9^c
Na-butyrate	44.7±0.2	175.1±0.6	492.9±2.9^a	963.1±4.7^a	1480±7.1^a	1915±7.3^a
Negative control	44.9±0.2	173.0±0.9	484.6±2.6^b	942.9±5.1^b	1460±7.1^a	1863±9.7^b
Probability	0.0881	0.1887	0.0439	0.0027	0.0001	0.0001

Feed consumption (g/bird/day)	1 week	2 weeks	3 weeks	4 weeks	5 weeks	Cumulative (g/bird)
Na-butyrate+CPI	22.7±0.48	52.1±0.94	109.6±2.32	125.7±2.53	160.9±2.68	3291±34.90
CPI	23.9±0.44	54.3±0.52	104.7±1.68	123.0±3.94	165.4±7.39	3298±78.45
Na-butyrate	23.6±0.27	54.4±0.44	106.4±1.86	127.1±2.23	163.7±2.18	3326±34.57
Negative control	23.5±0.41	54.1±0.75	105.4±1.18	122.4±2.79	165.7±3.52	3296±44.42
Probability	0.1961	0.0765	0.2432	0.6379	0.8677	0.9692

Feed conversion (g feed/g live body weightgain)	1 week	2 weeks	3 weeks	4 weeks	5 weeks	
Na-butyrate+CPI	0.918±0.025	1.067±0.025	1.339±0.026	1.518±0.018	1.779±0.023	
CPI	0.962±0.015	1.137±0.021	1.366±0.019	1.531±0.025	1.810±0.043	
Na-butyrate	0.929±0.007	1.108±0.013	1.341±0.019	1.474±0.019	1.737±0.018	
Negative control	0.956±0.017	1.121±0.023	1.364±0.025	1.462±0.021	1.770±0.028	
Probability	0.2209	0.1253	0.7488	0.0714	0.3987	

Weekly mortality rate (%)	1 week	2 weeks	3 weeks	4 weeks	5 weeks	Cumulative mortality rate
Na-butyrate+CPI	2.22±1.13	2.59±0.96	0.00±0.00	1.48±0.82	2.59±1.24	8.88±1.93
CPI	2.59±0.79	1.48±0.82	1.11±1.11	3.33±1.51	4.07±1.78	12.58±3.27
Na-butyrate	2.96±0.49	1.48±0.60	0.37±0.37	1.48±0.82	1.11±0.57	7.40±1.23
Negative control	2.22±0.82	1.85±0.83	1.11±0.57	1.85±0.99	3.70±1.10	10.73±1.60
Probability	0.9104	0.7441	0.5410	0.5727	0.3493	0.3650

**Means with different superscripts are significantly different (p≤0.05). CPI=*Clostridium perfringens* infected

relative weights of thymus or spleen, for 35-day-old male broilers (Table-4). On the other hand, birds that were infected with NE and consumed Na-butyrate diet had significantly the highest relative weights of the bursa of Fabricius, as compared to the other three groups.

Humoral anti-ND vaccine antibody titers

Serum antibody responses to vaccination against ND antigen that were determined at 2, 3, 4, and 5 weeks of age are presented in Table-5. NE infection significantly lowered HI titers against ND as compared to other groups at all studied intervals. NE infected, or non-infected birds that consumed Na-butyrate diet had significantly higher antibody titers, as compared to the groups that consumed basal ration.

DNA fragmentation using gel electrophoresis laddering assay

The results of gel electrophoresis laddering assay showed that the supplementation with NA-butyrate resulted in very low DNA damage which was relatively similar to the negative control birds (Figure-1). Where, the DNA bands resulted from the damaged DNA were very low in the supplemented birds with Na-butyrate. However, NE infected birds expressed more DNA bands compared with the control ones or

those supplemented with Na-butyrate. On the contrary, the damaged DNA due to *C. perfringens* infection from birds consumed Na-butyrate had decreased DNA fragmentation versus infected birds with *C. perfringens* alone (Figure-1).

Expression of immune protein encoding genes (alpha-toxin and GPD) and IGF-1 gene: The results revealed that the expression levels of alpha-toxin and GPD genes were significantly higher in birds infected with *C. perfringens* versus any of the other groups (Figures-2 and 3). However, the expression levels of alpha-toxin and GPD genes in birds supplemented with Na-butyrate were similar to the control birds. In addition, *C. perfringens* infection and supplementation with Na-butyrate showed expression levels of alpha-toxin and GPD genes significantly lower than the infected birds with *C. perfringens*alone; however, it was still significantly higher than the negative control group (Figures-2 and 3). The expression level of IGF-1 gene decreased significantly in NE infected birds as compared with that in the control ones (Figure-4). However, the expression level of the IGF-1 gene in birds supplemented with Na-butyrate was significantly higher than that in infected birds and relatively similar to that of the control group. In addition, the infection with *C. perfringens* and supplementation with Na-butyrate significantly increased the expression level of IGF-1 compared with that in birds infected with *C. perfringens* alone (Figure-4) provided that it was still significantly lower than the negative control group.

Discussion

Na-butyrate supplementation to the ration of non-infected broiler chickens for 35 days resulted in increased final body weight (52.4 g), decreased feed

Table-3: Effect of Na-butyrate feed supplementation on production number of CPI and non-infected broilers.

Treatment	Production number
Na-butyrate+CPI	264.4±6.06[ab]**
CPI	245.3±14.25[b]
Na-butyrate	285.0±6.90[a]
Negative control	262.0±8.28[ab]
Probability	0.0059

**Means with different superscripts are significantly different (p≤0.05). CPI=*Clostridium perfringens* infected

Table-4: Effect of Na-butyrate feed supplementation on relative weights of thymus, spleen and bursa of Fabriciusand intestinal length and diameter of CPI and non-infected broilers.

Treatment	Trait (%)				
	Thymus	Spleen	Bursa	Intestinal length (cm)	Intestinal diameter (cm)
Na-butyrate+CPI	0.780±0.04	0.205±0.005	0.265±0.024[a]*	196.5±1.82[bc]	0.960±0.018
CPI	0.700±0.02	0.210±0.007	0.210±0.007[b]	194.5±1.49[c]	0.955±0.021
Na-butyrate	0.740±0.03	0.220±0.009	0.220±0.009[b]	201.3±1.45[a]	0.990±0.010
Negative control	0.745±0.03	0.200±0.007	0.200±0.009[b]	199.5±1.02[ab]	0.985±0.015
Probability	0.3059	0.1430	0.0056	0.0083	0.3491

**Means with different superscripts are significantly different (p≤0.05). CPI=*Clostridium perfringens* infected

Table-5: Effect of Na-butyrate feed supplementation on weekly antibody titers against Newcastle virus vaccine of CPI and non-infected broilers.

Treatment	HI Titer			
	2 weeks	3 weeks	4 weeks	5 weeks
Na-butyrate+CPI	6.20±0.41[a]*	5.70±0.27[a]	5.10±0.33[a]	6.80±0.25[a]
CPI	4.00±0.59[b]	4.10±0.16[b]	3.30±0.21[b]	3.50±0.28[c]
Na-butyrate	6.20±0.27[a]	5.90±0.16[a]	6.00±0.25[a]	7.20±0.20[a]
Negative control	5.10±0.42[ab]	5.80±0.25[a]	5.88±0.52[a]	5.44±0.38[b]
Probability	0.0012	0.0001	0.0001	0.0001

*Means with different, superscripts, within age are significantly different (p≤0.05). CPI=*Clostridium perfringens* infected

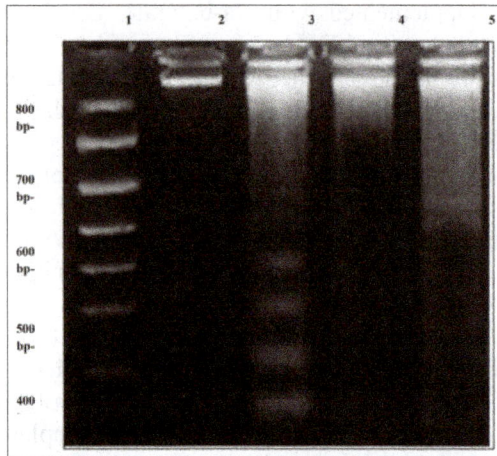

Figure-1: DNA fragmentation detected with agarose gel of DNA extracted from intestinal tissues of chicken by DNA gel electrophoresis laddering assay. Lane 1 represents DNA ladder. Lane 2 represents negative control chickens. Lane 3 represents chickens infected with *C. perfringens*. Lane 4 represents chickens treated with Na-butyrate. Lane 5 represents chickens infected with *C. perfringens* and treated with Na-butyrate.

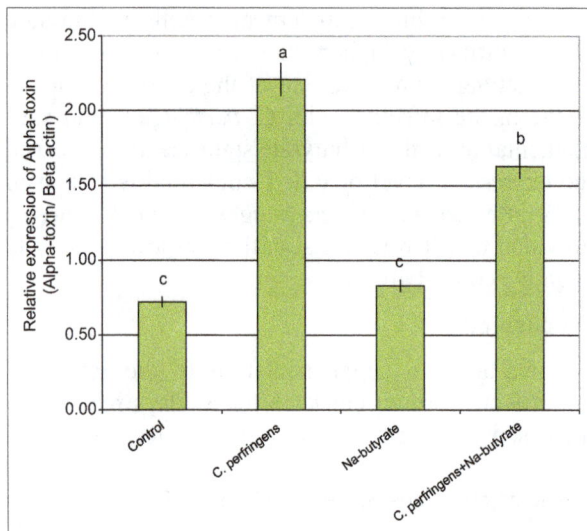

Figure-3: Semi-quantitative real time-polymerase chain reaction analysis of GPD-mRNAs in bursa tissues collected from chickens infected with *C. perfringens* and/or Na-butyrate.[a,b,c]Means with different letters, differ significantly (p≤0.05).

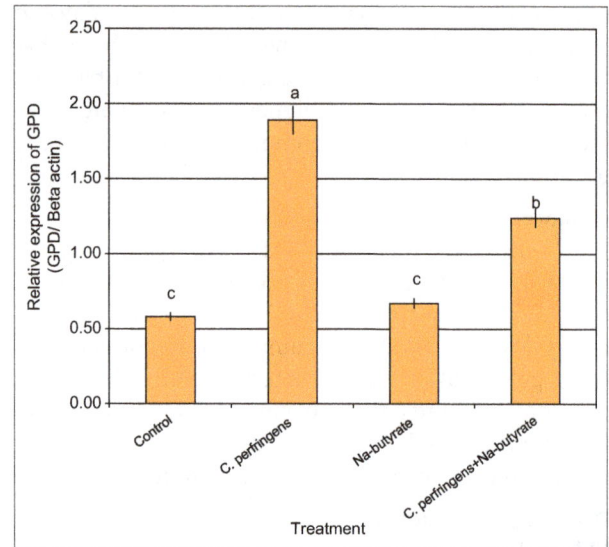

Figure-2: Semi-quantitative real time-polymerase chain reaction analysis of alpha-toxin-mRNAs in bursa tissues collected from chickens infected with *C. perfringens* and/or Na-butyrate.[a,b,c]Means with different letters, differ significantly (p≤0.05).

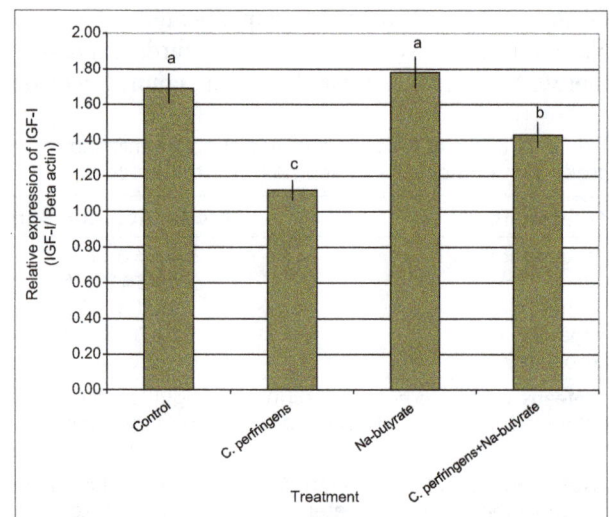

Figure-4: Semi-quantitative real time-polymerase chain reaction analysis of insulin-like growth factor-1 - mRNAs in liver tissues collected from chickens infected with *C. perfringens* and/or Na-butyrate.[a,b,c]Means with different letters, differ significantly (p≤0.05).

consumption (30 g), improved FCR (33 points), lowered cumulative mortality (3.33%) with increased production number (23.0), increased intestinal diameter (0.005 cm), and intestinal length (2 cm) and increased BF weight (2%) with higher HI antibody titers against ND vaccine as compared with their untreated negative controls. Addition of similar dose of Na-butyrate to the ration of NE infected birds resulted in increased final body weight (29.2 g), decreased feed consumption (6.5 g), improved FCR (31 points), lowered cumulative mortality (3.7%) with increased production number (19.1), increased intestinal diameter (0.005 cm), and intestinal length (1.8 cm) with significant increase in BF weight (5.5%) and higher HI

antibody titers against ND vaccine, as compared with the infected untreated group. Recently, several clinical studies indicated that butyric acid or its sodium salt mediated the immunity response [27]. The obtained results might attributed to the fact that organic acids have properties of lowering the intestinal pH, enhancing protein digestion, influencing intestinal cell morphology, stimulating pancreatic secretions, acting as a substrate for the intermediary metabolism, improving the retention of many nutrients (e.g. chelating minerals), increase intestinal integrity and influencing the electrolyte balance in the feed and intestine [28,29]. Taking in consideration that many countries have banned or limited the general use of antibiotics in feed as growth promoters (AGP) in animals [8]; the positive effect of Na-butyrate encapsulated in palm fat on performance variables could be used alternatively to AGP which confirms the results of Awaad *et al.* [30], who reported that usage of protected organic acids, in poultry nutrition, could be an efficacious tool to replace AGP. Moreover,Gauthier [29] concluded that organic acids could be a powerful tool in maintaining the health of poultry GIT, thus improving their production performances. Jankowskia *et al.* [31] reported that the use of butyric acid in poultry nutrition is quite well accepted due to the reduction of pH that limits the development of pathogens and helps in the digestion of proteins. They explained its mode of action as: Once Na-butyrate reaches the stomach of the bird, it quickly release sodium ion and, due to the low pH, butyrate is rapidly converted to the undissociated form, termed the butyric acid. This form is the one responsible for the antimicrobial activity, as the butyric acid is strongly lipophilic and can diffuse across the membranes of bacteria.

Experimental induction of NE in broiler chickens in the present investigation increased expression levels of alpha-toxin and GPD genes in the bursa tissues. Kulkarni *et al.* [21] found that expression of alpha-toxin and GPD genes were highly expressed in broilers infected with *C. perfringens*. On the other hand, the expression levels of these genes in broilers supplemented with Na-butyrate in the present work were similar to the negative control group. Moreover, treatment of broilers with Na-butyrate increased the expression level of IGF-1 and decreased the DNA fragmentation induced by NE infection. These results are in agreement with those reported by Jankowskia *et al.* [31]. Recent studies have shown that the effects of butyrate in the intestinal lumen are induced via the activation of specific receptors in the epithelial cells. When present in the lower part of the intestinal tract, butyrate can eliminate colonization of detrimental bacteria inhibiting the expression of the gene that is responsible for the invasion of the epithelial cells [21]. These previous findings could give us an explanation that why Na-butyrate enhanced the growth and inhibited the DNA fragmentation in the intestine (due to the butyric acid role which suppresses the infection that induced DNA damage).

Conclusion

The present investigation proved the effectiveness of Na-butyrate encapsulated in palm fat in improving the production performance variables, immune response, and intestinal morphology in experimentally induced NE as well as in non-infected chicken broilers. Na-butyrate supplementation alleviated the negative effects of NE infection on broiler alpha-toxin and GPD genes in the bursa tissues and increased the expression level of IGF-1 and decreased intestinal DNA fragmentation induced by NE infection.

Authors' Contributions

MGE carried out the DNA fragmentation and gene expression analyzes. A. Atta applied the immune status assessment. HBG and ME carried out the productive performance together with the statistical analysis of the obtained results. BS carried out the bacteriological work. MHHA planed the investigation. All authors participated in draft and revision of the manuscript. All authors read and approved the final manuscript.

Acknowledgments

The authors acknowledge NUTRI-AD International, Belgium for supplying the material of Na-butyrate (Admix® 30). They acknowledge the Animal Production Department, Faculty of Agriculture, Cairo University, Egypt, for financial support for carrying out the experimental work. They also acknowledge the Cell Biology Department, National Research Centre, Cairo, Egypt for carrying out the DNA fragmentation and gene expression work.

Competing Interests

The authors declare that they have no competing interests.

References

1. Aarestrup, F.M. (1999) Association between the consumption of antimicrobial agents in animal husbandry and the occurrence of resistant bacteria among food animals. *Int. J. Antimicrob. Agends.*, 12: 279-285.

2. Sengupta, N., Alam, S., Kumar, R. and Singh, L. (2011) Diversity and antibiotic susceptibility pattern of cultivable anaerobic bacteria from soil and sewage samples of India. *Infect. Genet. Evol.*, 11: 64-77.

3. Llanco, L.A., Nakano, V., Ferreiranda, A. and Avila-Campos, M. (2012) Toxinotyping and antimicrobial susceptibility of *Clostridium perfringens* isolated from broiler chickens with necrotic enteritis. *Int. J. Microbiol. Res.*, 4: 290-294.

4. Shojadoost, B., Andrew, R. and John, F. (2012) The successful experimental induction of necrotic enteritis in chickens by *Clostridium perfringens* a critical review. *Vet. Res.*, 43: 74-86.

5. Roediger, W.E. (1982) Utilization of nutrients by isolated epithelial cells of the rat colon. *Gastroenterology*, 83: 424-429.

6. Gálfi, P. and Neogrády, S. (2002) The pH-dependent inhibitory action of n-butyrate on gastrointestinal epithelial cell division. *Food Res. Int.*, 34: 581-586.

7. Leu, R., Hu, Y., Brown, I. and Young, G. (2009) Effect of high amylase maize starches on colonic fermentation and apoptotic response to DNA-damage in the colon of rats. *Nutr. Metab.*, 6: 11.

8. Young, G.P. and Gibson, P.R. (1995) Butyrate and the human cancer cell. Cambridge University Press, Cambridge.

9. LeLeu, R., Brown, I., Hu, Y., Morita, T., Esterman, A. and Young, G. (2007) Effect of dietary resistant starch and protein on colonic fermentation and intestinal tumourigenesis in rats. *Carcinogenesis*, 28: 240-245.

10. Fernández-Rubio, C., Ordónez, C., Abad-González, J., Garcia-Gallego, A., Pilar Honrubia, M., Jose Mallo, J. and Balana-Fouce, R. (2008) Butyric acid based feed additives help protect broiler chickens from *Salmonella enteritidis* infection. *Poult. Sci.*, 88: 943-948.

11. Candela, M., Maccaferri, S., Turroni, S., Carnevali, P. and

Brigidi, P. (2010) Functional intestinal microbiome, new frontiers in prebiotic design. *Int. J. Food Microbiol.,* 140: 93-101.

12. Elmenawey, M.A. and Gharib, H.B. (2013) Effects of monospecies and multispecies probiotics on productive performance, intestinal histomorphological parameters and immune response in broilers. *Egypt. J. Anim. Prod.,* 50: 93-102.

13. NRC. (1994) Nutrient Requirements of Poultry. 9th ed. National Academy Press, Washington, DC.

14. Timbermont, L., Lanckriet, A., Gholamiandehkordi, A., Pasmans, F., Martel, A., Haesebrouck, F., Ducatelle, R. and Van Immerseel, F. (2009) Origin of *Clostridium perfringens* isolates determines the ability to induce necrotic enteritis in broilers. *Comp. Immunol. Microbiol. Infect. Dis.,* 32: 503-512.

15. North, M.O. (1984) Broiler, roaster, and capon management. In: Commercial Chicken Production Manual. 3rd ed. Ch. 20. The AVI Publishing Company Inc., Westport Connecticut. p387.

16. Timmerman, H., Veldman, A., van den Elsen, E., Rombouts, F. and Beynen, A. (2006) Mortality and growth performance of broilers given drinking water supplemented with chicken-specific probiotics. *Poult. Sci.,* 85: 1383-1388.

17. Swayne, D.E., Glisson, J.R., Jackwood, M.W., Pearson, J.E. and Reed, W.M. (1998) A Laboratory Manual for the Isolation and Identification of Avian Pathogens. 4th ed. American Association of Avian Pathologists. Inc., Kennett Square, Pennsylvania, USA.

18. Gibb, R.K., Taylor, D., Wan, T., Oconnor, D., Doering, D. and Gercel-Taylor, C. (1997) Apoptosis as a measure of chemosensitivity to cisplatin and taxol therapy in ovarian cancer cell lines. *Gynecol. Oncol.,* 65: 13-22.

19. Ali, F.K., El-Shafai, S.A., Samhan, F.A. and Khalil, W.K.B. (2008) Effect of water pollution on expression of immune response genes of *Solea aegyptiaca* in Lake Qarun. *Afr. J. Biotechnol.,* 7: 1418-1425.

20. Elmegeed, G., Khalil, W., Mohareb, R., Ahmed, H., Abd-Elhalim, M. and Elsayed, G. (2011) Cytotoxicity and gene expression profiles of novel synthesized steroid derivatives as chemotherapeutic anti-breast cancer agents. *Bioorgan. Med. Chem.,* 19: 6860-6872.

21. Kulkarni, R., Parreira, V., Sharif, S. and Prescott, J. (2007) Immunization of Broiler chickens against *Clostridium perfringens* - Induced necrotic enteritis. *Clin. Vac. Immunol.,* 14: 1070-1077.

22. Hwang, H.S., Han, K.J., Ryu, Y.H., Yang, E.J., Kim, Y.S., Jeong, S.Y., Lee, Y.S., Lee, M.S., Koo, S.T. and Choi, S.M. (2009) Protective effects of electroacupuncture on acetyl-salicylic acid-induced acute gastritis in chicken. *World J. Gastroenterol.,* 15: 973-977.

23. Houshmand, M., Azhar, K., Zulkifli, I., Bejo, M. and Kamyab, A. (2011) Effects of nonantibiotic feed additives on performance, nutrient retention, gut pH, and intestinal morphology of broilers fed different levels of energy. *J. Appl. Poult. Res.,* 20: 121-128.

24. Bio-Rad Laboratories, Inc. (2006) Real-Time PCR Applications Guide. Bulletin 5279. Bio-Rad Laboratories, Inc., Hercules, CA.p101.

25. SAS Institute Inc. (2004) SAS/STAT® 9.1 User's Guide. SAS Institute Inc., Cary, NC.

26. Duncan, D.B. (1955) Multiple range and multiple F testes. *Biometrics,* 11: 7-42.

27. Vanhoutvin, S.A., Troost, F.J., Hamer, H.M., Lindsey, P.J., Koek, G.H., Jonkers, D.M., Kodde, A., Venema, K. and Brummer, R.J. (2009) Butyrate-induced transcriptional changes in human colonic mucosa. *PLoS One,* 4: e6759.

28. Zhang, W.H., Gao, F., Zhu, Q.F., Li, C., Jiang, Y., Dai, S.F. and Zhou, G.H. (2011) Dietary sodium butyrate alleviates the oxidative stress induced by corticosterone exposure and improves meat quality in broiler chickens.*Poult. Sci.,* 90: 2592-2599.

29. Gauthier, R. (2002) Intestinal health, the key to productivity (The case of organic acids). Scientific precongress Avicola IASA. XXVII Convencion ANECA-WPDC, Puerto Vallarta, Jal. Mexico, 30 April 2002.

30. Awaad, M.H.H., Atta, A.M., Elmenawey, M., Shalaby, B., Abdelaleem, G.A., Madian, K., Ahmed, K., Marzin, D., Benzoni, G. and Iskander, D.K. (2011) Effect of acidifiers on gastrointestinal tract integrity, zootechnical performance and colonization of *Clostridium perfringens* and aerobic bacteria in broiler chickens.*J. Am. Sci.,* 7: 618-628.

31. Jankowskia, J., Juśkiewiczb, J., Lichtorowicza, K. and Zdunčzykb, Z. (2012) Effects of the dietary level and source of sodium on growth performance, gastrointestinal digestion and meat characteristics in turkeys. *Anim. Feed Sci. Technol.,* 178: 74-83.

9

Diagnosis and prevalence of ovine pulmonary adenocarcinoma in lung tissues of naturally infected farm sheep

Ganesh G. Sonawane[1], Bhupendra Nath Tripathi[2], Rajiv Kumar[3] and Jyoti Kumar[4]

1. Animal Health Division, ICAR-Central Sheep and Wool Research Institute, Avikanagar, Malpura, Tonk, Rajasthan, India; 2. ICAR-National Research Centre on Equines, Hisar, Haryana, India; 3. Animal Biotechnology Section, ICAR-Central Sheep and Wool Research Institute, Avikanagar, Malpura, Tonk, Rajasthan, India; 4. Animal Health Division, ICAR-Central Sheep and Wool Research Institute, Avikanagar, Malpura, Tonk, Rajasthan, India.
Corresponding author: Ganesh G. Sonawane, e-mail: sganesh413@gmail.com,
BNT: bntripathi1@yahoo.co.in, RK: rajivbiotech028@gmail.com, JK: jyotivet@gmail.com

Abstract

Aim: This study was aimed to detect ovine pulmonary adenocarcinoma (OPA) in sheep flocks affected with pulmonary disorders at organized farm.

Materials and Methods: A total of 75 sheep died naturally were thoroughly examined for the lesions of OPA during necropsy. Tissue sections from affected portion of the lungs from each animal were collected aseptically and divided into two parts; one each for polymerase chain reaction (PCR) and another for histopathology.

Results: On PCR examination of lung tissues, six sheep (8%) were found to be positive for JSRV. Two of them were 3-6 months of age and did not show clinical signs/gross lesions of OPA. Four adult sheep positive on PCR revealed characteristic lesions of OPA on gross and histopathological examination.

Conclusion: In the absence of known specific antibody response to the infection with JSRV, there is no diagnostic serological test available. The PCR assay employed in this study on lung tissues, using primers based on the U3 region of the viral long terminal repeat for JSRV would be helpful in the screening of preclinical and clinical cases of OPA in sheep.

Keywords: diagnosis, lung tissues, ovine pulmonary adenomatosis, sheep.

Introduction

In Rajasthan sheep and goats are generally reared through an extensive system of rearing and are one of the major sources of sustainable livelihood of rural poor and have great economic value in terms of meat, wool and milk. In the present scenario, the demand for meat in India has increased rapidly, and emphasis has shifted from wool toward mutton as the main produce from sheep rearing [1]. Respiratory infections are quite common and responsible for 30-40% of mortality in sheep of various ages. Ovine pulmonary adenocarcinoma (OPA) has been identified in a wide variety of breeds in many countries around the world including India [2]. It is responsible for severe economic losses to the sheep industry in many sheep rearing countries and the subclinical form of the disease affects growth rate, carcass weight, and milk and wool production [3]. OPA is believed to be the most important disease that can affect international trade as determined by the Office International des Epizooties (OIE) [4]. In addition to its importance as a veterinary problem, OPA has wider relevance for fundamental studies on cancer because it has similar pathological and epidemiological features to bronchoalveolar carcinoma in humans, and is considered a useful animal model of pulmonary carcinogenesis. OPA is a contagious lung cancer of sheep previously known as sheep pulmonary adenomatosis and ovine pulmonary carcinoma [5]. OPA is caused by Jaagsiekte sheep retrovirus (JSRV), which induces oncogenic transformation of alveolar and bronchiolar secretory epithelial cells. In addition to sheep, goats and wild moufflon are also susceptible to the virus [6]. Natural cases of OPA occur in sheep at 2-4 years of age; the disease may affect lambs at the age of 2 months [7]. The incubation period in naturally infected animals is reported to be 6 months to 3 years. The clinical signs are progressive emaciation, weight loss and respiratory distress, particularly after exercise. Affected sheep often lag behind the flock. There is usually a thin mucus discharge from the nostrils, and if the head is lowered, a copious frothy exudate may pour from the nares. Moist rales may be heard on auscultation, but coughing is not usually prominent. The clinical signs are slowly progressive, ending in severe dyspnea. Death usually occurs in days to a few months, often from secondary bacterial pneumonia [7-9].

OPA can be transmitted via aerosols or droplets. The horizontal transmission has been demonstrated among sheep of all ages, but neonates seem to be particularly susceptible to infection. JSRV can be found in tumors, lung fluids, peripheral blood leukocytes and lymphoid organs and before the development of tumor, the virus can be detected in lymphoreticular cells [10]. There is no evidence that *in utero* transmission is statistically significant in the epidemiology of this disease; however, recent studies suggest that JSRV might be spread through milk or colostrum. JSRV does not survive for long periods in the environment [11].

Diagnosis of OPA is possible when clinical signs or tumors are observed [12], and the presence of JSRV can be confirmed in lung fluid or tumors by immunoblotting [13], ELISA [14] or polymerase chain reaction (PCR) [15-17]. However, it is more difficult to identify infected animals during the pre-clinical period due to the lack of detectable JSRV proteins outside the tumor [14] and of circulating JSRV-specific antibodies [18]. However, no routine assays for preclinical diagnosis of JSRV infection are available. In India, very few studies have been conducted for the detection of OPA and limited to the histopathological diagnosis only. OIE has mentioned PCR assays for the detection of JSRV in blood, bronchoalveolar lavage, lung, and lymph node tissues; however, we face difficulty in amplification of targeted gene from the lungs showing gross and histopathological OPA lesions. Therefore, the protocol for DNA extraction and PCR assay was slightly modified and optimized. In the absence of serological test and cell culture system for JSRV isolation, there is no confirmatory laboratory method for the antemortem diagnosis of OPA in affected animals and primary diagnosis can be made on the basis of flock history, clinical signs, and post-mortem lesions. The disease can be confirmed by histopathology and PCR examination. In our study, the aim was to confirm the existence and prevalence of OPA in naturally died animals exhibiting gross lesions in lungs related to OPA, therefore, histopathology and PCR used.

Materials and Methods

Ethical approval

Ethical approval was not necessary as samples were collected from dead animals.

Animals and necropsy

In this study, a total of 75 sheep died naturally were thoroughly examined for the pneumonic and OPA lesions during necropsy. The history was collected from the records of the farm under study and postmortem requisition forms received in the division. Detailed history on clinical signs including body weights, progressive emaciation, etc., was recorded before necropsy examination. Tissue sections from affected portion of the lungs from each animal were collected aseptically and divided into two parts; one each for PCR and another for histopathology. All tissues to be used for DNA extraction was transported to laboratory on ice and stored at −20°C until further use.

For histopathology, tissues were preserved in 10% neutral buffered formalin.

Histopathology

The formalin fixed tissues were cut into pieces of 2-3 mm thickness and washed thoroughly with water for several hours before putting in ascending grades of alcohol for dehydration. The dehydrated tissues were cleared in xylene and embedded with paraffin. Sections of 4-5 μm thickness were prepared from paraffin blocks and stained with hematoxylin and eosin [19].

DNA extraction and PCR

The genomic DNA was isolated from the lungs of 75 sheep using commercial DNA extraction kit (Himedia, India) as per the method described by the manufacturer. The primers (Jag F, 5'-TGGGAGCTCTTTGGCAAAAGCC-3', Jag R, 5'-CACCGGATTTTTACACAATCACCGG-3') flanking a region of 176 bp region of U3-LTR gene [10] and (F,- 5'TGTTCCAGTATGATTCCACCC-3'; R, 5'-ATAAGTCCCTCCACGATGCC-3') product size 388 bp, specific to ovine glyceraldehyde-3-phosphate dehydrogenase (GAPDH) gene [20] were synthesized commercially (Sigma–Aldrich) and used. The samples that were negative by the U3-PCR were tested by PCR for GAPDH to verify the integrity of the DNA [10].

The genomic DNA isolated from tissues were amplified in 50 μl reaction mixture containing 1× PCR buffer, 1.5 mM $MgCl_2$, 200 mM of dNTPs, 0.5 U of Taq polymerase (MBI Fermantas, MO, USA), 1 μM of primers (Jag F and Jag R), and 2 μl (0.6-0.8 μg) of purified genomic DNA solution. The PCR conditions consisted of initial denaturation at 94°C for 10 min, 40 cycles each of denaturation at 94°C for 1 min, annealing at 59°C for 1 min and synthesis at 72°C for 1 min, and final elongation at 72°C for 3 min. In every batch of PCR, negative (DNA from lungs tissues of healthy sheep amplified with ovine specific GAPDH primers) control was included. The PCR products were analyzed by visualization of desired size of DNA band in the ethidium bromide-stained agarose gel (2.0%). Unfortunately positive virus nucleic acids are not available with us, however, confirmed OPA positive animals (Based on gross and histopathology results) were considered as a positive control to screen other samples suspected to be positive for OPA.

Results

PCR examination

A total of 75 sheep died naturally were thoroughly examined for the lesions of OPA during necropsy. On PCR examination of lung tissues using U3-LTR gene, of 75, six (8%) sheep (four adult and two lambs) were found to be positive for JSRV (Figure-1). In rest of the animals, macroscopic and microscopic findings in the lungs were related to various types of pneumonia (congestion/hemorrhage, edema, consolidation and

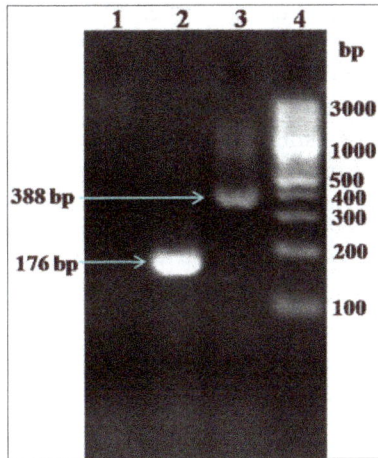

Figure-1: Polymerase chain reaction (PCR) amplification of U3 gene fragment of Jaagsiekte resolved on 2.0% agarose gel electrophoresis: Lane 1 - Non-template PCR control; Lane 2 - Amplification of JAG U3 gene; Lane 3 - Negative control (with healthy sheep lungs DNA and glyceraldehyde-3-phosphate dehydrogenase primers) and Lane 4: 100 bp plus DNA ladder (Fermentas, Cat SM0323).

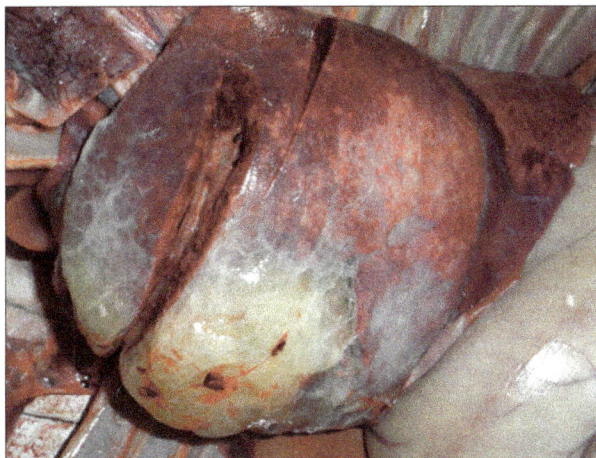

Figure-2: Ovine pulmonary adenocarcinoma affected sheep lung showing pearly-white, hard nodule.

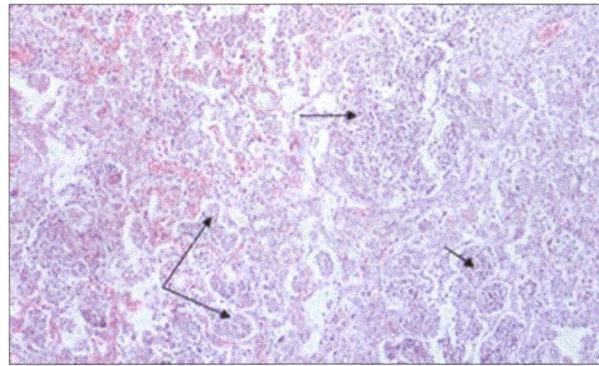

Figure-3: Lungs of ovine pulmonary adenocarcinoma polymerase chain reaction positive sheep showing proliferative changes in alveolar epithelial cells forming papillomatous projections into the alveoli (arrow) (H and E, 100×).

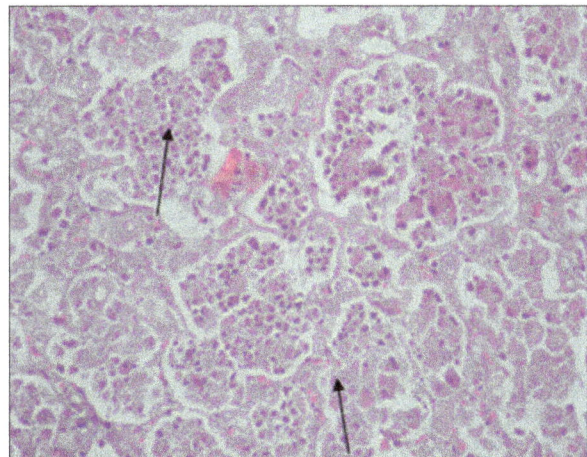

Figure-4: Alveolar epithelial cell proliferation and lymphocyte infiltration in the lungs of ovine pulmonary adenocarcinoma affected sheep (arrow) (H and E, 400×).

suppuration, etc.) and considered as other than OPA lesions. We feel it will be unrelated to mention findings of the each and every case in the present manuscript. GAPDH PCR product length in negative animals was same as in positive animals as expected.

Gross lesions

The adult PCR positive sheep revealed characteristic lesions of OPA on gross and histopathological examination. Clinical history of these animals revealed weakness, anorexia, panting, cough, and sneezing. Grossly, the lungs appeared grayish to light purple in color, which were enlarged in size and heavier. Consistency varied from granular to meaty. On the surface of the lungs slightly elevated variable-sized nodules ranging from 1.5 to 2 cm in diameter were observed. After cutting the surfaces revealed the presence of grayish exudates. In two sheep 2-3 cm pearly-white, hard nodules elevated from the surface of the parenchyma were observed particularly

in diaphragmatic lobes along with congestion in rest of the portions of the lungs (Figure-2). Clinical history of the PCR positive lambs revealed symptoms of pneumonia. Grossly, the lungs of these lambs showed lesions of pneumonia unrelated to the OPA.

Histopathology

Histological examination of lungs of adult PCR positive sheep revealed the characteristic proliferative changes in the alveoli. The alveoli revealed papillomatous proliferation forming well-marked papillae with distinct connective tissue cores giving adenomatous appearance. These papillomatous ingrowths partially or completely obstructed the alveolar lumen with projections into the alveoli (Figure-3). The bronchial and bronchiolar lining cells also revealed hyperplastic changes and rarely formed papillary projections which obstructed the bronchiolar lumen partially or completely. There was infiltration of numerous macrophages in the lumen and in the vicinity of proliferated alveoli was seen. In some of the lungs, interstitial spaces of the alveoli were found to be thickened with lymphocytes and plasma cells (Figure-4). A similar infiltration of mononuclear cells was also evident in peribronchial, peribronchiolar, and perivascular areas. In addition, the neutrophilic aggregates were observed in the lumen of several alveoli. The lungs of OPA negative control sheep did not reveal any histological alteration (Figure-5).

Discussion

OPA is a contagious viral disease of sheep that results in pulmonary neoplasia mainly in sheep and rarely in goats. The economic losses can be statistically significant up to 80% of the flock on first exposure to the infection and continuing losses may occur up to 20% each year in some flocks [21]. Eradication of the disease from a flock is difficult because no diagnostic test can detect animals in the preclinical stage. In this study, the prevalence of OPA was observed in 8% of sheep naturally died due to pulmonary affections.

The gross lesions observed in the lungs of adult sheep and microscopic proliferative changes observed in the alveolar and bronchiolar epithelium were consistent with the observations of the previous OPA studies [2,9,22]. There was infiltration of numerous macrophages in the lumen and in the vicinity of proliferated alveoli as previously reported by various workers in both natural and experimentally induced OPA [23,24]. The pathogenic role of macrophages in OPA has not been fully demonstrated, however, it was suggested that these cells may be useful in clearance of excess surfactant secreted by the neoplastic type II pneumocytes. It was also demonstrated that the tumor cells secrete a chemotactic factor that might be responsible for the recruitment of macrophages [25]. Infiltration of the inflammatory cells particularly neutrophils in the alveoli of affected lungs in present report may reflect secondary bacterial infection [24,26]. Further, OPA affected sheep lack circulating anti-JSRV antibodies and have an increased susceptibility to secondary bacterial infection, indicate that OPA affected sheep are immunocompromised [27].

Diagnostic accuracy of JSRV PCR using field data from 125 Scottish sheep flocks was studied by

Lewis *et al.* [28] using Primers P1 and P2 spanned a 229-bp region internal to the gag gene (position 1598 to 1826 of JSRV). Each blood sample of sheep was subsequently tested for the presence of JSRV proviral DNA using a hemi-nested PCR and the second round was a Taqman PCR using the carboxy-fluorescein (6-fluorescein amidite; FAM) labeled probe. It was found the PCR had a high true (analytical) sensitivity and that the low observed (diagnostic) sensitivity in individual samples was due to low concentrations of target DNA in the blood of clinically healthy animals. In this study, of six PCR positive sheep, two were 3-6 months of age and did not show clinical signs/gross lesions suggestive of OPA. Histologically, lungs of these sheep showed pneumonic lesions without evidence of OPA. The positivity of these sheep in early age reflects the sensitivity of the PCR assay used in this study. The high sensitivity for detection of OPA with improved PCR techniques has been previously reported in lymphoreticular system and peripheral blood mononuclear cells before the onset of neoplasia in experimentally inoculated lambs [27], during the pre-clinical period of the natural disease in the sheep flocks and in the in-contact sheep with no evidence of pulmonary neoplasia [29]. Our study was aimed to detect the existence of OPA in the naturally died sheep due to pneumonia in the farm under study. The gross and histopathological studies carried out to evaluate OPA lesions in the lungs. We optimized the PCR assay using published primer sequences specific for JSRV and used as a secondary confirmation test. The sensitivity and specificity of assay with these primer sequences have already been reported by previous workers [4]. The absence of gross and pathological lesions of OPA in the lungs may be due to non-development of tumor as the OPA lesions are thought to be age-dependent and clinical signs could be seen in those animals that have developed tumors [30]. In contrast to other ovine retroviral infections like Maedi-Visna, there is no known specific antibody response to infection by JSRV [18]. Therefore, there is no diagnostic serological test available [4]. Other diagnostic aids such as ultrasonography, lung biopsy, cytological and biochemical analysis of bronchoalveolar lavage, lacks sufficient sensitivity and specificity for diagnosis of early stages of the disease [3].

Conclusions

Based on the pathological investigation and PCR results, this study concludes that the OPA was prevalent in the sheep farm under study. PCR assay used on lung tissues would be helpful in the screening of preclinical and clinical cases of OPA on postmortem in sheep. However, there is need to develop PCR assays in clinical samples such as bronchoalveolar lavage, blood, colostrum, and milk in the OPA affected sheep flocks in India for early clinical diagnosis of OPA so as to reduce the incidence of the disease.

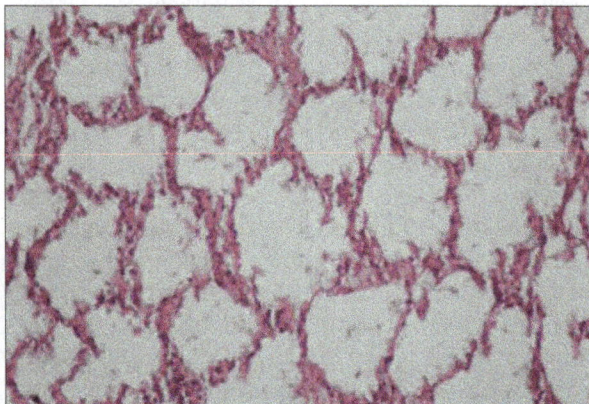

Figure-5: Lungs of polymerase chain reaction negative sheep for ovine pulmonary adenocarcinoma (negative control) (H and E, 400×).

Authors' Contributions

GGS and BNT designed the study. GGS, JK, and RK conducted the study, the study progress monitored by BNT. GGS prepared the original draft of the manuscript. All authors read, revised, and approved the final manuscript.

Acknowledgments

The authors thank the Director, ICAR-Central Sheep and Wool Research Institute, Avikanagar and Head, Division of Animal Health, ICAR-CSWRI, Avikanagar for providing necessary facility and support to carry out this research work.

Competing Interests

The authors declare that they have no competing interest.

References

1. Annual Report. (2012-13) Department of Animal Husbandry Dairying and Fisheries Ministry of Agriculture. Government of India, New Delhi.
2. Kumar, M.A., Kumar, R., Varshney, K.C., Palanivelu1, M., Sridhar, B.G. and Sivakumar, M. (2014) Incidence of ovine pulmonary adenocarinoma in southern parts of India: A slaughter house based study. *Indian J. Vet. Pathol.*, 38(3): 149-152.
3. Azizi, S., Tajbakhsh, E. and Fathi, F. (2014) Ovine pulmonary adenocarinoma in slaughtered sheep: Apathological and polymerase chain reaction study. *J.S.A. Vet. Assoc.*, 85: 1.
4. OIE. (2012) Manual of Diagnostic Tests and Vaccines for Terrestrial Animals. 7th ed. Available from: http://www.oie.int. accessed on 21-01-2016.
5. Fan, H., Palmarini, M. and DeMartini, J.C. (2003) Transformation and oncogenesis by jaagsiekte sheep retrovirus. *Curr. Top. Microbiol. Immunol.*, 275: 139-177.
6. Sanna, M.P., Sanna, E., De Las Heras, M., Leoni, A., Nieddu, A.M., Pirino, S., Sharp, J.M. and Palmarini, M. (2001) Association of jaagsiekte sheep retrovirus with pulmonary carcinoma in Sardinian moufflon (Ovis musimon). *J. Comp. Path.*, 125: 145-152.
7. Sharp, J.M. and DeMartini, J.C. (2003) Natural history of JSRV in sheep. *Curr. Top. Microbiol.*, 275: 55-80.
8. Griffiths, D.J., Martineau, H.M. and Cousens, C. (2010) Pathology and pathogenesis of ovine pulmonary adenocarcinoma. *J. Comp. Pathol.*, 142(4): 260-283.
9. Rama Devi, V., Yadav, E.J., Rao, T.S., Satheesh, K., Suresh, P., Manasa, B.B. (2014) Nucleotide sequencing and phylogenetic analysis using PCR amplicons of U3 gene of Jaagsiekte sheep retrovirus (JSRV) detected in natural cases of ovine pulmonary adenocarinoma in India. *Open J. Vet. Med.*, 4: 267-275.
10. Palmarini, M., Holland, M.J., Cousens, C., Dalziel, R.G. and Sharp, J.M. (1996) Jaagsiekte retrovirus establishes a disseminated infection of the lymphoid tissues of sheep affected by pulmonary adenomatosis. *J. Gen. Virol.* 77: 2991-2998.
11. Grego, E., De Meneghi, D., Alvarez, V., Benito, A.A., Minguijon, E., Ortin, A., Mattoni, M., Moreno, B., de Villareal, M.P, Alberti, A., Capucchio, M.T., Caporale, M., Juste, R., Rosati, S. and De Las Heras, M. (2008) Colostrum and milk can transmit jaagsiekte retrovirus to lambs. *Vet. Microbiol.*, 130: 247-257.
12. De las Heras, M., Gonzalez, L. and Sharp, J.M. (2003) Pathology of ovine pulmonary adenocarcinoma. *Curr. Top. Microbiol.* 275: 25-54.
13. Sharp, J.M. and Herring, A.J. (1983) Sheep pulmonary adenomatosis: Demonstration of a protein which crossreacts with the major core proteins of mason-pfizer monkey virus and mouse mammary tumour virus. *J. Gen. Virol.*, 64: 2323-2328.
14. Palmarini, M., Dewar, P., De las Heras, M., Inglis, N.F., Dalziel, R.G. and Sharp, J.M. (1995) Epithelial tumour cells in the lungs of sheep with pulmonary adenomatosis are major sites of replication for jaagsiekte retrovirus. *J. Gen. Virol.*, 76: 2731-2737.
15. Bai, J., Zhu, R.Y., Stedman, K., Cousens, C., Carlson, J., Sharp, J.M. and DeMartini, J.C. (1996) Unique long terminal repeat U3 sequences distinguish exogenous jaagsiekte sheep retroviruses associated with ovine pulmonary carcinoma from endogenous loci in the sheep genome. *J. Virol.*, 70: 3159-3168.
16. Palmarini, M., Cousens, C., Dalziel, R.G., Bai, J., Stedman, K., DeMartini, J.C. and Sharp, J.M. (1996) The exogenous form of Jaagsiekte retrovirus is specifically associated with a contagious lung cancer of sheep. *J. Virol.*, 70: 1618-1623.
17. De las Heras, M., Ortin, A., Salvatori, D., Perez de Villareal, M., Cousens, C., Ferrer, L.M., Cebrian, L.M., Garcia de Jalon, J.A., Gonzalez, L. and Sharp, J.M. (2005) A PCR technique for the detection of jaagsiekte sheep retrovirus in the blood suitable for the screening of ovine pulmonary adenocarcinoma in field conditions. *Res. Vet. Sci.*, 79: 259-264.
18. Ortin, A., Minguijon, E., Dewar, P., Garcia, M., Ferrer, L.M., Palmarini, M., Gonzalez, L., Sharp, J.M. and De las Heras, M. (1998) Lack of a specific immune response against a recombinant capsid protein of jaagsiekte sheep retrovirus in sheep and goats naturally affected by enzootic nasal tumour or sheep pulmonary adenomatosis. *Vet. Immunol. Immunopathol.*, 61: 229-237.
19. Luna, L.G. (1968) Manual of Histologic Staining Methods of the Armed Forces Institute of Pathology. McGraw-Hill, USA.
20. Tai, T.C., Lye, S.J. and Adamson, S.L. (1998) Expression of prostaglandin E2 receptor subtypes in the developing sheep brainstem. *Brain Res. Mol. Brain Res.*, 57: 161-166.
21. CFSPH, The Centre for Food Security and Public Health, Iowa State University. (2009) Ovine Pulmonary Adenocarcinoma. Available from: http://www.cfsph.iastate.edu. Accessed on 14-07-2015.
22. Khodakaram-Tafti, A. and Razavi, Z. (2010) Morphopathological study of naturally occurring ovine pulmonary adenocarcinoma in sheep in Fars province, Iran. *Iran. J. Vet. Res. S. Univ.*, 11: 134-138.
23. Synder, S.P., De Martini, J.C., Ameghino, E. and Caletti, E. (1983) Coexistence of pulmonary adenomatosis and progressive pneumonia in sheep in the central sierra of Peru. *Am. J. Vet. Res.*, 44: 1334-1338.
24. Garcia-Goti, M., Gonzalez, L., Cousens, C., Cortabarria, N., Extramiana, A.B., Minguijon, E., Ortin, A., De las Heras, M. and Sharp, J.M. (2000) Sheep pulmonary adenomatosis: Characterization of two pathological forms associated with jaagsiekte retrovirus. *J. Comp. Pathol.*, 122: 55-65.
25. Myer, M.S., Verwoerd, D.W. and Garnett, H.M. (1987) Production of a macrophage chemotactic factor by cultured jaagsiekte tumour cells. *Onderstepoort J. Vet. Res.*, 54: 9-15.
26. Sonawane, G.G., Singh, F., Tripathi, B.N., Dixit, S.K., Kumar, J. and Khan, A. (2012) Investigation of an outbreak in lambs associated with *Escherichia coli* O95 septicaemia. *Vet. Pract.*, 13: 72-75.
27. Holland, M.J., Palmarini, M., Garcia-Goti, M., Gonzalez, L., McKendrick, I., De las Heras, M. and Sharp, J.M. (1999) Jaagsiekte retrovirus is widely distributed both in T and B lymphocytes and in mononuclear phagocytes of sheep with naturally and experimentally acquired pulmonary adenomatosis. *J. Virol.*, 73: 4004-4008.
28. Lewis, F.I., Brulisauer, F., Cousens C., Mckendrick, I.J. and Gunn, G. (2011) Diagnostic accuracy of PCR for jaagsiekte

sheep retrovirus using field data from 125 Scottish sheep flocks. *Vet. J.*, 187: 104-108.

29. Gonzalez, L., Garcia-Goti, M., Cousens, C., Dewar, P., Cortabarria, N., Extramiana, A.B., Ortin, A., De Las Heras, M. and Sharp, J.M. (2001) Jaagsiekte sheep retrovirus can be detected in the peripheral blood during the

pre-clinical period of sheep pulmonary adenomatosis. *J. Gen. Virol.*, 82: 1355-1358.

30. Palmarini, M., Sharp, J.M., De las Heras, M. and Fan, H. (1999) Jaagsiekte sheep retrovirus is necessary and sufficient to induce a contagious lung cancer in sheep. *J. Virol.*, 73: 6964-6972.

10

Diagnosis of pathological conditions of kidney by two-dimensional and three-dimensional ultrasonographic imaging in dogs

Dinesh Dehmiwal[1], S. M. Behl[1], Prem Singh[1], Rishi Tayal[1], Madan Pal[1] and R. K. Chandolia[2]

1. Department of Veterinary Surgery and Radiology, Lala Lajpat Rai University of Veterinary and Animal Sciences, Hisar, Haryana, India; 2. Department of Veterinary Gynaecology and Obstetrics, Lala Lajpat Rai University of Veterinary and Animal Sciences, Hisar, Haryana, India.
Corresponding author: Dinesh Dehmiwal, e-mail: dd2012vets@gmail.com,
SMB: drsmbehl@gmail.com, PS: pswatch05@yahoo.co.in, RT: tayalrishi1@gmail.com,
MP: drmadanlega@gmail.com, RKC: rchandolia@yahoo.com

Abstract

Aim: The objective of the study was to obtain and compare two-dimensional (2D) and three-dimensional (3D) ultrasonographic images of the kidney in different disease conditions.

Materials and Methods: In this study, 11 clinical cases of different age groups of dogs suffering from kidney diseases were diagnosed by 2D and 3D ultrasonography at Teaching Veterinary Clinical Complex, Lala Lajpat Rai University of Veterinary and Animal Sciences, Hisar. The ultrasound (US) machine used for this study was 3D US machine (Nemio-XG: Toshiba, Japan) having four-dimensional (4D) volumetric probe. The images were acquired with 3-6 MHz 2D curvilinear transducer and 4.2-6 MHz 4D volumetric curvilinear transducer.

Results: Nephritis was diagnosed in four dogs aged between 5 months and 6 years. In all the cases of nephritis diffuse increase in echogenicity of kidney, parenchyma was observed. Two dogs with end-stage kidney disease were also diagnosed. In both 2D and 3D ultrasonography, the kidney size was decreased and architectural details were also lost in them. The cases of regional renal diseases diagnosed were hydronephrosis and nephrolithiasis. Dilated renal pelvis was the common finding in all the three cases of hydronephrosis in both 2D and 3D ultrasonogram. Nephroliths were observed in one case with the history of hematuria and oliguria. The multifocal renal disease diagnosed in this study was dysplastic polycystic kidney. In 2D ultrasonogram, six anechoic cavities appeared with thin strip of renal parenchyma. In 3D ultrasonogram, the cysts appeared as black anechoic areas.

Conclusion: The result of the current study showed that the clinical conditions of kidney such as nephritis, end-stage kidney, hydronephrosis, polycystic kidney, and nephrolithiasis can be diagnosed easily using 2D and 3D ultrasonography. Visualization of renal structures was clear in 2D ultrasonography in the conditions of nephritis and end-stage kidney. However, the conditions such as hydronephrosis, polycystic kidney, and nephrolithiasis were visualized clearly in both 2D and 3D ultrasonography equally.

Keywords: hydronephrosis, hyperechoic, hypoechoic, nephritis, ultrasonography.

Introduction

Ultrasound (US) imaging is usually one of the first studies performed to assess the kidneys because important anatomic information concerning the size, shape and internal architecture can be obtained even in the presence of impaired renal function or abdominal fluid [1].

The US is furthermore useful for guiding interventional procedures [2]. The three-dimensional (3D) ultrasonography, available in medicine for over 10 years enabled great advances in the area of diagnostic imaging. This technique facilitates the volumetric study of organs and structures, besides it, provide a third image plane, the coronal plane which allows more precisely volumetric calculation mainly those of irregular shapes.

The 3D ultrasonography is still a new technique in veterinary medicine, and few are the scientific papers that report its experimental use [3]. The objective of the study was to obtain and compare two-dimensional (2D) and three-dimensional (3D) ultrasonographic images of the kidney in different disease conditions.

Materials and Methods

Ethical approval

The study was conducted after the approval of Institutional Animal Ethics Committee.

Study site

The study was conducted in the Department of Veterinary Surgery and Radiology with the collaboration of Department of Veterinary Gynaecology and Obstetrics, College of Veterinary Sciences, Lala Lajpat Rai University and Animal Sciences (LUVAS), Hisar (Haryana).

Animals

The dogs (n=11) with pathological conditions of kidneys reported to Teaching Veterinary Clinical Complex (TVCC), College of Veterinary Sciences, LUVAS, Hisar (Haryana) were used for the study.

Ultrasonographic examination

The study was conducted on 11 clinical cases of different age groups of dogs suffering from kidney diseases brought to TVCC, LUVAS, Hisar. The dogs were sedated with xylazine at 1 mg/kg body weight for restraining. For scanning of kidneys, the area caudal to the 11th rib up to the pubis on either side of the midline, up to the level of transverse process of lumbar vertebrae was shaved properly. The dogs were controlled in lateral recumbency, i.e., left lateral recumbency for right kidney and right lateral recumbency for left kidney. The left kidney was scanned below the transverse process of first to third lumbar vertebrae and for the right kidney, in addition, an intercostal approach through the last or second last intercostal space was used to scan it in its transverse plane. Scanning area was shaved properly and enough gel was applied over the site and the surface of the transducer to get a better image. The US machine used for this study was 3D US machine (Nemio-XG: Toshiba, Japan) having four-dimensional (4D) volumetric probe. The images were acquired with 3-6 MHz two-dimensional (2D) curvilinear transducer and 4.2-6 MHz 4D volumetric curvilinear transducer.

Results

The various conditions of kidney diagnosed were nephritis (n=4), end-stage kidney (n=2), hydronephrosis (n=3), polycystic kidney (n=1), and nephrolithiasis (n=1).

Nephritis

Nephritis was diagnosed in four dogs aged between 5 months and 6 years. In the first case, a dog was brought to TVCC with the history of anorexia since 20 days, epistaxis, scanty urine with increased values of blood urea nitrogen (BUN) and creatinine. In 2D ultrasonogram (Figure-1a), there was a lack of distinction between cortex and medulla. The echogenicity of cortex and medulla was found to be increased. Renal margins were also not clearly demarcated. In 3D ultrasonogram (Figure-1b), the renal parenchyma appeared as a continuous structure without the distinction of cortex and medulla. The margins of kidney were more clearly demarcated in 3D. In the second case, a bitch was brought to TVCC with the history of continuous vomition, anorexia and not responding to the treatment. The 2D ultrasonogram revealed homogenous renal parenchyma without demarcation of cortex and medulla and increased echogenicity. The renal sinus appeared as a bright echogenic area. In 3D ultrasonogram, the renal parenchyma and renal margins were clearly visualized. In both 2D and 3D ultrasonography, the renal cortex and medulla were

not distinct. In the third case, a pup of 6 months age with the history of anorexia, intermittent vomition and stunted growth was brought to TVCC. In 2D ultrasonogram, the kidney appeared as a hyperechoic structure without demarcation of cortex and medulla. Renal margins were clearly visualized. In 3D ultrasonogram, the renal parenchyma was more clearly visualized. The other renal structures were poorly visualized. In the fourth case, a dog was brought to the TVCC with the history of anorexia, vomition and hematuria since 5 days. In 2D ultrasonogram (Figure-2a), the renal architecture was clearly visualized. The echogenic renal sinus and renal diverticulae were clearly visible. In 2D ultrasonogram, renomegaly was observed and the corticomedullary junction was also

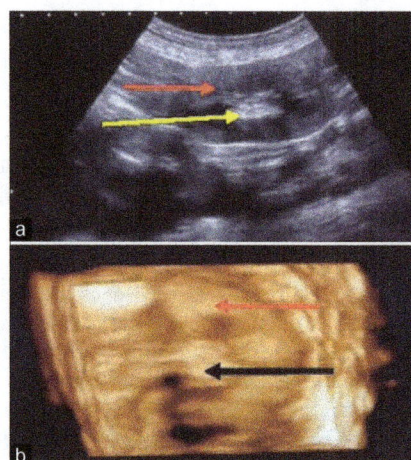

Figure-1: Nephritis (Case 1): (a) In two-dimensional ultrasonogram of kidney, the echogenicity of renal parenchyma has increased without differentiation of cortex and medulla (red arrow). Echogenic renal crest (yellow arrow), (b) in three-dimensional (3D) renal parenchyma without distinction of cortex and medulla (red arrow). Renal crest visible in the center (black arrow).

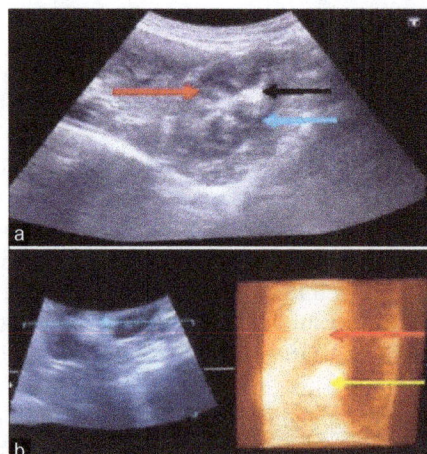

Figure-2: Nephritis (Case 4): (a) In two-dimensional ultrasonogram of kidney, the echogenic of renal diverticulae (red arrow), renal crest (black arrow) and corticomedullary junction (blue), (b) in three-dimensional ultrasonogram of kidney, homogeneous without differentiation of medulla (red arrow). Echogenic renal sinus in the center (yellow arrow).

clearly demarcated. In 3D ultrasonogram (Figure-2b), the renal parenchyma was visualized without clear demarcation of cortex and medulla. The echogenic renal sinus was visualized clearly. Renal margins were not clearly demarcated.

End-stage kidney

In this study, two cases of end-stage kidney were diagnosed with the help of ultrasonography. In the first case, a cocker spaniel dog of age 7 years was brought to the TVCC with the history of anorexia and vomition since 5 days. Furthermore, there was blood in the vomitus. The values of BUN and creatinine were 295 and 12.5 mg/dl, respectively. In 2D ultrasonogram (Figure-3a), the margins of kidney were not clear. The renal architecture was poorly visualized with no distinction of cortex and medulla. The renal parenchyma appeared as an area of mixed echogenicity with both hypoechoic and hyperechoic areas. Renal sinus was the most distinct structure in the whole kidney. In 3D ultrasonogram (Figure-3b) also the kidney architecture was poorly visualized. Kidney margins were also not clear. The renal sinus appeared as an echogenic area. Kidney parenchyma was visualized without distinction of cortex and medulla. In the second case, a dog of 13 years age was brought to the TVCC with the history of anorexia, continuous vomition since 6 days and urine incontinence since 1 week. The values of BUN and serum creatinine were 161 and 16 mg/dl, respectively. In both 2D and 3D ultrasonogram, there was no demarcation of kidney margins. The renal architecture was poorly visualized with no distinction of renal structures. The renal parenchyma appeared as a structure of mixed echogenicity. It was more clearly visualized in 3D ultrasonogram.

Hydronephrosis

In this study, hydronephrosis was observed in two cases of urinary tract obstruction and one case of ascites. In the first case, a dog was brought to the TVCC with the history of constipation, urine incontinence, and anorexia since 8 days. The values of BUN and serum creatinine were 326 and 13.3 mg/dl, respectively. In 2D ultrasonogram (Figure-4a), dilated anechoic renal pelvis was observed. Due to obstruction back pressure of urine causes atrophy of renal parenchyma. The renal cortex appeared thinner. There was acoustic enhancement distal to the dilated renal pelvis. The corticomedullary junction and interlobar vessels were not distinct. In 3D ultrasonogram (Figure-4b), the dilated renal pelvis was visualized clearly. The renal pyramids were also visualized. There was no distinction of cortex and medulla. The margins of kidney were also not clearly demarcated. In the second case, a dog of 6 year age was brought to the TVCC with the history of urine incontinence since 10 days. The values of BUN and creatinine were 142 and 18 mg/dl, respectively. The urinary bladder of dog was palpable from body wall. In 2D ultrasonogram, renal pelvis appeared dilated with anechoic

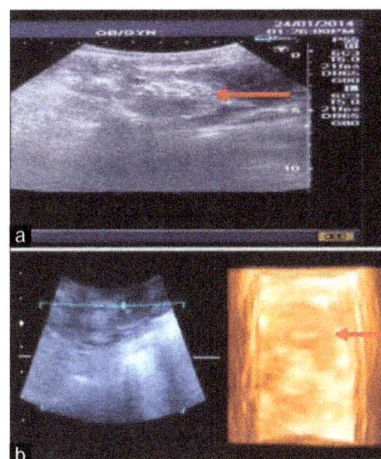

Figure-3: End-stage kidney (Case 1): (a) In two-dimensional ultrasonogram of kidney, small sized kidney appears without distinct margins (red arrow) and differentiation of cortex and medulla, (b) in three-dimensional ultrasonogram of kidney, small sized kidney appears without distinct margins (red arrow).

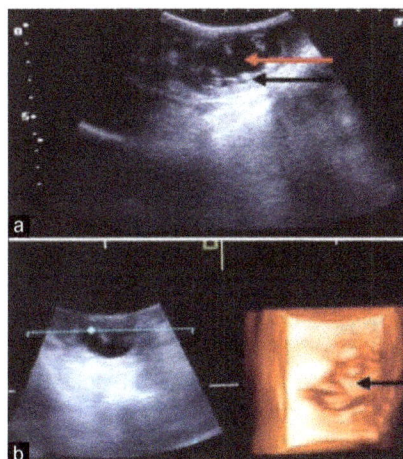

Figure-4: Hydronephrosis Case 1: (a) In two-dimensional ultrasonogram of kidney with dilated renal pelvis (red arrow). Atrophied renal parenchyma with loss of architectural details (black arrow), (b) in three-dimensional ultrasonogram dilated renal pelvis (red arrow).

lumen. Poor corticomedullary junction distinction and mixed echogenicity of renal parenchyma were observed. Kidney margins were clearly demarcated. In 3D ultrasonogram, the visualization of renal architecture was more clear. The dilated renal pelvis with anechoic lumen was clearly visualized. Kidney margins were also clearly visualized. In the third case, a Rottweller dog of 16 months age was brought to the TVCC with the history of anorexia since 2 months and blood in vomitus and urine. Body condition was very poor. The abdomen of dog was distended with the fluid of ascites. In 2D ultrasonogram (Figure-5a), all the visceral organs were clearly visualized due to fluid in the abdominal cavity. The kidney architecture was clearly visualized. The renal parenchyma appeared as a homogenous structure without distinction of cortex and medulla. Three focal hypoechoic areas were visualized in the medullary regions. Renal sinus was hyperechoic. The renal pelvis was not visualized. Hydronephrosis appeared due to fluid in the renal parenchyma and not due to ureteral obstruction. In 3D ultrasonogram (Figure-5b), focal hypoechoic areas appeared in the renal parenchyma. The renal architecture and renal margins were clearly demarcated. The cortex and medulla appeared distinct.

Nephrolithiasis

Nephroliths were observed in one case with the history of hematuria and oliguria. A Pomeranian dog of age 12 years was brought to the TVCC with the history of oliguria and blood mixed urine since 7 days. A radiograph revealed the cystoliths in the urinary bladder but no information about nephroliths was obtained. In 2D ultrasonogram (Figure-6a), the renal cortex and medulla were more echogenic than normal and corticomedullary junction was also poorly visualized. A small hyperechoic shadow of nephrolith near the diverticula was clearly visible. Renal diverticulae and kidney margins were clearly visualized.

In 3D ultrasonogram (Figure-6b), the renal architecture was more clearly visualized. The renal sinus and diverticulae were also more clear than 2D ultrasonogram. The nephroliths appeared as a small hyperechoic structure in the renal parenchyma.

Polycystic kidney

The multifocal renal disease diagnosed in this study was dysplastic polycystic kidney. A black Labrador dog of age 6 years was brought to the TVCC with the history of scanty feces, anorexia, scanty urination, and epistaxis. The BUN and creatinine values were 282.0 and 9.3 mg/dl, respectively. In 2D ultrasonogram (Figure-7a), six anechoic fluid filled structures were observed in the renal parenchyma. The cortex appeared thinner than normal. The margins of kidney were also not clearly seen. The acoustic enhancement distal to these fluid filled structures was also clearly visualized. Renal sinus and diverticulae were clearly visible. In 3D ultrasonogram (Figure-7b), the anechoic lumen of cysts was visualized but there boundary was not distinct. The renal sinus and diverticulae were more prominent than 2D ultrasonogram.

Discussion

US is the most commonly used imaging method for studying urinary tract disorders in dogs, as it is easy to perform, inexpensive and provides excellent contrast resolution in real-time [4]. A large number of studies have been carried out to access and enumerate sonographic features of the kidney, ureter, urinary bladder, and urethra both in healthy and diseased dogs. However, sonographic features of any urinary disease are not specific. Therefore, clinical and laboratory findings are required along with ultrasonography to arrive at a definitive diagnosis [5]. Diseases of the kidney diagnosed by ultrasonography can be divided into diffuse renal diseases, regional renal diseases, and focal or multifocal renal diseases. The diffuse

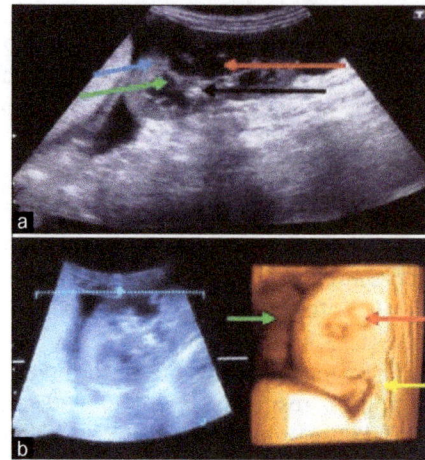

Figure-5: Hydronephrosis Case 3: (a) In two-dimensional ultrasonogram of kidney with dilated renal pelvis (red arrow). Atrophied renal parenchyma with loss of architectural details (black arrow), (b) in three-dimensional ultrasonogram fluid filled areas (red arrow), course of ureter (yellow arrow) and ascetic fluid outsite the kidney (green arrow).

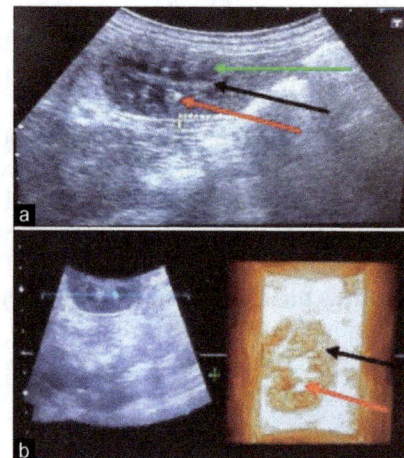

Figure-6: Nephrolithiasis: (a) In two-dimensional ultrasonogram of kidney the nephrolith is clearly visible (red arrow). The architectural details showing renal crest (black arrow) and divarticulae (green arrow), (b) in three-dimensional ultrasonogram of kidney the nephrolith (red arrow) and renal parenchyma (black arrow).

renal diseases diagnosed were nephritis and end-stage kidney. The regional renal diseases diagnosed were hydronephrosis and nephrolithiasis. The multifocal renal disease diagnosed was polycystic kidney [1].

Diffuse renal diseases observed in dogs are mainly glomerulonephritis, chronic interstitial nephritis, and end-stage kidney. They are most difficult to evaluate ultrasonographically as compared to regional and multifocal renal diseases and creates a diffuse increase in echogenicity of kidney parenchyma [6]. Verma et al. [5] also observed hyperechoic cortex and medulla in the case of nephritis. The ultrasonographic features are not specific to further differentiate between glomerulonephritis and interstitial nephritis. According to Finn-Bodner [6], the major ultrasonographic findings of glomerulonephritis are hyperechoic medulla and cortex or

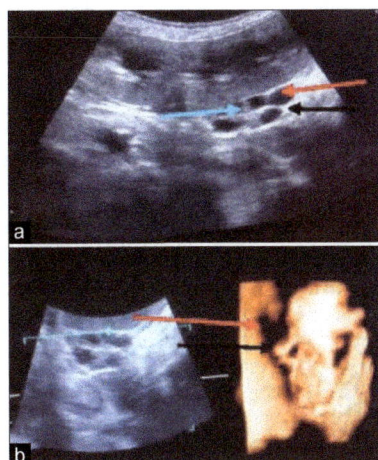

Figure-7: Polycystic kidney: (a) In two-dimensional ultrasonogram of kidney, six anechoic fluid filled structures (red arrow), thin renal parenchyma with indistinct kidney margins (black arrow) and renal divarticulae (blue arrow), (b) in three-dimensional ultrasonogram of kidney, anechoic fluid filled structures (red arrow), and renal diverticulae (black arrow).

diffuse increase in renal echogenicity. In interstitial nephritis, there is infiltration of inflammatory cells and exudates as well as the proliferation of fibrous tissue [7]. These results in increased echogenicity of renal parenchyma. Thus, the ultrasonographic features are not specific and require renal biopsy, hematological, biochemical, and urological observations for confirmatory diagnosis. Nephritis was diagnosed in four dogs aged between 5 months and 6 years. In all the cases, partial or full anorexia, intermittent vomition, dehydration, and lethargy were common signs. In two cases, the values of BUN and creatinine were very high. Hematuria was present in one case. In one of the case, there was a pup of 5 months age with partial anorexia, intermittent vomition, stunted growth, weakening of limbs and rough hair coat. Ultrasonography revealed increased echogenicity of renal parenchyma. This suggested the possibility of interstitial nephritis in the pup. The interstitial nephritis is associated with leptospirosis and infectious canine hepatitis in dogs [7]. The pup was vaccinated and the disease may be occurred due to vaccination failure.

End-stage kidney was the other diffuse renal disease diagnosed by ultrasonography in two dogs of age 13 and 7 years respectively. The values of BUN and creatinine were found to be increased in both the cases. Prolonged anorexia, persistent vomition, and oliguria were common clinical signs. One of the dogs was suffering from prostate enlargement and the other one was suffering from cystitis. The hemogram of dogs revealed anemia and neutrophilia. Erythropoietin deficiency may be the main cause of anemia, while azotemia may be the result of the loss of renal function and reduction in glomerular filtration rate [8]. In 2D ultrasonogram, margins of the kidney were not clear and decrease in the size of the kidney was observed. Finco *et al.* [9] observed that the decreased kidney size is related with chronic renal failure. The architectural details were also lost in both the cases. Similar findings were reported earlier by Verma *et al.* [5]. According to Felkai *et al.* [10], the loss of architectural details is a significant feature of chronic renal disease and occurs due to gradual loss of nephrons over a period of time. Thus, the ultrasonographic features along with clinical and laboratory findings were suggestive of end-stage kidney.

Regional renal diseases affect an anatomic or functional compartment of the kidney and are easier than diffuse renal diseases to diagnose by ultrasonography. They include pyelonephritis, hydronephrosis, nephrocalcinosis, nephrolithiasis, and hypercalcemic nephropathy. Urinary tract infection is common in dogs; especially in females is most often happening the result of ascending bacterial contamination of vulva, perivascular skin and vestibule [11]. In this study, the cases of regional renal diseases diagnosed were hydronephrosis (n=3) and nephrolithiasis (n=1). In both hydronephrosis and pyelonephritis renal pelvis dilatation occurs. According to Ackerman [12], Feeney and Walter [13] and Lamb [14] the hydronephrosis can create cyst-like expansion of the kidney. Pyelonephritis is unlikely to cause this extreme amount of pelvic dilatation. Thus, the differentiation of hydronephrosis and pyelonephritis is difficult with ultrasonography. According to Sastry and Rama Rao [7], hydronephrosis is the result of complete or partial obstruction of the urine flow from the affected kidney. Nyland *et al.* [1] reported that the renal pelvis should not be identifiable sonographically in normal dogs and cats. The urinary calculi, hemorrhagic cystitis, prostate enlargement, neoplasms and gravid uterus can cause urine obstruction and development of hydronephrosis. In this study, two cases of urinary tract obstruction and one case of ascites were observed with hydronephrosis. In 2D ultrasonogram, dilated renal pelvis was the common finding in all the three cases. In one case of urine obstruction the hydronephrosis was severe and kidney parenchyma becomes atrophied. In another case increased medullary echogenicity, poor differentiation between cortex and medulla and dilated renal pelvis were observed. Similar findings were observed by Verma *et al.* [5]. In 3D ultrasonogram, the dilated renal pelvis and renal diverticulae were more clearly visualized.

Nephroliths were observed in one case with the history of hematuria and oliguria. Radiograph revealed the cystoliths in the urinary bladder but no information about nephroliths was obtained. Ultrasonography is valuable for precise localization of radiographically visible mineral opacities in the region of the kidneys and ureters [15]. Nephroliths usually appear as intensely hyperechoic, discrete structures within the renal pelvis and collecting ducts [1]. Cystic calculi were also present in that case. In 2D ultrasonogram, the calculi appeared as a small hyperechoic structure near the caudal renal diverticula. No acoustic shadowing was observed. These findings were in agreement with the observations of Finn-Bodner [6] who opined that nephroliths may or may not create acoustic shadow. In 3D ultrasonogram, the nephrolith appeared as bright hyperechoic structure without changing their position.

The multifocal renal disease diagnosed in this study was dysplastic polycystic kidney. A black Labrador dog of age 6 years was brought to the TVCC with the history of scanty feces, anorexia, scanty urination and epistaxis. The 2D ultrasonogram revealed nephritis in left kidney and numerous cysts in right kidney. Six anechoic cavities appeared with thin strip of renal parenchyma. In 3D ultrasonogram, the cysts appeared as black anechoic areas. Konde [16] also described the renal cysts as circular anechoic structures with well-defined walls.

Conclusion

The result of the current study showed that the clinical conditions of kidney such as nephritis, end-stage kidney, hydronephrosis, polycystic kidney, and nephrolithiasis can be diagnosed easily using 2D and 3D ultrasonography. Visualization of renal structures was more clear in 2D as compared to 3D ultrasonography in the conditions of nephritis and end-stage kidney. However, the visualization of renal structures in conditions such as hydronephrosis, polycystic kidney and nephrolithiasis was clear in both 2D and 3D ultrasonography equally.

Authors' Contributions

DD, SMB, and PS have designed the study and planned the research experiment. DD performed the research experiments. PS, RT, and RKC supervised the research. MP helps in conducting experiments. All the authors read and approved the final manuscript.

Acknowledgments

The authors thank the Department of the Veterinary Gynaecology and Obstetrics for providing the US machine.

Competing Interests

The author declares that they have no competing interest.

References

1. Nyland, T.G., Widmer, W.R. and Matton, J.S. (2015) Urinary tract. In: Small Animal Diagnostic Ultrasound. 3rd ed. W.B. Saunders Company, Philadelphia, PA. p557-608.
2. Karpenstein, H., Klumpp, S., Seyrek-Inta, D. and Kramer, M. (2011) Ultrasonography of urinary tract diseases in the dog and cat. *Tierarztl Prax Ausg K Kleintiere Heimtier*, 39(4): 281-288.
3. Mendonça, D.S., Moron, R.F.F., Maldonado, A.L.L., Araujo, E., Nardozza, L.M.M. and Moron, A.F. (2012) Assessment of renal volume by three-dimensional ultrasonography in pregnant bitches: An experimental study using virtual organ computer-aided analysis. BMC Vet. Res., 8: 102.
4. Robotti, G. and Lanfranchi, D. (2013) Urinary tract diseases in dogs: US findings. A mini pictorial essay. *J. Ultrasound*, 16(2): 93-96.
5. Verma, P., Mohindroo, J., Singh, S.S. and Singh, C.B. (2006) Sonographic findings in affections of urinary system in dogs. *Indian J. Vet. Surg.*, 27(2): 104-107.
6. Finn-Bodner, S.T. (1995) In: Cartee, R.E., Selcer, B.A. and Hudson, J.A., editors. Practical Veterinary Ultrasound. Williams and Wilkins, Philadelphia, PA. p156-199.
7. Sastry, G.A. and Rama Rao, P. (2013) The urinary system. In: Veterinary Pathology. 7th ed. CBS Publishers, New Delhi. p377-400.
8. Plozin, D.J., Osborne, C.A., Jacob, F. and Ross, S. (2000) Chronic renal failure. In: Ettinger, S.J. and Feldmen, E.C. editors. In: Textbook of Internal Medicine. 5th ed., Vol. I. W.B. Saunders, Philadelphia, PA. p1634-1661.
9. Finco, D.R., Stiles, N.S., Kneller, S.K., Lewis, R.E. and Barret, R.B. (1971) Radiographic estimation of kidney size of the dog. *J. Am. Vet. Med. Assoc.*, 159: 995-1002.
10. Felkai, C.S., Voros, K., Vrabely, T. and Karsai, F. (1992) Ultrasonographic determination of renal volume in the dog. *Vet. Radiol. Ultrasound*, 33(5): 292-296.
11. Ramezani, N., Soroori, S., Jamshidi, S. and Molazem, M. (2012) Three-dimensional power doppler ultrasonographic evaluation of induced cystitis in dogs. *Iran. J. Vet. Surg.*, 7(1-2): 39-48.
12. Ackerman, N. (1991) Radiology and Ultrasound of Urogenital Diseases in Dogs and Cats. Iowa State University Press, Ames, IA. p1-25.
13. Feeney, D.A. and Walter, P.A. (1989) Ultrasonography of the Kidneys, Adrenal Glands and Urinary Bladder. American Institute of Ultrasound in Medicine Animal. Ultrasound Course Proceedings.
14. Lamb, C.R. (1990) Abdominal ultrasonography in small animals: Intestinal tract and mesentery, kidneys, adrenal glands, uterus and prostate. *J. Small Anim. Pract.*, 31: 295-304.
15. Heng, H.G., Rohleder, J.J. and Pressler, B.M. (2012) Comparative sonographic appearance of nephroliths and associated acoustic shadowing artifacts in conventional vs. Spatial compound imaging. *Vet. Radiol. Ultrasound*, 53(2): 217-20.
16. Konde, L.J. (1985) Sonography of the kidney. *Vet. Clin. North Am. Small Anim. Pract.*, 15(6): 1149-1158.

11

Molecular characterization and combined genotype association study of bovine cluster of differentiation 14 gene with clinical mastitis in crossbred dairy cattle

A. Sakthivel Selvan, I. D. Gupta, A. Verma, M. V. Chaudhari and A. Magotra

Molecular Genetics Laboratory, Dairy Cattle Breeding Division, National Dairy Research Institute, Karnal, Haryana, India.
Corresponding author: I. D. Gupta, e-mail: idgupta1959@gmail.com,
ASS: drasakthivel1987@gmail.com, AV: archana.ndri@gmail.com, MVC: mvet99@gmail.com,
AM: ankitoms@gmail.com

Abstract

Aim: The present study was undertaken with the objectives to characterize and to analyze combined genotypes of cluster of differentiation 14 (CD14) gene to explore its association with clinical mastitis in Karan Fries (KF) cows maintained in the National Dairy Research Institute herd, Karnal.

Materials and Methods: Genomic DNA was extracted using blood of randomly selected 94 KF lactating cattle by phenol-chloroform method. After checking its quality and quantity, polymerase chain reaction (PCR) was carried out using six sets of reported gene-specific primers to amplify complete KF CD14 gene. The forward and reverse sequences for each PCR fragments were assembled to form complete sequence for the respective region of KF CD14 gene. The multiple sequence alignments of the edited sequence with the corresponding reference with reported *Bos taurus* sequence (EU148610.1) were performed with ClustalW software to identify single nucleotide polymorphisms (SNPs). Basic Local Alignment Search Tool analysis was performed to compare the sequence identity of KF CD14 gene with other species. The restriction fragment length polymorphism (RFLP) analysis was carried out in all KF cows using *Helicobacter pylori 188I* (*Hpy188I*) (contig 2) and *Haemophilus influenzae I* (*HinfI*) (contig 4) restriction enzyme (RE). Cows were assigned genotypes obtained by PCR-RFLP analysis, and association study was done using Chi-square (χ^2) test. The genotypes of both contigs (loci) number 2 and 4 were combined with respect to each animal to construct combined genotype patterns.

Results: Two types of sequences of KF were obtained: One with 2630 bp having one insertion at 616 nucleotide (nt) position and one deletion at 1117 nt position, and the another sequence was of 2629 bp having only one deletion at 615 nt position. ClustalW, multiple alignments of KF CD14 gene sequence with *B. taurus* cattle sequence (EU148610.1), revealed 24 nt changes (SNPs). Cows were also screened using PCR-RFLP with *Hpy188I* (contig 2) and *HinfI* (contig 4) RE, which revealed three genotypes each that differed significantly regarding mastitis incidence. The maximum possible combination of these two loci shown nine combined genotype patterns and it was observed only eight combined genotypes out of nine: AACC, AACD, AADD, ABCD, ABDD, BBCC, BBCD, and BBDD. The combined genotype ABCC was not observed in the studied population of KF cows. Out of 94 animals, AACD combined genotype animals (10.63%) were found to be not affected with mastitis, and ABDD combined genotyped animals was observed having the highest mastitis incidence of 15.96%.

Conclusion: AACD typed cows were found to be least susceptible to mastitis incidence as compared to other combined genotypes.

Keywords: cluster of differentiation 14, combined genotypes, *Helicobacter pylori 188I*, *Haemophilus influenzae I*, mastitis, single nucleotide polymorphisms.

Introduction

In India, out of total milk production (132.4 MT), 45% milk (59.80 MT) is contributed by cattle, whereas out of total cattle milk production more than half (32.3 MT) is contributed by crossbred cattle [1]. The prevalence of bovine mastitis ranged from 29.34% to 78.54% in cows [2-4], and in the last five decades, economic losses due to mastitis have increased from 52.9 crores per annum in 1963 [5] to 7165.51 crores per annum in 2012 [6].

There is sizeable evidence that suggests resistance to non-infectious diseases such as bovine leukocyte adhesion deficiency [7], bovine chondrodysplastic dwarfism [8], and dermatophilosis [9] and infectious diseases such as tuberculosis, salmonellosis [10], Jhone's disease [11], brucellosis [12], bovine leukemia virus infection [13], foot and mouth disease [14], and mastitis [15] have genetic basis. Therefore, present efforts are directed toward approaches such as identification of resistance genes, quantitative trait loci, and markers for such diseases so that disease can be detected at an early stage or a disease-resistant animal can be selected for further breeding [16]. There are a number of reports for candidate gene association with mastitis in *Bos taurus* [17-21] and also for *Bos indicus* animals [22,23].

Cluster of differentiation 14 (CD14) is a 55-k Dalton glycosyl phosphatidylinositol-anchored surface glycoprotein that is expressed mainly on monocytes and macrophages, and weakly on polymorphonuclear neutrophils surface [24]. It also acts as opsonin receptor, thereby helps in recognition and destruction of invading agents such as bacteria. Because of this role, as suggested by Ogorevc *et al.* [20,25], CD14 gene is one of the excellent candidates for mastitis in cattle. Ibeagha-Awemu *et al.* [19] and Pal *et al.* [26] characterized CD14 gene in Canadian Holstein and Jersey and Vrindavani Crossbred cattle breeds, respectively, while Kumar *et al.* [27] found an association between genetic variants of CD14 gene with mastitis incidence in Sahiwal (*B. indicus*) cattle. However, there is no report on CD14 gene characterization, single nucleotide polymorphisms (SNPs) detection, and combined genotype study in Karan Fries (KF) cattle (*B. indicus* × *B. taurus*) which is one of the important crossbred cattle in India. Therefore, a study was planned to characterize and identify SNPs in complete CD14 gene and explore the possible association between genetic variants of CD14 gene in KF cattle (*B. indicus* × *B. taurus*) with clinical mastitis using combined genotyping.

Materials and Methods

Ethical approval

The experiment was approved by Institutional Animal Ethics Committee.

PCR-RFLP analysis

Blood samples were collected from randomly selected 94 KF cows maintained at cattle yard of National Dairy Research Institute, Karnal. Cows with history of incidences of clinical mastitis (affected ≥ once) and also non-affected cows were selected. Genomic DNA isolation was done by phenol-chloroform method as described by Sambrook and Russell [28] with minor modifications. Quality of genomic DNA was checked on 0.8% agarose gel electrophoresis. Quality and quantity of DNA were also estimated by nanodrop spectrophotometer method.

Six sets of forward and reverse gene-specific primers reported by Ibeagha-Awemu *et al.* [19] and Kumar *et al.* [27] were used to amplify complete KF CD14 gene. Primers were synthesized and procured from M/s. Eurofins Genomics India Pvt., Ltd., Bengaluru. The sequence of primers, their respective nucleotide numbers, target region, and amplicon sizes are given in Table-1.

The polymerase chain reaction (PCR) mixture was incubated in thermal cycler initially at 94°C for 2 min followed by 34 cycles of 94°C for 30 s, 60°C (contig 1, 4, 5, 6) or 59°C (contig 2, 3) for 30 s, 72°C for 40 s, and a final extension of 72°C for 10 min. The amplified PCR products were checked on 2% agarose gel to ensure amplification of target region. Amplified PCR products from all sets of primers were custom sequenced from both ends (5' and 3' ends) by M/s. SciGenom Labs Pvt., Ltd. Nucleotide sequences were visualized and edited using BioEdit software. The forward and reverse sequences for each PCR fragments were assembled to form a complete sequence for the respective region of KF CD14 gene. The multiple sequence alignments of the edited sequence with corresponding reference with reported *B. taurus* sequence (EU148610.1) were performed with ClustalW software to identify SNPs. Basic Local Alignment Search Tool (BLAST) analysis was performed to compare the sequence identity of KF CD14 gene with other species.

The restriction fragment length polymorphism (RFLP) analysis was carried out in all KF cows using *Helicobacter pylori 1881I* (*Hpy1881I*) (contig 2) and *Haemophilus influenzae I* (*HinfI*) (contig 4) restriction enzyme (RE). PCR amplified CD14 gene products of each animal were digested with 0.4 µl each of *Hpy1881I* and *HinfI* RE at 37°C for 16 h. Fragments of RE digestion were separated on 2.5% agarose gel and photographed using gel documentation system. Cows were grouped as mastitis affected and not affected and were assigned genotypes obtained by PCR-RFLP analysis.

Table-1: Sequence of the primers referred for amplification of complete CD14 gene in KF cattle.

Primer set	Sequence (5'-3')		Number of base pairs	Target region	Amplicon size (bp)
1	F	ATTACCTTCTTCTGCACCTCCA	22	−404-307	711
	R	GAAAGTGAAGTCGCTCAGTCCT	22	(Promoter)	
2	F	ACACACCTGGAGAAGGCAA	20	177-729	553
	R	TCCAAGGGCTAGTTCCAG AG	20	(Promoter*)	
3	F	CAATTCCTGGTCAGGGAACTAA	22	561-1173	613
	R	GGCAGCCTCTGAGAGTTTATGT	22	(Promoter*)	
4	F	CTTCCTGTTATAGCCCCTTTCC	22	1012-1843	832
	R	CACGATACGTTACGGAGACTGA	22	(Promoter*, Exon-1, Intron, Exon-2*)	
5	F	GGGTACTCTCGTCTCAAGGAAC	22	1722-2546	825
	R	CTGAGCCAATTCATTCCTCTTC	22	(Exon-2*)	
6	F	ACCTGACTCTGGACGGAAATC	21	2347-3093	747
	R	TAC AGGAGAGCAACCCTGAAA	21	(Exon-2*)	

*Overlapping and partial. CD14=Cluster of differentiation 14, KF=Karan Fries

Statistical analysis

Chi-square (χ^2) test was performed to test whether gene variants were independent. Further, restriction fragments were utilized to construct combined genotypes.

Results and Discussion

Two types of sequences of KF were obtained: One with 2630 bp having one insertion at 616 nucleotide (nt) position and one deletion at 1117 nt position, and the another sequence was of 2629 bp having only one deletion at 615 nt position. ClustalW, multiple alignments of KF CD14 gene sequence with *B. taurus* cattle sequence (EU148610.1) reported by Ibeagha-Awemu *et al.* [19], revealed 24 nt changes (SNPs) (Figure-1 and Table-2). Out of 24 SNPs compared with *B. taurus*, 13 SNPs were transition type of mutation, 8 SNPs were transversion type of mutation, 2 SNPs were deletion type of mutation, and 1 SNP was insertion type of mutation. 5 SNPs were in coding region resulting in synonyms amino acid change. Table-3 depicts comparative nucleotide sequences of Karan Fries (KF), *Bos taurus* and Sahiwal cattle showing nucleotide change of Guanine to adenine at position 2601. Crossbreeding and, species and breed variation of inheritance between KF (Tharparkar [*B. indicus*] × Holstein Friesian [*B. taurus*]), *B. taurus* may have been caused SNPs in KF cattle compared to reported CD14 gene sequence of *B. taurus* [19]. In BLAST analysis, KF cattle showed 86-99% sequence identity with several domestic animals (Table-4).

PCR-RFLP analysis revealed two polymorphic patterns in contig 2 and 4. *Hpy188I* had cutting site in contig 2 that exhibited three genotypes (band patterns) such as AA (305 and 248 bp), AB (305, 248, 138 and 110 bp), and BB (305, 248, 138, and 110 bp) genotypes. *HinfI* had cutting site in contig 4 that exhibited three genotypes (band patterns) such as CC (377, 272, and 183 bp), CD (377, 272, 225, 183, and 47 bp), and DD (377, 225, 183, and 47 bp) genotypes. So, there were three genotypes in contig 2 (AA, AB, and BB) and three genotypes in contig 4 (CC, CD, and DD).

Chi-square (χ^2) analysis revealed that all the genotypes of KF cattle differed significantly from each other regarding mastitis incidence. The genotypes of both contigs (loci) number 2 and 4 were combined with respect to each animal to construct combined genotype patterns. If animal number "1" was having genotype "AA" at locus number 2, whereas genotype "CD" at locus number 4 then that animal will have combined genotype pattern "AACD." In this way, combined genotypes were constructed. The maximum possible combination of these two loci shown

Table-2: Summary of nucleotide changes in CD14 gene of KF as compared to *B. taurus* (EU148610.1).

Region	Position	KF	*B. taurus* (Ibeagha et al., 2008)
Promoter	269	A	G
	271	C	T
	273	A	C
	276	C	G
	277	A	G
	281	C	T
	357	T	G
	418	C	A
	431	A	G
	458	G	C
	615	Deletion	A
	616	A (insertion)	-
	778	T	C
	922	A	G
	1117	Deletion	T
Exon 1	1239	G	T
	1291	C	T
Intron	1359	C	G
	1361	A	G
Exon 2	1811	A	G
	1909	G	A
	2276	T	C
Exon 2, 3'UTR	2601	A	G
	2621	G	T

B. taurus=Bos taurus, CD14=Cluster of differentiation 14, KF=Karan Fries

Table-3: Comparative nucleotide sequences of Karan Fries (KF), *Bos taurus* and Sahiwal cattle showing nucleotide change at position 2601 (G>A).

KF_2630	GCCTTCTACCCCATCCT	2610
KF_2629	GCCTTCTACCCCATCCT	2610
Bos taurus	GCCTTCTGCCCCATCCT	2610
Sahiwal	GCCTTCTGCCCCATCCT	2610

Table-4: Identity of CD14 gene of KF (*B. indicus×Bos taurus*) with other species.

Accession no.	Species	Homology (%)
EU148610.1	*B. taurus*	99
DQ457089.1	*B. bubalis*	98
NM_001077209.1	*O. aries*	97
DQ457090.1	*C. hircus*	93
AY753180.1	*S. scrofa*	86

B. taurus=Bos taurus, B. bubalis=Bubalus bubalis, O. aries=Ovis aries, C. hircus=Capra hircus, S. scrofa=Sus scrofa, CD14=Cluster of differentiation 14, KF=Karan Fries

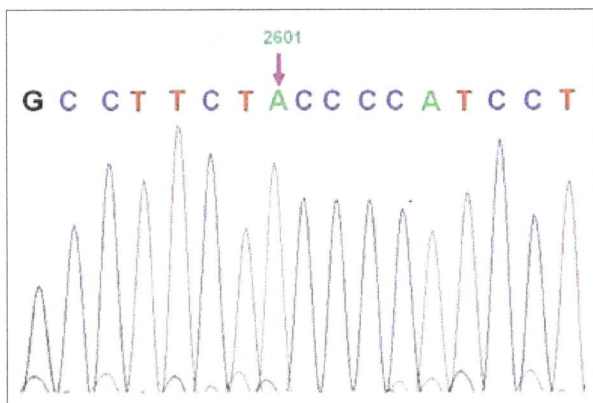

Figure-1: Chromatogram showing nucleotide change at position 2601 (G>A).

Table-5: Frequency of combined genotype of CD14 gene in KF cattle.

Combined genotype	Total animals	Mastitis affected					Mastitis not affected			
		Number of animals	Percentage				Number of animals	Percentage		
			Within each genotype	Among mastitis affected (n=59)	Within herd (n=94)			Within each genotype	Among mastitis not affected (n=35)	Within herd (n=94)
AACC	04	02	50.0	03.39	02.13		02	50.0	05.71	02.13
AACD	20	10	50.0	16.94	10.63		10	50.0	28.57	10.63
AADD	16	8	50.0	13.55	08.51		8	50.0	22.85	08.51
ABCC					Not observed					
ABCD	10	9	90.0	15.25	09.57		1	10.0	02.85	01.06
ABDD	21	15	71.4	25.42	15.96		6	28.57	17.14	06.38
BBCC	03	1	33.3	01.69	01.06		2	66.66	05.71	02.12
BBCD	06	6	100.0	10.16	06.38		-	-		
BBDD	14	8	57.1	13.55	08.51		6	42.85	17.14	06.38
Total	94	59	-	100.00	62.77		35	-	100.00	37.23

CD14=Cluster of differentiation 14, KF=Karan Fries

nine combined genotype patterns, and it was observed only eight combined genotypes out of nine: AACC, AACD, AADD, ABCD, ABDD, BBCC, BBCD, and BBDD with 4, 20, 16, 10, 21, 3, 6, and 14 numbers of animals in each combined genotype, respectively (Table-5). The combined genotype ABCC was not observed in the studied population of KF cows.

Association analysis of combined genotyped cows of CD14 gene with clinical mastitis

In Table-5, out of the four animals of combined genotypes "AACC," 50% animals were mastitis affected and 50% animals were mastitis not affected. Among 59 animals (mastitis affected) and 94 animals (total animals analyzed for combined genotype study), 3.39% and 2.13% animals, respectively, were of "AACC" combined genotype. Similarly, among 35 animals (mastitis not affected) and 94 animals (total animals analyzed for combined genotype study), 5.71% and 2.13% animals, respectively, were of "AACC" combined genotype.

Among 94 cows studied for combined genotype analysis, 59 were mastitis affected. When the frequencies of combined genotypes of CD14 gene, fragments in KF cows were analyzed within each genotype: 100%, 90%, and 71.4% of animals in BBCD, ABCD, and ABDD genotype were observed having mastitis incidence, respectively. While among 59 mastitis affected KF cows, combined genotype ABDD was observed having the highest mastitis incidence (25.42%), i.e., 15 out of 59 animals. Out of 59 cows, around 64%, i.e., 38 cows with combined genotypes ABCD, ABDD, BBCD, and BBDD were mastitis affected which is in accordance with previous reports by Selvan *et al.* [29] where cows with AB and BB genotypes and by Selvan *et al.* [30] where cows with CD and DD genotypes were mastitis affected. Further, on comparison within herd (94 animals), combined genotype ABDD was observed having the highest mastitis incidence of 15.96%. Similar comparison was done for non-mastitis affected animals (35 animals). Out

of 94 animals, AACD combined genotype animals (10.63%) were found to be not affected with mastitis (Table-5). Hence, it can be inferred that animals with ABDD genotypic combination are more susceptible to mastitis, and on the other hand, AACD typed animals are least susceptible to incidence of mastitis as compared to other combined genotypes.

Conclusions

It may be possible that cows with AACD combined genotype might have a higher percentage of leukocytes expressing CD14 molecules on their surface which may increase the speed of response to pathogen attack [31,32]. Further research will be needed to conclude the relationships among CD14 genotypes, combined genotypes, concentration of CD14 in mammary tissues, and clinical mastitis.

Authors' Contributions

IDG conceived and designed the work. ASS conducted experiment. ASS and MVC done analysis, association study and AM assisted in writing of the manuscript. IDG and AV helped in revision of the manuscript. All authors read and approved the final manuscript.

Acknowledgments

The authors are thankful to Head DCB Division, for providing necessary research facilities. The authors also thankful to the Director (NDRI) for financial assistance provided during the research work.

Competing Interests

The authors declare that they have no competing interest.

References

1. BAHS. (2014) Basic Animal Husbandry Statistics. Government of India, Ministry of Agriculture, Department of Animal Husbandry, Dairying and Fishries, Krishi Bhawan, New Delhi.

2. Sharma, S.D. and Rai, P. (1977) Studies on the incidence

of bovine mastitis in Uttar Pradesh. *Indian. Vet. J.,* 54: 435-439.

3. Ebrahimi, A., Kheirabadi, K.H.P. and Nikookhah, F. (2007) Antimicrobial susceptibility of environmental bovine mastitis pathogen in west central Iran. *Pak. J. Biol. Sci.,* 10: 3014-3016.

4. Sharma, N. and Maiti, S.K. (2010) Incidence, etiology and antibiogram of subclinical mastitis in cows in durg, Chhattisgarh. *Indian J. Vet. Res.,* 19: 45-54.

5. Dhanda, M.R. and Sethi, M.S. (1962) Investigation of mastitis in India. ICAR Research, Series No. 35, New Delhi, India.

6. NDRI News Letter. (2012) 17(1). Available from: http://www.ndri.res.in. Accessed on 15-01-2016.

7. Shuster, D.E., Kehrli, M.E.Jr., Ackermann, M.R. and Gilbert, R.O. (1992) Identification and prevalence of a genetic defect that causes leukocyte adhesion deficiency in Holstein cattle. *Proc. Natl. Acad. Sci.,* 89: 9225-9229.

8. Takeda, H., Takami, M., Oguni, T., Tsuji, T., Yoneda, K., Sato, H., Ihara, N., Itoh, T., Kata, S.R. and Mishina, Y. (2002) Positional cloning of the gene LIMBIN responsible for bovine chondrodysplastic dwarfism. *Proc. Natl. Acad. Sci.,* 99, 10549-10554.

9. Maillard, J.C., Berthier, D., Chantal, I., Thevenon, S. and Sidibe, I. (2003) Selection assisted by BoLA-DR/DQ haplotype against susceptibility to bovine dermatophilosis. *Genet. Select. Evol.,* 35(1): S193-S200.

10. Qureshi, S., Larivière, L., Sebastiani, G., Clermont, S., Skamene, E., Gros, P. and Malo, D. (1996) A high-resolution map in the chromosomal region surrounding the LPS locus. *Genomics,* 31: 283-294.

11. Pinedo, P.J., Donovan, A., Rae, O. and DeLapaz, J. (2009) Association between paratuberculosis infection and general immune status in dairy cattle. In: Proceedings of the 10th International Colloquium on Paratuberculosis. Vol. 1. p127.

12. Kumar, N., Mitra, A., Ganguly, I., Singh, R., Deb, S.M., Srivatsava, S.K. and Sharma, A. (2005) Lack of association of brucellosis resistance with (GT) (13) microsatellite allele at 3'UTR of NRAMP1 gene in Indian zebu (Bos indicus) and crossbred (Bos indicus X Bos taurus) cattle. *Vet. Microbiol.,* 111: 139-143.

13. Juliarena, M.A., Poli, M., Ceriani, C., Sala, L., Rodríguez, E., Gutierrez, S., Dolcini, G., Odeon, A. and Esteban, E.N. (2009) Antibody response against three widespread bovine viruses is not impaired in Holstein cattle bovine leukocyte antigen (BoLA) DRB3.2 carrying alleles associated with bovine leukemia virus resistance. *J. Dairy Sci.,* 92(1): 375-381.

14. Garcia-Briones, M.M., Russell, G.C., Oliver, R.A., Tami, C., Taboga, O., Carrillo, E., Palma, E.L., Sobrino, F. and Glass, E.J. (2000) Association of bovine DRB3 alleles with immune response to FMDV peptides and protection against viral challenge. *Vaccine,* 19: 1167-1171.

15. Beecher, C., Daly, M., Childs, S., Berry, D.P., Magee, D.A., McCarthy, T.V. and Giblin, L. (2010) Polymorphisms in bovine immune genes and their associations with somatic cell count and milk production in dairy cattle. *BMC Genet.,* 11: 99-108.

16. Rainard, P. and Riollet, C. (2006) Innate immunity of the bovine mammary gland. *Vet. Res.,* 37: 369-400.

17. Rupp, R., Hernandez, A. and Mallard, B.A. (2007) Association of bovine leukocyte antigen (BoLA) DRB 3.2 with immune response, mastitis and production and type traits in Canadian Holsteins. *J. Dairy Sci.,* 90: 1029-1038.

18. Wang, X., Xu, S., Xue, S., Ren, H. and Chen, J. (2007) Genetic polymorphism of TLR4 gene and correlation with mastitis in cattle. *J. Genet. Genom.,* 34(5): 406-412.

19. Ibeagha-Awemu, E.M., Lee, J.W. and Ibeagha, A.E. (2008) Bovine CD14 gene characterization and relationship between polymorphisms and surface expression on monocytes and polymorphonuclear neutrophils. *BMC Genet.,* 9: 50-60.

20. Ogorevc, J., Kunej, T., Razpet, A. and Dovc, P. (2009) Database of cattle candidate genes and genetic markers for milk production and mastitis. *Anim. Genet.,* 40: 832-851.

21. Yuan, Z., Chu, G., Dan, Y., Li, J., Zhang, L., Gao, X., Gao, H., Li, J., Xu, S. and Liu, Z. (2012) BRCA1: A new candidate gene for bovine mastitis and its association analysis between single nucleotide polymorphisms and milk somatic cell score. *Mol. Biol. Rep.,* 39: 6625-6631.

22. Soumya, N.P., Gupta, I.D., Verma, A., Raja, K.N., Chauhan, I. and Chaudhari, M.V. (2013) Identification of CARD-15 gene polymorphism in Sahiwal cattle. *Indian. J. Anim. Res.,* 47(1): 83-86.

23. Wakchaure, S.R., Gupta, I.D., Verma, A., Kumar, S.R. and Kumar, D. (2012) Study of toll like receptors 4 (TLR 4) gene in cattle: A review. *Agric. Rev.,* 33(3): 220-225.

24. Antal-Szalmas, P., Van Strjp, J.A.G., Weersink, A.J.L., Verhoef, J. and Van Kessel, K.P.M. (1997) Quantitation of surface CD 14 on human monocytes and neutrophils. *J. Leukoc. Biol.,* 61: 721-728.

25. Ogorevc, J., Kunej, T. and Dovc, P. (2008) An integrated map of cattle candidate genes for mastitis: A step forward to new genetic markers. *Acta Agric. Slov.,* 2: 85-91.

26. Pal, A., Sharma, A., Bhattacharya, T.K., Chatterjee, P.N. and Chakravarty, A.K. (2011) Molecular characterization and SNP detection of CD14 gene of crossbred cattle. *Mol. Biol. Int.,* DOI: 10.4061/2011/507346.

27. Kumar, V., Gupta, I.D., Verma, A., Kumar, S.R. and Chaudhari, M.V. (2014) CD14 gene polymorphism using *HINFl* restriction enzyme and its association with mastitis in Sahiwal cattle. *Indian J. Anim. Res.,* 48(1): 11-13.

28. Sambrook, J. and Russell, D.W. (1989) Preparation and analysis of eukaryotic DNA. In: Molecular Cloning: A Laboratory Manual. 3rd ed. Cold Spring Harbor Laboratory Press, New York. p6.1-6.62.

29. Selvan, A.S., Gupta, I.D., Verma, A., Chaudhari, M.V., Kanungo, S. and Kumar, S.R. (2014a) Characterization of promoter region of CD14 gene and association with clinical mastitis in Karan Fries cattle. *Indian. J. Anim. Res.,* 48(6): 545-547.

30. Selvan, A.S., Gupta, I.D., Verma, A., Chaudhari, M.V. and Kumar, V. (2014b) Cluster of differentiation 14 gene polymorphism and its association with incidence of clinical mastitis in Karan fries cattle. *Vet. World,* 7(12): 1037-1040.

31. Paape, M.J., Shafer-Weaver, K., Capuco, A.V., Van Oostveldt, K. and Burvenich, C. (2000) Immune surveillance of mammary tissue by phagocytic cells. *Adv. Exp. Med. Biol.,* 480: 259-277.

32. Akira, S., Uematsu, S. and Takeuchi, O. (2006) Pathogen recognition and innate immunity. *Cell,* 124: 783-801.

12

Comparison of Surti goat milk with cow and buffalo milk for gross composition, nitrogen distribution, and selected minerals content

Dhartiben B. Kapadiya[1], Darshna B. Prajapati[1], Amit Kumar Jain[1], Bhavbhuti M. Mehta[1],
Vijaykumar B. Darji[2] and Kishorkumar D. Aparnathi[1]

1. Department of Dairy Chemistry, SMC College of Dairy Science, Anand Agricultural University, Anand, Gujarat, India;
2. Department of Agricultural Statistics, BA College of Agriculture, Anand Agricultural University, Anand, Gujarat, India.
Corresponding author: Kishorkumar D. Aparnathi, e-mail: kd_aparnathi@yahoo.co.in,
DBK: dhartikapadiya@gmail.com, DBP: darshna367@gmail.com, AKJ: amitkr10@gmail.com,
BMM: bhavbhuti5@yahoo.co.in, VBD: vbdarjee@yahoo.com

Abstract

Aim: The study was undertaken to find out the gross composition, nitrogen distribution, and selected mineral content in Surti goat milk, and its comparison was made between cow and buffalo milk.

Materials and Methods: Goat milk samples of Surti breed and buffalo milk samples were collected during the period from July to January 2014 at Reproductive Biology Research Unit, Anand Agricultural University (AAU), Anand. Cow milk samples of Kankrej breed were collected from Livestock Research Station, AAU, Anand. Samples were analyzed for gross composition such as total solids (TS), fat, solid not fat (SNF), protein, lactose, and ash. Samples were also analyzed for nitrogen distribution such as total nitrogen (TN), non-casein nitrogen (NCN), non-protein nitrogen (NPN), and selected minerals content such as calcium, magnesium, phosphorous, and chloride. Total five replications were carried out.

Results: Goat milk had the lowest TS, fat, protein, and lactose content among all three types of milk studied in the present investigation. On the other hand, the highest TS, fat, protein, and lactose content were found in buffalo milk. Buffalo milk had the highest SNF, calcium, magnesium, and phosphorous content, which was followed by goat milk and lowest in cow milk. The SNF, protein, TN, and calcium content of goat milk were statistically non-significant (p<0.05) with cow milk. The lactose content of goat milk was significantly lower (p>0.05) than that of the cow milk as well as buffalo milk. The goat milk had the highest ash and NCN content, which were followed by buffalo milk and lowest in cow milk. However, the differences in ash, NPN, and phosphorous content of three types of milk studied, *viz.*, goat milk, cow milk, and buffalo milk were found statistically non-significant (p<0.05). The NCN content of buffalo milk was statistically non-significant (p<0.05) with cow milk as well as goat milk. The NCN and magnesium content of goat milk were significantly higher (p>0.05) than that of the cow milk. The magnesium content of goat milk was statistically non-significant (p<0.05) with buffalo milk. The chloride content of goat milk was significantly higher (p>0.05) than that of the buffalo milk as well as cow milk.

Conclusion: It can be concluded from the study that the goat milk has lower TS, fat, lactose, protein content, TN as well as NPN but higher ash and NCN content compared to cow milk and buffalo milk. The goat milk has lower calcium, phosphorous compared to buffalo milk while it has higher calcium, phosphorous compared to cow milk, and it has higher magnesium, chloride content compared to cow milk and buffalo milk.

Keywords: gross composition, nitrogen distribution and mineral content, Surti goat milk.

Introduction

Milk is considered as nearly complete human food and it is considered as the first food for the newly born offspring. There are numerous studies throughout the world and thousands of references available, especially with regard to milk consumed by humans. However, the literature data mainly concern cow and buffalo milk and to a lesser extent, goat and sheep milk.

Goat milk offers a wide variety of health benefits such as better digestibility [1], more alkalinity [2], less αs1 casein than cow's milk and is, therefore, less allergenic [3]. Goat milk also has antioxidant, antimicrobial, and medicinal property [4,5]. Goat milk contains a higher carotene (pro-vitamin A) having cancer-preventing properties. It is also useful in the treatment of ulcers due to its more effective acid buffering capacity [6]. Goat milk has a stronger flavor due to the liberation of short-chain fatty acids during rough handling, which gives off a goaty smell [7,8]. Unlike cow milk, which is slightly acidic, goat milk is alkaline in nature, which is very useful for people with acidity problems [2].

Goat milk is more digestible because of its small-sized globules, uniform protein, fat distribution, and less lactose. Modified goat milk can also be used in baby feeding [1]. Goat milk provides a healthy and a balanced diet for the children who are allergic to cow milk, as the symptoms may disappear with goat milk consumption [3]. Nutritional value of milk is closely related with its composition, which is highly affected by factors such as breed, feed, stage of lactation, and season [3,9]. Particularly during lactation, there are significant changes in the amount and composition of goat milk [10]. Various symptoms are reduced due to protein allergy, inability to digest lactose (particularly with lactose intolerance people) by taking goat's milk.

The vitamin and mineral contents of goat's milk and cow's milk are fairly similar, though goat's milk contains more calcium, vitamin B6, vitamin A, potassium, niacin, copper, and the antioxidant selenium. Goat milk is an excellent source of calcium, phosphorus, and potassium. It is also a good source of magnesium, sodium, and iron [3,11]. Calcium helps to protect against colon cancer, improves blood clotting ability, and helps to maintain healthy blood pressure and to prevent muscle cramps/contractions. Goat milk is a good source of calcium, containing approximately 13% more calcium than cow's milk. Magnesium is particularly beneficial to the heart, helping to maintain a regular heartbeat, preventing the formation of blood clots and raising good cholesterol levels. It also works with calcium and vitamin D to maintain healthy bones. Goat milk has a higher content of magnesium than cow's milk. Phosphorus works in conjunction with calcium and vitamin D that can not only build and maintain strong bones but also plays a role in activities of the brain, kidney, heart, and blood. Goat milk has a higher phosphorous content than cow's milk [12,13]. The value of goat milk in human nutrition has so far received very little academic attention.

Estimated population of Milch goat for the Gujarat state during the year 2010-2011 was estimated at 27,181 hundred, which was 0.63% increased over previous year's estimate (during 2009-2010) of 27,011 hundred. The total estimated milk production of goat for the state during 2010-2011 works out to be 235.61 thousand tons, which was increased 1.89% over the previous year's estimate (during 2009-2010) of 231.24 thousand tons. Estimated number of productive goats in Anand during 2010-2011 was 374 hundred [14].

The Food Safety and Standards Authority of India (FSSAI), Ministry of Health and Family Welfare, and Government of India were interested to develop new standards of milk and required to generate a standard database on milk and milk products. The data on gross composition, nitrogen distribution, mineral content, and related information of milk of various species and breed of animals were lacking. Moreover, there were no reported values on these aspects of goat milk in Anand/Gujarat. Therefore, there was a need to undertake a systematic study to generate data. This work provides basic database for gross composition and nitrogen distribution pattern and selected mineral

content of milk of Surti goat. This information will be beneficial to goat keepers, industrial personnel, and various government agencies as well as to society.

Materials and Methods
Ethical approval

Ethical approval was not applicable for this study. However milk samples were collected as per standard milking techniques.

Milk samples

Goat milk samples of Surti breed and buffalo milk samples were collected during the period from July to January 2014, at Reproductive Biology Research Unit, Anand Agricultural University (AAU), Anand. Cow milk samples of Kankrej breed were collected from Livestock Research Station, AAU, Anand, and used for investigation. Raw milk samples were collected at milking time in a clean and dry container. The samples were transported to the laboratory. Total five replications were carried out.

Chemical and glassware

During the entire study, chemicals used for chemical analysis for various properties were of analytical grade.

Gross chemical composition of milk

Total solids (TSs) in all the milk samples were determined gravimetrically by the procedure as described in Bureau of Indian Standards (BIS) handbook [15]. The milk fat content in all the milk samples was estimated by following the Gerber method as described in BIS handbook [15]. Solid not fat (SNF) content of goat, cow, and buffalo milk was calculated by subtracting percent fat content of milk samples from their respective percent TS content of the milk. The protein content of all the milk samples was determined using the micro Kjeldahl method of nitrogen estimation as described in BIS Handbook [15]. The percent total protein was obtained by multiplying the percent nitrogen by a factor of 6.38. The lactose content of all the milk samples was determined using Lane-Eyon Method described in BIS handbook [15]. The procedure outlined in BIS handbook [15] was followed for determination of ash content in all the milk samples.

Nitrogen distribution

Total nitrogen (TN) content of all the milk samples was determined using the micro Kjeldahl method of nitrogen estimation as described in BIS handbook [15]. Non-casein nitrogen (NCN) content and non-protein content of all the milk samples were determined using Rowland's analytical scheme for nitrogen fractions of milk as described in a laboratory manual on chemical analysis of milk protein by Kumar *et al.* [16].

Selected minerals content

Calcium and magnesium were determined simultaneously in milk by complexometric method of Davies and White [17] using disodium salt of ethylenediaminetetraacetic acid. Phosphorous was determined by the colorimetric method of Fiske and Subbarow [18]. The chloride content of all the milk sample of milk was determined by Hammer and Bailey [19] using $AgNO_3$.

Statistical analysis

The collected data were subjected to statistical analysis. Data were analyzed by completely randomized design and critical difference test at 5% level of significance (p<0.05) as per the procedure mentioned by Steel and Torrie [20].

Results

The gross composition of goat, cow, and buffalo milk is mentioned in Table-1. The range of TS content in goat milk was 12.32-13.02% with a mean value of 12.76%. Similarly, in cow milk, range of TS was 13.29-14.20% with a mean value of 13.79%. On the other hand, TS content ranged between 17.88% and 19.18% with a mean value of 18.45% in buffalo milk. Thus, TS content of goat milk was significantly lower (p>0.05) than that of the cow milk as well as buffalo milk. The range of fat content in goat milk was 3.4-4.2% with a mean value of 3.84%. Similarly, in cow milk, range of fat was 4.2-5.5% with a mean value of 4.88%. On the other hand, fat content ranged between 7.9% and 8.8% with a mean value of 8.30% in buffalo milk. The fat content of goat milk was significantly lower (p>0.05) than that of the cow milk as well as buffalo milk. The range of SNF content in goat milk was 8.37-8.82% with a mean value of 8.57%. Similarly, in cow milk, range of SNF was measured to be 8.37-8.83% with a mean value of 8.54%. On the other hand, SNF content ranged between 9.04% and 9.68% with a mean value of 9.48% in buffalo milk. The SNF content of goat milk was statistically non-significant (p<0.05) with cow milk. The range of protein content in goat milk was 3.18-3.49% with a mean value of 3.42%. Similarly, in cow milk, range of protein was 3.19-3.62% with a mean value of 3.49%. On the other hand, protein content ranged between 4.11% and 4.74% with a mean value of 4.48% in buffalo milk. The protein content of goat milk was

statistically non-significant (p<0.05) with cow milk. The range of lactose content was 3.78-4.45% with a mean value of 4.16% in goat milk. Similarly, in cow milk, range of lactose was 4.45-5.31% with a mean value of 4.76%. On the other hand, lactose content ranged between 4.67% and 5.27% with a mean value of 4.86% in buffalo milk. The lactose content of goat milk was significantly lower (p>0.05) than that of the cow milk as well as buffalo milk. The range of ash content was 0.76-1.06% with a mean value of 0.89% in goat milk. Similarly, in cow milk, range of ash was 0.73-0.79% with a mean value of 0.76%. On the other hand, ash content ranged between 0.69% and 0.89% with mean value of 0.81% in buffalo milk. The goat milk had the highest ash content, which was followed by buffalo milk and cow milk had the lowest ash content.

The nitrogen distribution of goat, cow, and buffalo milk is mentioned in Table-2. The range of TN content was 0.498-0.548% with a mean value of 0.536% in goat milk. Similarly, in cow milk, range of TN was 0.499-0.568% with a mean value of 0.547%. On the other hand, TN ranged between 0.644% and 0.743% with a mean value of 0.702% in buffalo milk. The TN content of buffalo milk was significantly higher (p>0.05) than that of the cow milk and goat milk. The range of NCN content determined was 0.132-0.167% with a mean value of 0.153% in goat milk. Similarly, in cow milk, range of NCN was 0.103-0.136% with a mean value of 0.124%. On the other hand, NCN ranged between 0.118% and 0.157% with a mean value of 0.140% in buffalo milk. The NCN content of buffalo milk was statistically non-significant (p<0.05) with cow milk as well as goat milk. The range of non-protein nitrogen (NPN) content was 0.019-0.036% with a mean value of 0.029% in goat milk. Similarly, in cow milk, range of NPN was 0.036-0.074% with a mean value of 0.054%. On the other hand, NPN ranged between 0.023% and 0.082% with a mean value of 0.051% in buffalo milk. The differences in NPN content of three types of milk studied, *viz.*, goat milk, cow milk, and buffalo milk were found statistically non-significant (p<0.05).

Table-1: Gross composition of goat, cow, and buffalo milk.

Types of milk	Parameters (%)					
	Fat	SNF	TS	Protein	Lactose	Ash
Goat	3.84±0.37[a]	8.57±0.18[a]	12.76±0.29[a]	3.42±0.14[a]	4.16±0.31[a]	0.89±0.12[a]
	(3.4-4.2)	(8.37-8.82)	(12.32-13.02)	(3.18-3.49)	(3.78-4.45)	(0.76-1.06)
Cow	4.88±0.53[b]	8.54±0.17[a]	13.79±0.36[b]	3.49±0.18[a]	4.76±0.35[b]	0.76±0.02[a]
	(4.2-5.5)	(8.37-8.83)	(13.29-14.20)	(3.19-3.62)	(4.45-5.31)	(0.73-0.79)
Buffalo	8.30±0.37[c]	9.48±0.25[b]	18.45±0.56[c]	4.48±0.29[b]	4.86±0.24[b]	0.81±0.08[a]
	(7.9-8.8)	(9.04-9.68)	(17.88-19.18)	(4.11-4.74)	(4.67-5.27)	(0.69-0.89)
SEM	0.19	0.09	0.19	0.09	0.14	0.04
CD	0.59	0.28	0.58	0.29	0.42	-
Test	*	*	*	*	*	NS
CV %	7.51	2.31	2.79	5.60	6.60	10.14

[a-c]Values with different letters within a column are significantly different at 5% level of significant (i.e., p<0.05).
SEM=Standard error of mean, CD=Critical difference, CV=Coefficient of variance, NS=Not significant, SNF=Solid not fat, TS=Total solids

The selected mineral content of goat, cow, and buffalo milk is mentioned in Table-3. The calcium content determined in five replications ranged between 117.88 and 141.46 mg/100 ml with a mean value of 129.08 mg/100 ml in goat milk. Similarly, in cow milk, range of calcium was 111.99-129.67 mg/100 ml with a mean value of 120.24 mg/100 ml. On the other hand, calcium content ranged between 167.98 and 185.66 mg/100 ml with a mean value of 178.59 mg/100 ml in buffalo milk. The calcium content of buffalo milk was significantly higher (p>0.05) than that of the goat milk as well as cow milk. The magnesium content was determined between 18.48 and 21.16 mg/100 ml with a mean value of 19.94 mg/100 ml in goat milk. Similarly, in cow milk, range of magnesium was 9.73-16.54 mg/100 ml with a mean value of 12.65 mg/100 ml. On the other hand, magnesium content ranged between 14.59 and 21.40 mg/100 ml with a mean value of 18.29 mg/100 ml in buffalo milk. The magnesium content of goat milk was significantly higher (p>0.05) than that of the cow milk. The magnesium content of goat milk was statistically non-significant (p<0.05) with buffalo milk. The range of phosphorous content was 75.85-126.19 mg/100 ml

with a mean value of 98.91 mg/100 ml in goat milk. Similarly, in cow milk, range of phosphorous was 78.57-97.64 mg/100 ml with a mean value of 88.08 mg/100 ml. On the other hand, phosphorous ranged between 95.22 and 124.72 mg/100 ml with a mean value of 109.22 mg/100 ml in buffalo milk. The differences in phosphorous content of three types of milk studied were found statistically non-significant (p<0.05). The chloride content was between 0.15 and 0.17% with a mean value of 0.16% in goat milk. Similarly, in cow milk, range of chloride was 0.11-0.14% with a mean value of 0.13%. On the other hand, chloride content ranged between 0.10% and 0.12% with a mean value of 0.11% in buffalo milk. The chloride content of goat milk was significantly higher (p>0.05) than that of the buffalo milk as well as cow milk.

Discussion

Goat milk has health beneficial properties. The information on composition, nitrogen distribution, and selected mineral content of Surti goat milk produce in Gujarat is not available. Moreover, there is a need to take systematic study on comparative analysis of goat, cow, and buffalo milk for their composition, nitrogen distribution, and selected minerals content.

Shettar [21] reviewed that the TS content of Marwari, Assam local breed, Beetal × Assam local crossbred, and Jakhrana goats as 14.57%, 15.77%, 14.92%, and 13.55%, respectively. Soliman [22] analyzed goat milk and found that it contained 12.62% TS. Mahmood and Usman [12] reported that TS content of goat milk was 12.84%. TSs content in milk of various breeds of cow such as Ayrshire, Brown Swiss, Guernsey, Holstein, Jersey, and Zebu was 13.1%, 13.3%, 14.4%, 12.2%, 15.0%, and 14.7% and fat content in the same was 4.1%, 4.0%, 5.0%, 3.5%, 5.5%, and 4.9%, respectively [23]. The average TSs and fat content ranged between 16.39-18.48% and 6.57-7.97% in buffalo milk [24]. The data obtained in present study for average percent TS content of goat milk were lower than reported in the literature for milk obtained from goat in India. Similarly, the

Table-2: Nitrogen distribution of goat, cow, and buffalo milk.

Types of milk	Parameters (%)		
	TN	NCN	NPM
Goat	0.536±0.021[a] (0.498-0.548)	0.153±0.015[a] (0.132-0.167)	0.029±0.007[a] (0.019-0.036)
Cow	0.547±0.028[a] (0.499-0.568)	0.124±0.013[b] (0.103-0.136)	0.054±0.014[a] (0.036-0.074)
Buffalo	0.702±0.046[b] (0.644-0.743)	0.140±0.020[c] (0.118-0.157)	0.051±0.024[a] (0.023-0.082)
SEM	0.015	0.007	0.007
CD	0.05	0.022	-
Test	*	*	NS
CV%	5.62	11.64	37.003

[a-c]Values with different letters within a column are significantly different at 5% level of significant (i.e., p<0.05). SEM=Standard error of mean, CD=Critical difference, CV=Coefficient of variance, NS=Not significant, TN=Total nitrogen, NCN=Non-casein nitrogen, NPM=Non-protein nitrogen

Table-3: Selected mineral content of goat, cow, and buffalo milk.

Types of milk	Parameters			
	Calcium (mg/100 ml)	Magnesium (mg/100 ml)	Phosphorous (mg/100 ml)	Chloride (%)
Goat	129.08±9.41[a] (117.88-141.46)	19.94±1.02[a] (18.48-21.16)	98.91±19.89[a] (75.85-126.19)	0.16±0.01[a] (0.15-0.17)
Cow	120.24±7.04[a] (111.99-129.67)	12.65±2.84[b] (9.73-16.54)	88.08±7.62[a] (78.57-97.64)	0.13±0.01[b] (0.11-0.14)
Buffalo	178.59±6.79[b] (167.98-185.66)	18.29±2.52[a] (14.59-21.40)	109.22±12.16[a] (95.22-124.72)	0.11±0.06[c] (0.10-0.12)
SEM	3.50	1.01	6.33	0.003
CD	10.80	3.12	-	0.011
Test	*	*	NS	*
CV%	5.49	13.37	14.34	5.880

[a-c]Values with different letters within a column are significantly different at 5% level of significant (i.e., p<0.05). SEM=Standard error of mean, CD=Critical difference, CV=Coefficient of variance, NS=Not significant

data obtained for average TS content of cow and buffalo milk were also in general agreement with those reported in the literature for cow and buffalo milk, respectively. Arora *et al.* [25] analyzed Indian goat milk and found 3.73% fat, 3.02% protein, and 4.45% lactose. Shettar [21] reviewed that the milk of Jakhrana goats had 8.60±0.10% SNF. Mahmood and Usman [12] reported the fat content of goat milk as 3.97%. Park *et al.* [26] reported 9.0% SNF, 3.6% fat, and 0.7% ash in cow milk. Protein and lactose content in milk of various breeds of cow such as Ayrshire, Brown Swiss, Guernsey, Holstein, Jersey, and Zebu were found as 3.6%, 3.6%, 3.8%, 3.1%, 3.9%, and 3.9% and 4.7%, 5.0%, 4.9%, 4.9%, 4.9%, and 5.1%, respectively [23]. Rao and Nagarcenkar [27] reviewed average SNF, protein, lactose, and ash percent in Murrah (Indian) milk were 10.2%, 4.5%, 5.1%, and 0.8%, respectively. Sachdeva *et al.* [28] found that the milk of Barbari and Jamnapari goat milk had ash 0.82% and 0.9%. Hanl *et al.* [24] reported range of fat content between 6.57% and 7.97% in buffalo milk. Rao and Nagarcenkar [27] reviewed average protein and SNF percent in the milk of Sichun buffaloes. The values reported were 5.2% and 10.0%, respectively. The data obtained in the present study for average percent fat, SNF, protein, and ash content of goat milk were in general agreement with those reported in the literature for milk obtained from goat in India. The data were also in general agreement with those reported for goat milk obtained from exotic goat. Similarly, the data obtained for average percent ash content of cow and buffalo milk were also in general agreement with those reported in the literature for cow and buffalo milk, respectively.

Milk from Beetal goats contained less TN and NCN than milk from the Jamnapari, Barbari, and Bengal breeds (TN 0.518 vs. 0.532-0.534% and NCN 0.122 vs. 0.125-0.128%) [29]. Jenness [30] analyzed six samples from pygmy goats and reported average nitrogen distribution as 0.840% TN, 0.182% NCN, and 0.053% NPN. The reported range from literature about nitrogen distribution in pooled cow milk for TN was 0.43-0.70% [11]. Li *et al.* [31] studied nitrogen distribution of cow milk and reported 0.08-0.16% NCN and 0.023-0.042% NPN in cow milk. The distribution of nitrogen in different fractions of pooled Indian buffalo milk was studied by Sindhu and Singhal [32] and results obtained for TN, NCN, and NPN were 0.600%, 0.140%, and 0.035%, respectively. The data obtained in the present study for average percent TN and NCN content of goat milk were in general agreement with those reported in the literature for milk obtained from goat in India. The data were also in general agreement with those reported for goat milk obtained from exotic goat. Similarly, the data obtained for average percent TN and NCN content of cow and buffalo milk were also in general agreement with those reported in the literature for cow and buffalo milk, respectively. The data obtained in the present study for average percent

NPN content of goat milk were in general agreement with those reported in the literature for goat milk. The data obtained for average percent NPN content of cow and buffalo milk were slightly higher in general agreement with those reported in the literature for cow and buffalo milk, respectively. In the literature, percent NPN content in goat milk is reportedly higher than that in buffalo milk as well as cow milk. However, in the present study, goat milk was found to contain lower NPN compared to buffalo milk as well as cow milk. The comparative composition of proteins and their components in the milk of goats and cows have been reviewed by Jenness [33] and Haenlein [34], identifying many unique differences between the two species, and showing a wide diversity due to genetics of different breeds within each species, influences of stage of lactation, feeding, climate, and subclinical mastitis. Goat milk proteins are similar to the major cow milk proteins in their general classifications of α-, β-, κ-caseins, β-lactoglobulin, α-lactalbumin, but they differ widely in genetic polymorphisms and their frequencies in goat populations [35].

Soliman [22] studied goat milk and found the average value of calcium as 130.28 mg/100 g. Pal *et al.* [36] reported the magnesium and phosphorous content of goat milk as 20 mg/100 g and 130 mg/100 g. Pal *et al.* [36] reported calcium, magnesium, and phosphorous content of cow milk as 120 mg/100 g, 12 mg/100 g, and 95 mg/100 g. Soliman [22] studied cow milk and found the average value of calcium as 119.90 mg/100 g and average value of magnesium as 13.42 mg/100 g. The average calcium content of buffalo milk was reported to be 180 mg/100 g [37]. Magnesium and phosphorous content of buffalo milk ranged between 16 and 30 mg/100 g and 89-137 mg/100 g, respectively [38,39]. The data obtained in the present study for average calcium, magnesium, and phosphorous content of goat milk were in general agreement with reported in the literature for milk obtained from goat. Similarly, the data obtained for average calcium, magnesium, and phosphorous content of cow and buffalo milk were also in general agreement with reported in the literature for cow and buffalo milk, respectively. Shettar [21] reviewed chloride content in the milk of Marwari goat as 0.24±0.02%. The average chloride content of goat milk and cow milk were reported as 150 mg/100 g and 100 mg/100 g [26]. The chloride content of buffalo milk was 57-106 mg/100 g [19,38]. The data obtained in the present study for average percent chloride content of goat milk were in general agreement with those reported in the literature for goat milk. Similarly, the data obtained for average percent chloride content of cow and buffalo milk were higher than with those reported in the literature for cow and buffalo milk, respectively.

Conclusion

Although goat milk has more health beneficial properties, the data on indigenous goat milk are very scanty and fragmented. Moreover, FSSAI is interested to develop new standards database on milk and milk products of various species and breed of animals. There were no reported values on these aspects of Surti goat milk as well as no comparison was made so far with that of cow and buffalo milk in Anand/ Gujarat. It can be concluded from the study that the Surti goat milk has lower TS, fat, lactose, protein, TN, and NPN but higher ash as well as NCN content compared to cow milk and buffalo milk. The goat milk has lower calcium, phosphorous compared to buffalo milk while it has higher calcium, phosphorous compared to cow milk, and it has higher magnesium, chloride content compared to cow milk and buffalo milk.

Authors' Contributions

KDA supervised the experiment. DBK conducted the experiment and the laboratory analysis of the samples. DBK along with AKJ analyzed the data. DBK and BMM prepared the manuscript. VBD has helped in statistical analysis of the data. DBK, AKJ, BMM, DBP, and KDA reviewed the manuscript. All authors read and approved the final manuscript.

Acknowledgments

The authors acknowledge Anand Agricultural University, Anand for providing fund support to carry out this research work.

Competing Interests

The authors declare that they have no competing interests.

References

1. Desjeux, T.F. (1993) Nutritional value of goat's milk. *Lait*, 73(5): 573-580.
2. Saini, A.L. and Gill, R.S. (1991) Goat milk: An attractive alternate. *Indian Dairyman*, 42: 562-564.
3. Merin, U., Rosenthal, I. and Maltz, E. (1988) The composition of goat milk as affected by nutritional parameters. *Milchwissenschaft*, 43(6): 363-365.
4. Lopez, A., Collins, W.F. and Williams, H.L. (1985) Essential elements, cadmium and lead in raw and pasteurized cow and goat milk. *J. Dairy Sci.*, 68(8): 1878-1886.
5. Rincon, F., Moreno, R., Zurera, G. and Amaro, M. (1994) Mineral composition as a characteristic for the identification of animal origin of raw milk. *J. Dairy Res.*, 61(1): 151-154.
6. Boros, V., Herian, K. and Krcal, Z. (1989) Variations in mineral content of goat milk during lactation. *Prum. Potravin*, 40: 312-314.
7. Babayan, V.K. (1981) Medium chain length fatty acid esters and their medical and nutritional application. *J. Am. Oil Chem. Soc.*, 59: 49-51.
8. Haenlein, G.F. (1993) Producing quality goat milk. *Int. J. Anim. Sci.*, 8: 79-84.
9. Haenlein, G.F. (1980) Mineral nutrition of goats. *J. Dairy Sci.*, 63(10): 1729-1748.
10. Guzeler, N., Say, D. and Kaçar, A. (2010) Compositional changes of Saanen X Kilis goats' milk during lactation. *GIDA*, 35(5): 325-330.
11. Sahai, D. (1996) Buffalo Milk-Chemistry and Processing Technology. Shalini International Publications, Karnal, India.
12. Mahmood, A. and Usman, S. (2010) A comparative study on the physicochemical parameters of milk samples collected from buffalo, cow, goat and sheep of Gujarat, Pakistan. *Pak. J. Nutr.*, 9(12): 1192-1197.
13. Haenlein, G.F.W. (1992) Role of goat meat and milk in human nutrition. Proceeding Vth International Conference. Goats, ICAR Publishers, New Delhi, India. p575-580.
14. 28th Survey Report on Estimates of Major Livestock Products of Gujarat State (2011) Directorate of Animal Husbandry Krishibhavan, Sector 10-A Gandhinagar. p31-40.
15. BIS Handbook. (1981) SP: 18 (Part. I). ISI Handbook of Food Analysis. Part. XI. Dairy Products. Indian Standards Institution, New Delhi.
16. Kumar, R., Sangwan, R. and Mann, B. (2012) A Laboratory Manual on Chemical Analysis of Milk Protein. National Dairy Research Institute, Karnal, India. p27-29.
17. Davies, D.T. and White, J.C.D. (1962) The determination of calcium and magnesium in milk and milk diffusate. *J. Dairy Res.*, 29: 285-296.
18. Fiske, C.H. and Subbarow, Y. (1925) The colourimetric determination of phosphorous. *J. Biol. Chem.*, 66(2): 375-400.
19. Hammer, B.W. and Bailey, D.E. (1917) A rapid volumetric method for approximate estimation of chloride in milk. Research Bulletin No. 41. Agricultural Experiment Station Iowa State College of Agriculture and Mechanic Arts.
20. Steel, R. and Torrie, J.H. (1960) Principles and Procedures of Statistics. McGraw-Hill Book Co., Inc., New York.
21. Shettar, V.B. (2013) Goat Milk Composition. Available from: http://www.ietd.inflibnet.ac.in/jspui/bitstream/10603/6780/9/09_chapter%205. Accessed on 15-02-2014.
22. Soliman, Z.A. (2005) Comparison of chemical and mineral content of milk from human, cow, buffalo, camel and goat in Egypt. *Egypt J. Hosp. Med.*, 21: 116-130.
23. Altman, P.L. and Dittmer, D.S. (1961) Blood and Other Body Fluids. Federation of American Societies for Experimental Biology, Washington, DC. p1-540.
24. Hanl, X., Lee, F.L., Zhang, L. and Guo, M.R. (2012) Chemical composition of water buffalo milk and its low-fat symbiotic yogurt development. *Funct. Foods Health Dis.*, 2(4): 86-106.
25. Arora, R., Bhojak, N. and Joshi, R. (2013) Comparative aspacts of goat and cow milk. *Int. J. Eng. Sci. Invent.*, 2(1): 07-10.
26. Park, Y.W., Juarez, M., Ramos, M. and Haenlein, G.F.W. (2007) Physico-chemical characteristics of goat and sheep milk. *Small Rumin. Res.*, 68(1-2): 88-113.
27. Rao, M.K. and Nagarcenkar, R. (1977) Potentialities of the buffalo. *World Rev. Anim. Prod.*, 13: 53-62.
28. Sachdeva, K.K., Sengar, O.P.S., Singh, S.N. and Lindahl, I.L. (1974) Studies on goats. 2. Effect of plane of nutrition on milk production and composition. *Milchwissenschaft*, 29: 471-475.
29. Baghel, M.S. and Gupta, M.P. (1980) Breed variation on the nitrogen distribution in goat milk. *Indian J. Dairy Sci.*, 33(4): 505-507.
30. Jenness, R. (1974) The Composition of Milk in Lactation: A Comprehensive Treatise. Academic Press, New York. p3-107.
31. Li, H., Ma, Y., Li, Q., Wang, J., Cheng, J., Xue, J. and Shi, J. (2011) The chemical composition and nitrogen distribution of Chinese Yak (Maiwa) Milk. *Int. J. Mol. Sci.*, 12(8): 4885-4895.
32. Sindhu, J.S. and Singhal, O.P. (1988) Qualitative aspects of Buffalo milk constituents for product technology. Vol. 2. Proceeding 2nd World Buffalo Congress. I.C.A.R., New Delhi. p263-287.
33. Jenness, R. (1980) Composition and characteristics of goat milk: Review. *J. Dairy Sci.*, 63(10): 1605-1629.
34. Haenlein, G.F.W. (2001) Past, present, and future perspectives of small ruminant research. *J. Dairy Sci.*, 84(9): 2097-2115.

35. Grosclaude, F. (1995) Genetic polymorphisms of milk proteins. In: Proceedings of the IDF Seminar on Implications of Genetic Polymorphism of Milk Proteins on Production and Processing of Milk, Zurich, Switzerland. Vol. 3. International Dairy Federation Publication. p28-29.

36. Pal, U.K., Mandal, P.K., Rao, V.K. and Das, C.D. (2011) Quality and utility of goat milk with special reference to India: An overview. *Asian J. Anim. Sci.,* 5(1): 56-63.

37. Grifiths, M. (2010) Improving the Safety and Quality of Milk. 6th ed. Woodhead Publishing, Ltd., CRC Press, New York, Washington, DC. p405.

38. Dastur, N.N. (1956) Buffaloes' milk and milk products. *Dairy Sci. Abstr.,* 18: 967-1008.

39. Laxminarayana, H. and Dastur, N.N. (1968) Buffaloes' milk and milk products. *Dairy Sci. Abstr.,* 30: 177-186.

13

Effect of heat stress on reproductive performances of dairy cattle and buffaloes

Soumya Dash, A. K. Chakravarty, Avtar Singh, Arpan Upadhyay, Manvendra Singh and Saleem Yousuf

Dairy Cattle Breeding Division, ICAR-National Dairy Research Institute, Karnal, Haryana, India.
Corresponding author: Soumya Dash, e-mail: soumya.agb@gmail.com,
AKC: ak_chakravarty@yahoo.co.in, AS: avtar54@gmail.com, AU: upadhyay.arpan@gmail.com,
MS: manav21vet@gmail.com, SY: saleemyousuf57155@gmail.com

Abstract

Heat stress has adverse effects on the reproductive performances of dairy cattle and buffaloes. The dairy sector is a more vulnerable to global warming and climate change. The temperature humidity index (THI) is the widely used index to measure the magnitude of heat stress in animals. The objective of this paper was to assess the decline in performances of reproductive traits such as service period, conception rate and pregnancy rate of dairy cattle and buffaloes with respect to increase in THI. The review stated that service period in cattle is affected by season of calving for which cows calved in summer had the longest service period. The conception rate and pregnancy rate in dairy cattle were found decreased above THI 72 while a significant decline in reproductive performances of buffaloes was observed above threshold THI 75. The non-heat stress zone (HSZ) (October to March) is favorable for optimum reproductive performance, while fertility is depressed in HSZ (April to September) and critical HSZ (CHSZ) (May and June). Heat stress in animals has been associated with reduced fertility through its deleterious impact on oocyte maturation and early embryo development. The management strategies *viz.*, nutrition modification, environment modification and timed artificial insemination protocol are to be strictly operated to ameliorate the adverse effects of heat stress in cattle and buffaloes during CHSZ to improve their fertility. The identification of genes associated with heat tolerance, its incorporation into breeding program and the inclusion of THI covariate effects in selection index should be targeted for genetic evaluation of dairy animals in the hot climate.

Keywords: buffaloes, cattle, heat stress zone, reproductive traits, temperature humidity index.

Introduction

The cattle and buffaloes are known for their milk production and they contribute approximately 96% to total milk production in India. Though milk production in India has been reached to 132.4 million tonnes in 2012-13 with a growth rate of 3.5%, but there is high demand of milk [1] and it is projected that by 2030 India will be able to produce 200 million tonnes of milk [2]. This target will be achieved if there is the optimum balance between productivity and fertility. Fertility is a very broad term which is influenced by various factors including genetic, nutritional, hormonal, physiopathology, management and environment or climate. The fertility traits in dairy animals show a very low heritability value, and this indicates that most of the variations in the fertility are determined by non-genetic factors or environmental effects [3]. The main natural physical environmental factors affecting livestock system includes air temperature, relative humidity (RH), solar radiation, atmospheric pressure and wind speed (WS) [4]. All these environmental factors are pooled to produce heat stress on animals, which is defined as any combination of environmental variables producing conditions that are higher than the temperature range of the animal's thermoneutral zone (TNZ) [5]. Heat stress has an adverse effect on reproduction traits of dairy cattle [6,7] and buffaloes [8]. The negative influence of heat stress on reproduction traits of cattle and buffaloes can be quantified through formulating temperature humidity index (THI). The THI is a single value which incorporates the both of the air temperature and RH in the index [9]. Heat load index (HLI) is another index to measure the level of heat stress in feedlot cattle through incorporating the RH, wind speed and black-globe temperature (BGT) [10]. A negative correlation exists between reproduction traits of cattle and buffaloes with THI and animals experience the adverse effects of heat stress when the THI crosses a threshold level. The conception rate in lactating dairy cows declines with THI more than 72-73 in cattle [11,12] and 75 in buffalo [13]. The significant (p≤0.05) decline in the first service pregnancy rate of dairy cattle was observed at THI level above 72 [14] and heat stress was one of the major factors for a significant reduction in a pregnancy rate of crossbred cows in India [15]. The buffaloes are also susceptible to heat stress with respect to decline in fertility above THI level 75 in a subtropical climate [8]. This review was aimed to determine the influence of heat stress in relation with THI on reproductive performances of cattle and buffaloes.

Global Warming and its Impact on Animal Reproduction

Global warming has a great impact on the reproductive activity of cattle and buffaloes. Global warming has risen the surface temperature about 0.7°C since the early 20th century. It is anticipated that the temperature rise will be 1.8-4°C by 2100 [16]. The Intergovernmental Panel on Climate Change also indicated that the developing countries tend to be more vulnerable to extreme climatic events as they largely depend on climate sensitive sectors like agriculture and forestry. The greenhouse gas emission from agriculture sector is the most important factor for global warming, and livestock sector share 18% of total greenhouse gas emissions. The productive and reproductive performances of cattle and buffaloes are likely to be aggravated due to climate change and global warming. Assessment of the potential direct impacts of climate change on the reproduction of buffaloes indicate that there is increasing trend in incidences of silent estrus, the decline in reproductive activity and conception of buffaloes due to increase in air temperature during summer [17-19].

Different Heat Stress Models for Formulating THI and HLI

Hahn et al. [4] demonstrated the main natural physical environmental factors affecting livestock system includes air temperature, RH, WS, solar radiation, precipitation, atmospheric pressure, ultraviolet light and dust. This leads to the establishment of thermal indices which can better reflect the thermal stress of the animal. Hence, a variety of indices is used to estimate the degree of heat stress affecting performance traits viz., production traits, reproduction traits and growth traits in cattle and buffaloes. The most common among these indices is the THI. A number of methods have been developed over the years to formulate the THI, which is applied to measure the level of heat stress on animals (Table-1). The THI is the common measure of heat stress for humans through combining the dry bulb and wet bulb temperature [9]. Thereafter, formulas for calculation of THI were extended by including RH or dew point temperature [20,21].

All these THI models were used in a study conducted by Dash et al. [24] at Karnal in India. Month wise average THI values with seven different THI models during 20 years from 1993 to 2012 were presented in Figure-1. The maximum THI values were observed in the month of June as 87.41, 81.90, 89.58 and 81.60 with THI model 1, 3, 5 and 6, respectively. For other THI models (2, 4 and 7), maximum THI values were found in the month of July as 82.70, 82.97 and 82.99, respectively. The minimum THI values were found in the month of January for all the THI models (1-7) as 63.12, 52.06, 57.07, 54.82, 64.89, 56.71 and 54.80, respectively. After a thorough analysis of all the seven THI models with pregnancy rate of Murrah buffaloes, the THI model 1 [(0.4 × (T_{db} + T_{wb})] × 1.8 + 32 + 15) was identified as the best THI model for studying the effects of heat stress on pregnancy rate of buffaloes [24]. Bohmanova et al. [25] compared all the seven THI models and drawn the conclusion that there is variation in use of THIs according to the climatic condition. The THI which put more weight on the humidity is more appropriate for humid climates, whereas the indices with the more weight on ambient temperature work best under semiarid climates.

Various modifications to the THI have been proposed through formulating the HLI. Gaughan et al. [10] developed the HLI based on the weather parameters viz., RH, WS and BGT in feedlot cattle during hot weather. The HLI consists of two parts based on BGT threshold of 25°C as follows:

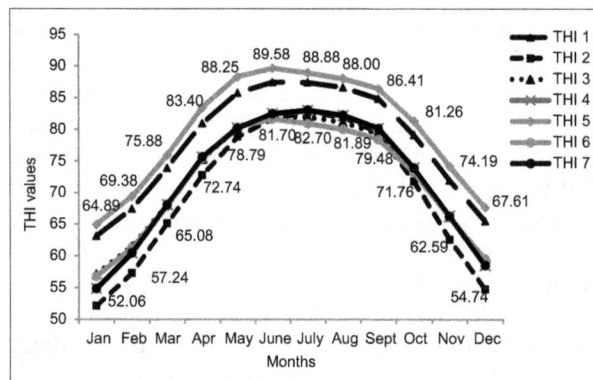

Figure-1: Monthly average temperature humidity index (THI) values with seven different THI models. Data are from Dash et al. [24].

Table-1: Different heat stress models for formulating temperature humidity indices.

Heat stress models	Formulae	References
THI 1	[0.4×(T_{db}+T_{wb})]×1.8+32+15	[9]
THI 2	(0.35×T_{db}+0.65×T_{wb})×1.8+32	[22]
THI 3	(T_{db}+T_{wb})×0.72+40.6	[20]
THI 4	(1.8×T_{db}+32)−(0.55−0.0055×RH)×(1.8×T_{db}−26)	[20]
THI 5	(0.55×T_{db}+0.2×T_{dp})×1.8+32+17.5	[20]
THI 6	T_{db}+(0.36×T_{dp})+41.2	[21]
THI 7	(0.8×T_{db})+[(RH/100)×(T_{db}−14.4)]+46.4	[23]

T_{db}=Dry bulb temperature, T_{wb}=Wet bulb temperature, RH=Relative humidity, THI=Temperature humidity index

$HLI_{BGT>25} = 8.62 + (0.38 \times RH) + (1.55 \times BGT) - (0.5 \times WS) + e (2.4 - WS)$

Where e is the base of the natural logarithm

$HLI_{BGT<25} = 10.66 + (0.28 \times RH) + (1.3 \times BGT) - WS$

The THI and HLI are considered as the appropriate guides to quantify the heat stress on animals. When an animal is exposed to THI or HLI above the threshold, then the core body temperature increases and the longer the duration of exposure above the threshold, the greater is the heat stress to animals.

Thermo-neutral zone (TNZ) and heat stress zone (HSZ)

The environmental stress is aggravated due to global warming accompanied with periods of extreme weather. If there are high temperature and humidity in the environment, then it is very difficult for the animal to dissipate heat and the animal undergoes heat stress. Heat stress is the state at which mechanisms get activated to maintain an animal's body thermal balance when exposed to uncomfortable elevated temperature. Heat stress is defined as any combination of environmental parameters producing conditions that are higher than the temperature range of the animal's TNZ [5]. The TNZ explains about the inter-relationship between the animal and the environment and it is defined as the range within which metabolic rate is minimal, and a healthy animal can make physical adaptation to maintain the normal body temperature with minimal change in metabolic activity. In general, the TNZ is surrounded by lower critical temperature and higher critical temperature (Figure-2). The upper critical temperature has been defined in dairy cows as 25-26°C [26].

When the environmental temperature moves away from the upper critical temperature, the detrimental effects of heat stress in terms of reduction of milk production, changes in milk composition and lower reproductive performances are observed in cattle and buffaloes. Various authors developed different zones whether the animals are comfortable or susceptible to heat stress based on the THI values.

Dairy cattle

Armstrong [27] categorized THI values into five different classes as no stress with THI value <72, mild stress (72-78), moderate stress (79-88), severe stress (89-98) and dead cows with THI >98 (Table-2). Similarly, The Livestock Weather Safety Index quantified environmental conditions using the THI as formulated by Thom [9] and it described the HSZ into four categories with different range of THI under each category like normal (≤74), alert (74< THI <79), danger stress (79≤ THI <84) and emergency stress (THI ≥84) in livestock. McDowell *et al.* [28] developed three different classes of THI as comfortable (≤70), stressful (71-78) and extreme distress (>78). Moran [29] described five categories of THI as no stress (<72), mild stress (72-78), severe stress (78-89), very severe stress (89-98) and dead cows (>98). The importance of classifying the THI into different classes involves the determination comfortable zone or HSZ where the animals have been exposed to heat stress. The acute exposure to extreme heat load is associated with disturbance to a physiological mechanism to the body like rapid respiration and excessive saliva production along with significant depression in reproductive performances in animals [30].

Buffalo

Dash *et al.* [31] studied the reproductive performance of Murrah buffaloes in relation with THI

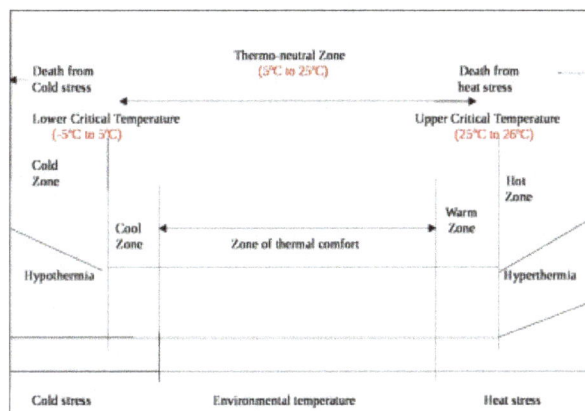

Figure-2: Thermoneutral zone in cattle.

Table-2: Classification of zones based on THI values in cattle with THI model [27].

THI	Stress level	Symptoms in cattle	Symptoms in buffalo
<72	None	Optimum productive and reproductive performance	Optimum productive and reproductive performance
72-78	Mild	Dairy cows seek for shade, increase in respiration rate and dilation of blood vessels	Elevation in rectal temperature and respiration rate
79-88	Moderate	Increase in respiration rate and saliva secretion. Reduction in feed intake and water consumption. Body temperature is increased and reproductive performances are severely affected in cattle	Respiration rate is significantly increased. Dry matter intake of buffalo is decreased and ratio of forage to concentrate intake is decreased. Water intake in buffalo is significantly increased
89-98	Severe	There is rapid increase in respiration and excessive saliva production. The reproductive performances in animals are significantly decreased	Excessive panting and restlessness are observed. Rumination and urination are lowered along with a negative impact on reproductive performances in buffaloes
>98	Danger	Heat stress is extreme and cows may die	Heat stress is extreme and buffaloes may die

THI=Temperature humidity index

values and identified three different zones as non-HSZ (NHSZ), HSZ and critical HSZ (CHSZ). The months from October to March were included under NHSZ with THI values 56.71-73.21 and months from April to September were incorporated under HSZ with THI values 75.39-81.60 while the months of May and June were identified as the CHSZ within the HSZ with THI values 80.27-81.60 (Table-3).

Effect of heat stress on reproductive performances of cattle and buffaloes

The productive and reproductive performances of dairy cattle and buffaloes varied according to the prevailing climate of their inhabitation. The major climatic zones include tropical, subtropical and temperate. The temperate zone is the most ideal for higher productivity in dairy animals. Therefore, this review focused the effect of heat stress on different fertility traits of cattle and buffaloes *viz.*, service period, conception rate and pregnancy rate in tropical/subtropical as well as temperate climate.

Effect of heat stress on service period in tropical or subtropical climate

Dairy cattle

The heat stress is considered as one of the main factors affecting reproductive performances in dairy cattle. High temperature in summer months combined with a high level of RH has adverse effects on reproductive performance in cows. In Thailand, the lowest THI of 72 was observed in December and highest mean THI was observed in April as 80. The cows which calved in February had the longest service period as 299±11 days while cows that calved in the months of October or November had a significantly shorter mean service reported as 133±7 days [32]. Boonkum *et al.* [33] also found the greatest service period of 154-day in Thai crossbred Holstein cows for calving in March and the lowest service period of 128-day for calving in the month of October. In summary, calving month greatly affects the phenotypic variation in service period of Thai Holstein crossbred cattle. The season of calving had highly significant (p<0.01) effect on service period of Sahiwal cattle. The cows calved during summer months had longest service period of

Table-3: Classification of zones based on THI values in buffalo [31].

Zones	Months	THI	
		Average	Range
NHSZ	October, November, December, January, February, March	64.08	56.71-73.21
HSZ	April, May, June, July, August, September	79.42	75.39-81.60
CHSZ	May, June	80.83	80.27-81.60

NHSZ=Non-heat stress zone, CHSZ=Critical heat stress zone, HSZ=Heat stress zone, THI=Temperature humidity index

159±3 days, whereas autumn calvers had the shortest service period of 148±4 days [34]. Heat stress controls the mechanism of hypothalamic-hypophyseal-ovarian axis in animals. The heat stress causes hyper-prolactinemia, reduction in luteinizing hormone frequency, poor follicle maturation and decreased oestradiol production leading to ovarian inactivity in cattle [35].

Effect of heat stress on service period in temperate climate

The non-return rate (NR) is currently used in as a measure of reproductive ability in cattle. When the cow does not return to further insemination in the same lactation, then the success in conception is assumed. Ravagnolo and Misztal [6] reported that NR45 of Holstein cattle showed a decrease rate of 0.005 per unit increase in THI on the day of insemination at THI >68 and NR45 was significantly lower and more susceptible to elevation in THI for first parity cows than second, third and fourth lactation cows (0.008 vs. 0.005 decrease). The seasonal trend for service period is observed in cattle. The service period in Holstein cows was longest (166 days) for March/April calving and shortest (130 days) for September calving [36]. The conclusion is drawn from the above research is that the service period of cows was longest for spring and shortest for fall calvings. High temperature combined with a high level of humidity in spring and summer season results in physiological disorders, affecting the digestive system, acid-base chemistry, blood hormones and finally resulting in longer service period in cows.

Buffalo

The month wise average service period of Murrah buffaloes was analyzed with the monthly average THI values [13]. The average service period of Murrah buffaloes was prolonged (180 days) in the month May with the corresponding THI value of 80.27. On the contrary, the lowest average service period (119 days) was observed at average THI 67.80 in the month of March. The service period of buffaloes was found increased with increase in average THI above 75 [13]. The cooler months with lower THI values caused decrease in service period while the months with higher THI values above threshold level 75 were associated with increase in service period in Murrah buffaloes.

Effect of heat stress on conception rate in tropical or subtropical climate

Dairy cattle

A significant change in conception rate of cattle was observed in response to the major climatic variables like temperature and humidity, which are combined to form the THI and the THI is popularly used to assess the fertility in bovines. Lactating dairy cows are particularly sensitive to heat stress because of high metabolic heat production inside the body associated with increased milk production. The negative effects of heat stress on conception rate of cattle are most evident when THI level crosses a threshold level. When the THI on the day of service is more than 72, it decreases the conception rate of dairy cows in Australia. The high heat load 3-5 weeks before service and 1 week after service was associated with reduced conception rate in cattle [11].

Effect of heat stress on conception rate in temperate climate

The conception rate of lactating dairy cows is highly affected by heat stress. Garcia-Ispierto et al. [7] reported that negative effects of heat stress on conception rate of Holstein cows seem to appear when THI ≥75 on 3 days prior to artificial insemination and the effects of heat stress are more evident in the form of declining conception rate from 30.6% to 23% when THI was above 80 in North-Eastern Spain. The threshold THI for the influence heat stress on conception rate of lactating dairy cows in Germany was 73 and the greatest negative impact of heat stress on conception rate was observed 21-1 day before breeding [12]. The conception rate in Holstein cows was found lowered following services performed in hot months. Nabenishi et al. [37] observed that conception rate of lactating dairy cows during the hot period (July to September) was significantly lower (p<0.01) with 29.5% as compared to the conception rate of 38.2% during the cool period (October to June). The reductions in conception rates in hot periods are due to the combined effects of environmental heat, which produces an alteration in the synthesis of reproductive hormones [4]. The heat stress during the summer season is able to change the follicular microenvironment of highly productive dairy cows, and the detrimental effect of heat stress is associated with physiological processes of the establishment and maintenance of pregnancy after fertilization [35].

Buffalo

The incidence of seasonal reproductive behavior is a more common in buffaloes. Buffaloes are sexually activated by decreased day length and temperature [38]. The highest breeding frequency in buffaloes is found during the winter and the lowest in the summer season. Abayawansa et al. [39] reported that maximum percentage of buffaloes exhibited postpartum estrous during the month of September followed by October and minimum during April and May due to high maximum air temperature. Silent estrus is the most important limiting factor especially during hot months which leads to poor reproductive efficiency in buffaloes [40]. Dash [13] studied in detail regarding the monthly average conception rate of Murrah buffaloes with monthly average THI values over a year. The highest average conception rate was observed as 78% in the month of October while the lowest was 59% in the month of August. The threshold THI for conception rate was identified as 75 for the reason that with increase in average THI above threshold 75, the decline in overall conception rate was observed in Murrah buffaloes [13]. Heat stress results in a significant reduction in conception rate during the hot and humid-hot months when the monthly average THI is higher than 75 in buffaloes.

Effect of heat stress on pregnancy rate in tropical or subtropical climate

Dairy cattle

Pregnancy rate is defined as the percentage of non-pregnant cows that become pregnant during each 21-day period. Now the pregnancy rate is more preferred compared to service period as an indicator of reproductive success because pregnancy rate can be easily defined and available soon. The pregnancy rate of animals is declined with respect to increase in THI above a threshold level. McGown et al. [14] reported that an increase in THI above 72 which corresponds to temperature 25°C and RH 50% resulted in a significant decrease in the first service pregnancy rate of Holstein cattle in Queensland, Australia. Another finding indicates that the month of insemination significantly (p<0.05) influenced the pregnancy rate in Holstein cows. A substantial decline in pregnancy rate was observed from 34.1% to 15.7% with increase in mean THI from 69 in May to 74 in July in a subtropical climate of Egypt [41]. The conception and the pregnancy rate of the Holstein dairy cattle were negatively affected by higher THI level under Egyptian subtropical conditions. The conception and the pregnancy rate of the Holstein cattle decreased from 35.8% and 29.4%, respectively, at low THI (<THI 70) to 16.1% and 12.1%, respectively, at high THI level of 80-85 [42]. The significant (p<0.05) reduction in a pregnancy rate of crossbred dairy cattle due to heat stress was also evident in India. When the dairy cattle was in TNZ, the pregnancy rate of was estimated as 32.6%, but it was significantly decreased to 20.5% when the animals came into HSZ [15]. In summer, risks for ovulatory failure, impaired oocyte quality or embryonic development, reduced progesterone production and increased embryo mortality may be the possible reasons for dramatic decline in fertility in animals [35].

Effect of heat stress on pregnancy rate in temperate climate

The highest pregnancy rate of Holstein-Friesian dairy cattle was observed in September-November as 32% while the lowest pregnancy rate of 24% in March-May in South-Eastern United States [43]. The lower pregnancy rate is due to the delay of rebreeding cows in the summer months with a high level of heat stress. Amundson et al. [44] observed the negative associations of THI with pregnancy rate of Bos taurus crossbred cows in all three breeding seasons from 0 to 21 days, 0 to 42 days, and 0 to 60 days, respectively. However, the change was more pronounced during the first 21 days of the breeding season with a −2.06% change in pregnancy rate for each unit of change in THI value.

Buffalo

The THIs play an important role in the reproductive functions of buffaloes and it is suggested that

THI >75 has a negative effect on reproductive performances of buffaloes in the tropical areas of Amazon basin in Brazil [45]. In a similar manner, a distinct relationship was observed between THI and pregnancy rate in Murrah buffaloes. The average pregnancy rate of Murrah buffaloes was found declining from 0.41 to 0.25 with the onset of THI ≥75 [8]. When the monthly average pregnancy rate of Murrah buffaloes was analyzed with monthly average THI values, then the lowest average pregnancy rate was observed as 0.25 in the month of July with corresponding THI 80.88 and the highest average pregnancy rate was obtained as 0.58 in the month of November at average THI value 66.09 [8]. The threshold THI for pregnancy rate in buffaloes was determined as 75 above which the detrimental effects of heat stress are affecting fertility are observed in buffaloes.

Impact of heat stress on oocyte and embryo quality

Heat stress has adverse effects on reproductive performances of cattle and buffaloes. The Higher ambient temperature during the summer has been associated with reduced fertility in dairy cattle through its deleterious impact on oocyte maturation and early embryo development [35]. There are several possible mechanisms by which heat stress can prevent the growth of oocytes. The foremost is the reduction on the synthesis of preovulatory surge in luteinizing hormone and estradiol. Hence, there is poor follicle maturation and this leads to ovarian inactivity in cattle [46]. Heat stress also delays follicle selection and reduces the degree of dominance of the dominant follicle. Heat stress decreases blood progesterone concentration, which is a major cause for abnormal oocyte maturation, implantation failure and finally early embryonic death in dairy cattle [47]. During heat stress, the intrauterine environment of the cow is compromised. Hence, there is decrease in blood flow to the uterus and elevated uterine temperature. These changes increase the chances of early embryonic loss and suppress embryonic development [48]. The exposure of females to heat stress conditions during days 0-3 of pregnancy or days 0-7 of pregnancy reduced embryonic survival. Heat stress has a deleterious effect on the oocyte quality in buffaloes. Follicular growth and atresia during anestrus are attributed to the inadequate secretion of gonadotropins by the hypophysis [18]. There is decrease in the concentration of oestradiol-17 beta in summer which reduces the intensity of estrus manifestation and results in silent heat in buffaloes [40]. The mean plasma prolactin concentration was significantly higher in summer than winter which may cause acyclicity or infertility in buffaloes [49].

Mitigation Strategies to Combat Heat Stress

There is huge economic loss due to heat stress in livestock. In India, there loss of 1.8 million tonnes of milk a year due to heat stress among cattle and buffaloes, which is attributable to approximately Rs. 2661 crore [50]. Poor nutrition, inappropriate management and environmental factors have a significant negative influence on reproductive efficiency of cattle [51,52]. Basically three mitigation strategies are applied to combat the negative influences of heat stress on animals which are described in the followings:

- Development of genetically heat tolerant dairy breeds
- Nutrition modification
- Environment modification
- Timed artificial insemination (TAI) protocol.

Development of genetically heat tolerant dairy breeds

Selection for higher milk yield in cows has led to increased metabolic heat production and this causes more susceptibility of the animal towards heat stress. The productivity and heat tolerance are antagonistic. The continual selection for production ignoring heat tolerance results in decreasing heat tolerance. There is the presence of considerable variation for heat tolerance between breeds and even between individuals within a breed. The identification and selection of heat tolerant dairy animals is useful to maintain both the high productivity and survivability when exposed to heat stress conditions. Therefore, the inclusion of THI covariate effects in the selection index should be targeted for genetic evaluation of dairy animals especially in the hot climate [53].

Improving animal adaptation to climate stress can be achieved in two ways such as through selection of the animals in heat stressed conditions and through introgressing heat adaptation genes from a local breed into a commercial herd [54]. The genes responsible for traits like coat color and hair length confer heat shock resistance in cells [55]. Hair coat characteristics like hair coat thickness and hair weight per unit surface are important determinant of non-evaporative heat loss from the body. The slick hair gene has been identified for increased thermal resistance due to its association with increased sweating rate and a lower metabolic rate in animals [56]. The slick hair gene responsible for slick hair coat improves heat tolerance capacity when introduced into temperate climate cattle breeds [57]. There are some other genes viz., ATP1A1 gene and heat shock protein (HSP) genes have been identified which confer thermal resistance and adaptation to thermal stress in cattle [58,59]. The ATP1A1 gene is known as Na+/K+ -ATPase subunit alpha-1. This gene is well recognized as a candidate for heat shock response because of its association to oxidative stress in cattle [58]. The bovine Na+/K+ -ATPase protein complex consists of α and β subunits. The ATP1A1 gene encodes the α1 isoform, the major isoform of α subunit of Na+-K+ ATPase pump. ATP1A1 gene has been mapped on B. taurus chromosome number 3 and is consisting of 22 introns, 23 exons. ATP1A1 gene is responsible for establishing the electrochemical gradient of Na+ and K+ across the plasma membrane, which is essential in the maintenance of body fluid and cellular homeostasis. The ATPA1 gene, ATPB2 gene and osteopontin were found to have significant association with thermo-tolerance in buffaloes [60]. The cellular heat shock response is another component of adaptation to heat stress. During hyperthermia, heat stress activates heat shock transcription factor-1 and this enhances expression of HSPs coupled with decreased expression and synthesis of other proteins, and HSP induced activation of immune system. The role of HSP is to activate the immune and endocrine system and also to alter the physiological state referred to as acclimation. The detailed understanding of genes in regulating the heat shock response in animals would be helpful to improve their thermal tolerance via gene manipulation [61]. The HSP70 family genes were found highly expressed in summer in Sahiwal and Tharparkar cattle and buffalo in India which enhances their thermotolerance and adaptive capacity to dry/hot humid environment [62].

The identification of major genes associated with thermo-tolerance that reduces the effects of heat stress in cattle and buffaloes and its subsequent incorporation into breeding program through marker assisted selection should be the breeding strategy for enhancing both the reproductive ability and adaptability to the warm climate. The crossbred cattle are better adapted and have better reproductive performance than purebred exotic cattle [63]. The thermal tolerance and reproductive performances of exotic cattle breeds can be improved by crossbreeding them with local cattle breeds.

Nutrition modification

When the cows are under heat stress, there is decrease in dry matter intake along with crude protein intake and due to reduced feed intake, there is negative energy balance in the body of heat stressed cows and buffaloes. Due to increase in core body temperature and inefficient heat dissipation processes, energy requirements for maintenance is found to be increased. Therefore, the measures to increase the nutrient density include feeding of high quality forage, concentrates and use of supplemental fats in the diet of animals. The feed additives are also very useful to stabilize the rumen environment from dietary modifications and also improve the energy utilization [64]. The dry matter digestibility and protein/energy ratio were also found to be decreased in heat stress conditions. Feeding of good quality low-degradable protein has shown to improve milk production in heat stressed cows. So both quantity and form of protein play important role during feeding of the heat stressed cows and buffaloes. Feeding supplemental niacin is also helpful in reducing the effects of heat stress in cattle. Supplementation with antioxidants during the heat stress period is another way to improve fertility through a decrease of oxidative stress in buffaloes [65].

Environment modification

The months of May and June were found very critical for the optimum reproductive performances in dairy animals. There was reduction in breeding values of reproductive traits in buffaloes during the CHSZ of May and June [66]. Therefore, in order to prevent the effects of heat stress, the modification of the surrounding environment is the key management practices to be followed in the dairy herd. Primary methods for altering the environment can be classified into two categories; first is the provision of shade and the other is evaporative cooling strategies with water. Provision of shade protects the cows and buffaloes from direct effects of solar radiation. Trees are an excellent source of shade combined with beneficial cooling as moisture evaporates from the leaves and animals also preferentially seek for tree shade over artificial shade structures [28]. Artificial shades are quite useful for heat stressed animals in confinement or in intensive situations. Shade is effective in protecting cows from solar radiation, but does not alter the air temperature or RH around the cows.

Though the evaporative cooling strategies are costly, but they are more useful to alleviate the heat stress in animals. Evaporative cooling systems use the energy from the air to evaporate water and evaporation of water into warm air reduces the air temperature. The milk production and reproductive performances of dairy cattle were improved using an evaporative cooling system [67]. Fogging systems use very fine droplets of water and these water droplets are immediately dispersed into the air stream and quickly evaporate, thus cooling the surrounding air. Misting systems generate larger droplets than fogging systems, but cool the air by the same principle. The sprinklers are different from foggers and misters. The sprinklers do not cool the air rather than the large droplet arising from them wet the hair coat and skin of the cows and buffaloes and then water evaporates to cool the hair and skin. This system is a very effective in combination with air movement. The mechanical air cooling is possible by using the evaporative cooling pad and fan system which are very useful in reducing the rectal temperature and respiratory rate in cows and buffaloes.

Timed artificial insemination (TAI) protocol

Heat stress reduces the length and intensity of estrus and hence the incidences of anestrous and silent ovulation are increased. The use of TAI protocol is practiced for accurate estrus detection and timely insemination in order to improve fertility in summer. Hormonal treatments have been developed to synchronize the time of ovulation, allowing the use of fixed TAI that does not require detection of estrus. The TAI protocol is commonly referred to as ovsynch and this consists of hormonal treatments of gonadotropin-releasing hormone (GnRH) (day 0), prostaglandin F2α (day 7) and GnRH (day 9) and artificial insemination is being performed 16-20 h after second GnRH treatment [68]. The ovysynch protocol can successfully synchronize ovulation in buffaloes and can also increase conception rate when combined with

TAI [69]. The CIDRsynch and Presynch protocols are also applied to improve conception rate and pregnancy rate of Holstein cows under subtropical environmental conditions [70]. This TAI protocol can be able to reduce losses in reproductive efficiency in cattle and buffaloes caused by poor estrus detection in summer.

Conclusion

The heat stress has adverse effects on the reproductive performances of cattle and buffaloes. The THI is the most commonly used index to measure the level of heat stress in animals. The reproductive traits of cattle are susceptible to the negative impacts of heat stress with increase in THI above 72, while the buffaloes are more prone to heat stress when the THI level surpasses 75. The months from April to September under HSZ show the average THI level above 75. This necessitates the adoption of proper management interventions in the form of nutrition modification and environment modification in order to ameliorate the effects of heat stress on cattle and buffaloes during April to September. The heat tolerant dairy animals should be selected which can enhance both the reproductive ability and adaptability to the warm climate.

Authors' Contributions

SD prepared the initial version of the manuscript. AU, MS and SY assisted in literature collection. SD, AKC and AS revised the manuscript and made final critical scientific corrections. All authors read and approved the final manuscript.

Acknowledgments

The authors are thankful to the Head, DCB Division for providing necessary information. The authors are also thankful to the Director, ICAR-NDRI for final for providing all possible kind of assistance for the preparation of the manuscript.

Competing Interests

The authors declare that they have no competing interests.

References

1. BAHS, Basic Animal Husbandry Statistics. (2014) Department of Animal Husbandry, Dairying and Fisheries, Ministry of Agriculture, Government of India.

2. NDRI Vision 2030. National Dairy Research Institute, Karnal, Haryana, India.

3. Thiruvenkadan, A.K., Panneerselvam, S., Rajendran, R. and Murali, N. (2010) Analysis on the productive and reproductive traits of Murrah buffalo cows maintained in the coastal region of India. *Appl. Anim. Husb. Rural Dev.,* 3: 1-5.

4. Hahn, G.L., Mader, T.L. and Eigenberg, R.A. (2003) Perspectives on development of thermal indices for animal studies and management. In: Proceeding Symposium. Interactions between Climate and Animal Production. EAAP Technical Series No. 7; p31-44.

5. Buffington, D.E., Collazo-Arochu, A., Canton, H.H., Pritt, D., Thatcher, W.W. and Collier, R.J. (1981) Black globe-humidity index (BGHI) as comfort equation for cows. *Trans. Am. Soc. Agric. Eng.* 34: 711.

6. Ravagnolo, O. and Misztal, I. (2002) Effect of heat stress on non return rate in Holsteins: Fixed-model analyses. *J. Dairy Sci.,* 85: 3101-3106.

7. Garcia-Ispierto, I., Lopez-Gatius, F., Bech-Sabat, G., Santolaria, P., Yaniz, J.L., Nogareda, C., De Rensis, F. and Lopez-Bejar, M. (2007) Climate factors affecting conception rate of high producing dairy cows in northeastern Spain. *Theriogenology,* 67: 1379-1385.

8. Dash, S., Chakravarty, A.K., Sah, V., Jamuna, V., Behera, R., Kashyap, N. and Deshmukh, B. (2015) Influence of temperature and humidity on pregnancy rate of Murrah buffaloes. *Asian-Aust. J. Anim. Sci.,* 28(7): 943-950.

9. Thom, E.C. (1959) The discomfort index. *Weatherwise,* 12: 57-59.

10. Gaughan, J.B., Mader, T.L., Holt, S.M. and Lisle, A. (2008) A new heat load index for feedlot cattle. *J. Anim. Sci.,* 86: 226-234.

11. Morton, J.M., Tranter, W.P., Mayer, D.G. and Jonsson, N.N. (2007) Effect of environmental heat on conception rates in lactating dairy cows: Critical periods of exposure. *J. Dairy Sci.,* 90: 2271-2278.

12. Schuller, L.K., Burfeind, O. and Heuwieser, W. (2014) Impact of heat stress on conception rate of dairy cows in the moderate climate considering different temperature humidity index thresholds, periods relative to breeding, and heat load indices. *Theriogenology,* 81: 1050-1057.

13. Dash, S. (2013) Genetic evaluation of fertility traits in relation to heat stress in Murrah buffaloes. M.V.Sc. Thesis, ICAR-NDRI (Deemed University), Karnal, Haryana, India.

14. McGowan, M.R., Mayer, D.G., Tranter, W., Shaw, M., Smith, C. and Davison, T.M. (1996) Relationship between temperature humidity index and conception efficiency of dairy cattle in Queensland. *Proc. Aust. Soc. Anim. Prod.,* 21: 454.

15. Khan, F.A., Prasad, S. and Gupta, H.P. (2013) Effect of heat stress on pregnancy rates of crossbred dairy cattle in Terai region of Uttarakhand, India. *Asian Pac. J. Reprod.,* 2(4): 277-279.

16. IPCC, (Intergovernmental Panel on Climate Change). (2014) Climate Change: Synthesis Report; Summary for Policymakers. Available from: https://www.ipcc. ch/pdf/ assessment-report/ar5/syr/AR5_SYR_FINAL_SPM.pdf. Last accessed on 25-12-2015.

17. Singh, G., Totey, S.M. and Talwar, G.P. (1989) *In vitro* fertilization of buffalo (*Bubalus bubalis*) oocytes matured *in vitro*. *Theriogenology,* 31(1): 255.

18. Das, G.K. and Khan, F.A. (2010) Summer anoestrus in buffalo - A review. *Reprod. Domest. Anim.,* 45: e483-e494.

19. Upadhyay, R.C., Rita Rani, A., Singh, S.V., Mohanty, T.K. and Gohain, M. (2012) Impact of climate change on reproductive functions of Murrah buffaloes. *J. Anim. Plant Sci.,* 22(3): 234-236.

20. National Research Council. (1971) A Guide to Environmental Research on Animals. National Academy of Sciences, Washington, DC.

21. Yousef, M.K. (1985) Stress Physiology in Livestock. CRC Press, Boca Raton, FL, USA.

22. Bianca, W. (1962) Relative importance of dry- and wet-bulb temperatures in causing heat stress in cattle. *Nature,* 195: 251-252.

23. Mader, T.L., Davis, M.S. and Brown-Brandl, T. (2006) Environmental factors influencing heat stress in feedlot cattle. *J. Anim. Sci.,* 84: 712-719.

24. Dash, S., Chakravarty, A.K., Singh, A., Sah, V., Shivahre, P.R. and Panmei, A. (2015) Identification of best temperature humidity index model for pregnancy rate of Murrah buffaloes in a subtropical climate. *Indian J. Dairy Sci.,* 68(1): 45-49.

25. Bohmanova, J., Misztal, I. and Cole, J.B. (2007) Temperature-humidity indices as indicators of milk production losses due to heat stress. *J. Dairy Sci.,* 90: 1947-1956.

26. Berman, A., Folman, Y.M., Kaim, M., Mamen, Z., Herz, D., Wolfenson, A. and Graber, Y. (1985) Upper critical

temperatures and forced ventilation effects for high-yielding dairy cows in a tropical climate. *J. Dairy Sci.,* 68: 488-495.

27. Armstrong, D.V. (1994) Heat stress interactions with shade and cooling. *J. Dairy Sci.,* 77: 2044-2050.

28. McDowell, R.E., Hooven, N.W. and Camoens, J.K. (1976) Effects of climate on performance of Holsteins in first lactation. *J. Dairy Sci.,* 59: 965-973.

29. Moran, J. (2005) Tropical Dairy Farming: Feeding Management for Small Holder Dairy Farms in the Humid Tropics. Landlinks Press, Colling Wood. p312.

30. Kadzere, C.T., Murphy, M.R., Silanikove, N. and Maltz, E. (2002) Heat stress in lactating dairy cows: A review. *Livest. Prod. Sci.,* 77: 59-91.

31. Dash, S., Chakravarty, A.K., Singh, A., Behera, R., Upadhyay, A. and Shivahre, P.R. (2014) Determination of critical heat stress zone for fertility traits using temperature humidity index in Murrah buffaloes. *Indian J. Anim. Sci.,* 84(11): 1181-1184.

32. Kaewlamun, W., Chayaratanasin, R., Virakul, P., Andrew, A.P., Humblot, P., Suadsong, S., Tummaruk, P. and Techakumphu, M. (2011) Differences of periods of calving on days open of dairy cows in different regions and months of Thailand. *Thai J. Vet. Med.,* 41(3): 315-320.

33. Boonkum, W., Misztal, I., Duangjinda, M., Pattarajinda, V., Tumwasorn, S. and Buaban, S. (2011) Genetic effects of heat stress on days open for Thai Holstein crossbreds. *J. Dairy Sci.,* 94: 1592-1596.

34. Kumar, A. and Gandhi, R.S. (2011) Evaluation of pooled lactation production and reproduction traits in Sahiwal cattle. *Indian J. Anim. Sci.,* 81(6): 600-604.

35. Wolfenson, D., Roth, Z. and Meidan, R. (2000) Impaired reproduction in heat-stressed cattle: Basic and applied aspects. *Anim. Reprod. Sci.,* 60-61: 535-547.

36. Oseni, S., Mistzal, I., Tsuruta, S. and Rekaya, R. (2004) Genetic components of days open under heat stress. *J. Dairy Sci.,* 87: 3022-3028.

37. Nabenishi, H., Ohta, H., Nishimoto, T., Morita, T., Ashizawa, K. and Tsuzuki, Y. (2011) Effect of the temperature humidity index on body temperature and conception rate of lactating dairy cows in southwestern Japan. *J. Reprod. Dev.,* 57: 450-456.

38. Zicarelli, L. (2010) Enhancing reproductive performance in domestic dairy water buffalo (*Bubalus bubalis*). *Soc. Reprod. Fertil. Suppl.,* 67: 443-455.

39. Abayawansa, W.D., Prabhakar, S., Singh, A.K. and Brar, P.S. (2011) Effect of climatic changes on reproductive performance of Murrah buffaloes in Punjab: A retrospective analysis. *Indian J. Anim. Sci.,* 81(4): 334-339.

40. Singh, M., Chaudhari, B.K., Singh, J.K., Singh, A.K. and Maurya, P.K. (2013) Effects of thermal load on buffalo reproductive performance during summer season. *J. Biol. Sci.,* 1(1): 1-8.

41. El-Wishy, A.B. (2013) Fertility of Holstein cattle in a subtropical climate of Egypt. *Iran. J. Appl. Anim. Sci.,* 3(1): 45-51.

42. El-Tarabany, M.S. and El-Bayoumi, K.M. (2015) Reproductive performance of backcross Holstein x Brown Swiss and their Holstein contemporaries under subtropical environmental conditions. *Theriogenology,* 83: 444-448.

43. Oseni, S., Misztal, I. and Tsuruta, S. (2005) Genetic parameters for pregnancy rate in Holstein cattle under seasonal heat stress. *Nig. J. Genet.,* 19: 43-57.

44. Amundson, J.L., Mader, T.L., Rasby, R.J. and Hu, Q.S. (2006) Environmental effects on pregnancy rate in beef cattle. *J. Anim. Sci.,* 84: 3415-3420.

45. Vale, W.G. (2007) Effects of environment on buffalo reproduction. *Ital. J. Anim. Sci.,* 6(2): 130-142.

46. Hansen, P.J. (2007) Exploitation of genetic and physiological determinants of embryonic resistance to elevated temperature to improve embryonic survival in dairy cattle during heat stress. *Theriogenology,* 68(1): S242-S249.

47. Khodaei-Motlagh, M., Shahneh, A.Z., Masoumi, R. and

Derensis, F. (2011) Alterations in reproductive hormones during heat stress in dairy cattle. *Afr. J. Biotechnol.,* 10(29): 5552-5558.

48. De Rensis, F. and Scaramuzzi, R.J. (2003) Heat stress and seasonal effects on reproduction in the dairy cow: A review. *Theriogenology,* 60: 1139-1151.

49. Roy, K.S. and Prakash, B.S. (2007) Seasonal variation and circadian rhythmicity of the prolactin profile during the summer months in repeat-breeding Murrah buffalo heifers. *Reprod. Fertil. Dev.,* 19: 596-605.

50. Upadhayay, R.C. (2010) Annual Milk Production Loss Due to Global Warming. Animal Physiology. National Dairy Research Institute (NDRI), Press Trust of India, New Delhi.

51. Fair, T. (2010) Mammalian oocyte development: Checkpoints for competence. *Reprod. Fertil. Dev.,* 22: 13-20.

52. Walsh, S.W., Williams, E.J. and Evans, A.C.O. (2011) A review of the causes of poor fertility in high milk producing dairy cows. *Anim. Reprod. Sci.,* 123: 127-138.

53. Bernabucci, U., Biffani, S., Buggiotti, L., Vitali, A., Lacetera, N. and Nardone, A. (2014) The effects of heat stress in Italian Holstein dairy cattle. *J. Dairy Sci.,* 97: 471-486.

54. Renaudeau, D., Collin, A., Yahav, S., de Basilio, V., Gourdine, J.L. and Collier, R.J. (2012) Adaptation to hot climate and strategies to alleviate heat stress in livestock production. *Animal,* 6(5): 707-728.

55. Hansen, P.J. and Arechiga, C.F. (1999) Strategies for managing reproduction in the heat stressed dairy cow. *J. Anim. Sci.,* 51(1): 36-50.

56. Dikmen, S., Alava, E., Pontes, E., Fear, J.M., Dikmen, B.Y., Olson, T.A. and Hansen, P.J. (2008) Differences in thermoregulatory ability between slick-haired and wild-type lactating Holstein cows in response to acute heat stress. *J. Dairy Sci.,* 91: 3395-3402.

57. Berman, A. (2011) Invited review: Are adaptations present to support dairy cattle productivity in warm climates? *J. Dairy Sci.,* 94: 2147-2158.

58. Liu, Y.X., Zhou, X., Li, D.Q., Cui, Q.W. and Wang, G.L. (2010) Association of ATP1A1 gene polymorphism with heat tolerance traits in dairy cattle. *Genet. Mol. Res.,* 9(2): 891-896.

59. Loredana, B., Patrizia, M., Valentina, P., Nicola, L., Alessandro, N. and Umberto, B. (2011) Cellular thermotolerance is associated with heat shock protein 70.1 genetic polymorphisms in Holstein lactating cows. *Cell Stress Chaperones.,* 16(4): 441-448.

60. Jayakumar, S. (2014) Molecular characterization of thermoregulatory genes in Murrah buffaloes. Ph. D. Thesis, ICAR-NDRI (Deemed University), Karnal, Haryana, India.

61. Collier, R.J., Collier, J.L., Rhoads, R.P. and Baumgard, L.H. (2008) Genes involved in the bovine heat stress response. *J. Dairy Sci.,* 91: 445-454.

62. Kumar, A., Ashraf, S., Goud, T.S., Grewal, A., Singh, S.V., Yadav, B.R. and Upadhyay, R.C. (2015) Expression profiling of major heat shock protein genes during different seasons in cattle (*Bos indicus*) and buffalo (*Bubalus bubalis*) under tropical climatic condition. *J. Therm. Biol.,* 51: 55-64.

63. El-Tarabany, M.S. and Nasr, M.A.F. (2015) Reproductive performance of Brown Swiss, Holstein and their crosses under subtropical environmental conditions. *Theriogenology,* 84: 559-565.

64. Zimbelman, R.B., Baumgard, L.H. and Collier, R.J. (2010) Effect of encapsulated niacin on evaporative heat loss and body temperature in moderately heat-stressed lactating Holstein cows. *J. Dairy Sci.,* 93(6): 1986-1997.

65. Megahed, G.A., Anwar, M.M., Wasfy, S.I. and Hammadeh, M.E. (2008) Influence of heat stress on the cortisol and oxidant-antioxident balance during oestrous phase in buffalo-cows (*Bubalus bubalis*): Thermo-protective role of antioxidant treatment. *Reprod. Domest. Anim.,* 43: 672-677.

66. Dash, S., Chakravarty, A.K., Singh, A., Shivahre, P.R.,

Upadhyay, A., Sah, V. and Singh, K.M. (2015) Assessment of expected breeding values for fertility traits of Murrah buffaloes under subtropical climate. *Vet. World,* 8(3): 320-325.

67. Ryan, D.P., Boland, M.P., Kopel, E., Armstrong, D., Munyakazi, L., Godke, R.A. and Ingraham, R.H. (1992) Evaluating two different evaporative cooling management systems for dairy cows in a hot, dry climate. *J. Dairy Sci.,* 75: 1052-1059.

68. Ambrose, D.J., Colazo, M.G. and Kastelic, J.P. (2010) The applications of timed artificial insemination and timed embryo transfer in reproductive management of dairy cattle. *R. Bras. Zootec.,* 39: 383-392.

69. Hoque, M.N., Talukder, A.K., Akter, M. and Shamsuddin, M. (2014) Evaluation of ovsynch protocols for timed artificial insemination in water buffaloes in Bangladesh. *Turk. J. Vet. Anim. Sci.,* 38: 418-424.

70. El-Tarabany, M.S. and El-Tarabany, A.A. (2015) Impact of thermal stress on the efficiency of ovulation synchronization protocols in Holstein cows. *Anim. Reprod. Sci.,* 160: 138-145.

14

Hypoglycemic, hypolipidemic and antioxidant effects of pioglitazone, insulin and synbiotic in diabetic rats

K. Kavitha[1], A. Gopala Reddy[1], K. Kondal Reddy[2], C. S. V. Satish Kumar[1], G. Boobalan[1] and K. Jayakanth[1]

1. Department of Veterinary Pharmacology and Toxicology, College of Veterinary Science, Hyderabad - 500 030, Telangana, India; 2. Department of Livestock Products Technology, College of Veterinary Science, Hyderabad - 500 030, Telangana, India.
Corresponding author: K. Kavitha, e-mail: kavithakalyan_23@yahoo.co.in,
AGR: gopalareddy123@rediffmail.com, KKR: kkkredddy5@rediffmail.com, CSVSK: satish513512@gmail.com,
GB: bhupalvets@gmail.com, KJ: dr.koppakajayakanth@gmail.com

Abstract

Aim: The objective of the study was to assess the effect of combination treatment of insulin, pioglitazone and synbiotic on streptozotocin (STZ)-induced diabetic rats.

Materials and Methods: Diabetes mellitus was induced chemically by intraperitoneal administration of STZ (40 mg/kg b.wt) to male Sprague-Dawley rats. The rats were divided randomly into six groups of six rats in each. Group 1 was maintained as a normal control. Group 2 was maintained as diabetic control; Group 3 was treated with insulin; Group 4 with insulin + synbiotic; Group 5 with insulin + pioglitazone; and Group 6 with insulin + synbiotic + pioglitazone. All the animals were treated for 60 days.

Results: Body weights, and concentration of reduced glutathione (GSH), and high-density lipoproteins cholesterol were significantly ($p<0.05$) reduced, whereas the concentration of blood glucose, total cholesterol, triglycerides, protein carbonyls and thiobarbituric acid reacting substances, and the activity of GSH peroxidase were significantly ($p<0.05$) elevated in Group 2 at the end of 8th week as compared to Group 1. The treatment Groups 3, 4, 5 and 6 revealed improvement in all the parameters, and the highest improvement was observed in combination Group 6.

Conclusion: From this study, it is concluded that combination of insulin, pioglitazone and synbiotic is useful in treating diabetes.

Keywords: diabetes, insulin, oxidative stress, pioglitazone, synbiotic.

Introduction

Diabetes mellitus (DM) is a metabolic disease characterized by insulin resistance, dyslipidemia, and hyperglycemia. Insulin resistance and beta-cell dysfunction are the pathophysiological hallmarks of Type 2 DM [1]. Increase in oxidative stress and changes in antioxidant capacity, induced by high glucose, play a central role in complications of diabetes [2]. Pioglitazone is a potent insulin sensitizer, binds to the peroxisome proliferator-activated receptor gamma (PPARγ) and enhances the sensitivity of liver, muscle and adipose tissue to insulin by promoting the uptake of glucose. It has been reported that pioglitazone improves plasma lipid profile and blood pressure, which are very beneficial for the diabetic patients associated with cardiovascular diseases [3].

Prebiotics is food ingredients, such as dietary fibers consisting of non-starch polysaccharides and lignin that are non-digestible and promote the growth of specific bacteria within the intestinal tract that confer health benefits in the host. They are used in medicine as a means of providing short chain fatty acids (SCFA), maintaining bowel function, building colonization resistance against pathogens, and treating antibiotic-associated diarrhea as well as inflammatory bowel disease [4]. Prebiotic increases the endogenous intestinotrophic proglucagon-derived peptide (GLP-2) production and consequently improves gut barrier functions during obesity and diabetes [5]. Probiotics are live microbial organisms confers health benefits to the host by interacting with intestinal mucosal barrier and potentially contributes to the homeostasis of mucosal immunity. *Lactobacillus* and *Bifidobacteria* species are the most common genera used in fermentation of foodstuffs as probiotics. Synbiotic is a combination of probiotic and prebiotic administered together. The administration of synbiotic may be beneficial as adjunct therapy in the treatment of diabetes [6].

The aim of the present study was to assess the combined effect of insulin, pioglitazone and synbiotic on blood glucose concentration, lipid profile, and antioxidant profile in diabetic rats.

Materials and Methods

Ethical approval

An experimental protocol was conducted on rats with the approval from Institutional Animal Ethics Committee (No. 2/I/2013).

Drugs and chemicals

Insulin (Insuman Basal-Aventis) was administered as a subcutaneous injection. Pioglitazone (Dr. Reddy's, India) was administered as a suspension in freshly prepared in 0.5% w/v carboxymethyl cellulose. Synbiotic, a combination of probiotic (*Bifidobacterium bifidum* 231) was procured from Department of Livestock Products Technology, College of Veterinary Science, Hyderabad, India, and prebiotic (fructo oligosaccharide [FOS]) from Xena Bioherbals, India were administered in normal saline.

Animals

A total of 36 male Sprague-Dawley rats were procured from the National Centre for Laboratory Animal Sciences, National Institute of Nutrition, Hyderabad, India. The rats were equally divided into six groups and acclimatized for a period of 2-week. Streptozotocin (STZ) at 40 mg/kg body weight was administered intraperitoneally to induce diabetes in five groups. A control group was administered with the normal saline. Blood samples were collected after 72 h and serum was separated to estimate serum glucose level. Rats with blood glucose value of >200 mg/dl were included in the study.

Experimental design

All the rats in groups were maintained as per the following treatment schedule for 8 weeks. Group 1: Non-diabetic control; Group 2: STZ (40 mg/kg i/p single dose)-induced diabetic control; Group 3: Insulin (4 U/kg once daily for 8 weeks) treatment in diabetic rats; Group 4: Insulin + synbiotic treatment (combination of *B. bifidum* 231 at 1.4×10^{11} CFU/rat/day intragastrically twice daily and FOS at 0.8 g/rat/day once daily for 8 weeks) in diabetic rats; Group 5: Insulin + pioglitazone (10 mg/kg once daily for 8 weeks) treatment in diabetic rats; and Group 6: Insulin + pioglitazone + synbiotic treatment in diabetic rats. The doses were selected based on in-house experimental data and literature search.

Blood and tissue collection

Blood was collected once in 2 weeks into serum vacutainers through retro-orbital plexus. The serum was separated and stored at $-20°C$ and tested for estimation of glucose (fortnightly), and total cholesterol (TC), triglycerides (TGs), and high-density lipoprotein cholesterol (HDL-C) concentration by using kits (Sigma Diagnostics Pvt. Ltd., India) at the end of the 4th and 8th week. Body weights of all groups were recorded at fortnight intervals. At the end of the study, six rats from each group were sacrificed and kidneys were collected, snap frozen and stored at $-20°C$ for further estimation of reduced glutathione (GSH) [7], GSH peroxidase (GPx) [8], thiobarbituric acid reacting substances (TBARS) [9], and protein carbonyls [10] in kidney homogenates.

Statistical analysis

The data were analyzed by one-way ANOVA using statistical package for social sciences (SPSS; version 16.0). Differences between means were tested using Duncan's multiple comparison tests and a significance was set at $p < 0.05$.

Results

The mean body weight in diabetic control Group 2 was significantly ($p < 0.05$) lower as compared to all the other groups on day 30 and 60. The body weights in the Groups 3-6 were significantly ($p < 0.05$) higher as compared to Group 2 at the end of day 30 and 60. The Groups 5 and 6 showed a significant ($p < 0.05$) increase in the body weights among all the treated groups at the end of the 60th day (Table-1). The serum glucose concentration (mg/dl) in the Group 1 was significantly ($p < 0.05$) lower, whereas Group 2 showed significantly ($p < 0.05$) higher concentration as compared to other groups throughout the experiment. All the treated Groups (3-6) showed significant ($p < 0.05$) decrease in glucose concentration on day 30 and 60 as compared to Group 2; the decrease was the highest in Groups 5 and 6 (Table-1).

The concentration of TC and TG (mg/dl) in Group 2 was significantly ($p < 0.05$) higher on day 30 and 60, as compared to Group 1. The values of the above variables in the treatment Groups (3-6), were significantly ($p < 0.05$) reduced at the end of the 60th day as compared to Group 2. The HDL-C concentration (mg/dl) was significantly ($p < 0.05$) lower in Group 2 as compared to Group 1 on day 30 and 60, while the treatment Groups 3, 4, 5 and 6 showed significant ($p < 0.05$) increase in HDL-C (Table-2).

The parameters of oxidant-antioxidant status in kidney revealed significant ($p < 0.05$) increase in the activity of GPx, and the concentration of TBARS and protein carbonyls, while the concentration of GSH was significantly ($p < 0.05$) lowered in Group 2. The values of these parameters revealed an improvement in the treatment Groups 3, 4, 5 and 6 at the end of the 60th day (Table-3).

Discussion

The cytotoxic action of STZ is mediated by the formation of free radicals such as superoxide and hydroxyl radicals that can cause rapid destruction of β-cells of the pancreas, resulting in partial or complete loss of insulin production, thereby resulting in the development of hyperglycemia and its complications, if untreated [11]. Body weights were significantly decreased in diabetic control may be due to catabolic processes involved in DM.

Thiazolidinediones like pioglitazone binds to PPARγ receptor promotes glucose uptake by increasing expression of insulin receptor substrate-2 and

Table-1: Body weight (g) and serum glucose concentration (mg/dl) in different groups of rats.

Groups (G)	Body weight (g)		Serum glucose (mg/dl)	
	30th day	60th day	30th day	60th day
G 1	347.17±8.73d	406.83±6.31e	80.67±2.21a	83.17±1.83a
G 2	235.17±6.65a	203.33±4.14a	299.00±1.06d	312.17±5.75e
G 3	302.83±9.77b	330.67±10.36b	241.50±3.93c	211.17±3.19d
G 4	307.17±7.21bc	332.50±7.83b	240.50±2.78c	200.70±3.97cd
G 5	313.33±3.02bc	351.17±3.89c	238.17±3.51bc	191.17±6.30c
G 6	326.33±5.13c	381.00±3.15d	229.33±5.87b	165.50±3.13b

Values are mean±SE (n=6); Duncan's multiple comparison test, means with different alphabets as superscripts differ significantly (p<0.05). SE=Standard error

Table-2: Serum lipid profile in different groups of rats.

Groups (G)	TC (mg/dl)		TGs (mg/dl)		HDL-C (mg/dl)	
	30th day	60th day	30th day	60th day	30th day	60th day
G 1	135.29±1.00a	138.29±1.00a	77.10±0.27a	76.03±0.66a	55.33±0.22f	57.69±0.49f
G 2	280.95±1.35e	309.53±1.31f	113.75±0.30e	123.56±0.30e	41.23±0.86a	42.01±0.94a
G 3	159.43±2.14d	151.81±0.70e	94.34±0.57d	89.70±0.27d	43.36±0.44b	45.11±0.49b
G 4	153.80±1.29c	147.17±0.47d	90.03±0.28c	86.31±0.60c	45.36±0.32c	47.16±0.43c
G 5	154.34±1.39c	143.29±1.03c	82.38±0.64b	81.14±0.77b	47.02±0.47d	49.89±0.45d
G 6	149.44±0.65b	139.17±1.35b	83.34±0.94b	77.01±0.46a	48.92±0.24e	54.34±0.76e

Values are mean±SE (n=6); Duncan's multiple comparison test, means with different alphabets as superscripts differ significantly (p<0.05). SE=Standard error, TC=Total cholesterol, TG=Triglycerides, HDL-C=High density lipoprotein cholesterol

Table-3: Anti-oxidant profile in kidney homogenates in different groups of rats.

Groups (G)	GPx (U/mg protein)	TBARS (nmol of MDA/mg protein)	Protein carbonyls (nmol carbonyls/mg protein)	GSH (nmol/mg protein)
	60th day	60th day	60th day	60th day
G 1	0.61±0.02a	3.53±0.06a	2.42±0.07a	30.51±0.24f
G 2	1.26±0.03f	8.59±0.09f	6.34±0.11f	15.05±0.31a
G 3	1.06±0.02e	6.16±0.05e	3.58±0.06e	23.30±0.39b
G 4	0.92±0.02d	4.91±0.05d	3.49±0.03cd	24.80±0.45c
G 5	0.85±0.02c	4.61±0.05c	3.31±0.06bc	26.52±0.38d
G 6	0.74±0.02b	4.37±0.06b	3.23±0.03b	27.64±0.26e

Values are mean±SE (n=6); Duncan's multiple comparison test, means with different alphabets as superscripts differ significantly (p<0.05). SE=Standard error, GPx=Glutathione peroxidase, TBARS=Thiobarbituric acid reacting substances, GSH=Glutathione

glucose transporter 4 protein in insulin sensitive tissues *viz.* adipose tissue, muscle and liver, results decrease in postprandial and fasting plasma glucose levels [12]. Pioglitazone increase body weight through *in vivo* up-regulation of genes including phosphoenolpyruvate carboxykinase, glycerol-3-phosphate dehydrogenase, and acetyl-CoA synthetase facilitating adipocyte lipid storage pathways [13].

Treatment with synbiotic reduce elevated blood glucose levels may be by stimulation of peripheral tissues glucose uptake, alteration of insulin metabolism and inhibition of glucose reabsorption by the kidneys, resulting in the elimination of glucose in the urine as reported by Roselino *et al.* [14]. Treatment with a combination of insulin, pioglitazone and synbiotic improved the body weights, and significantly lowered serum glucose concentration compared to other treated groups.

Rise in plasma TG and TC, and fall in HDL-C in diabetic animals is due to increased lipolysis in adipose tissue, and decreased the activity of insulin-dependent lipoprotein lipase leading to elevated blood levels of fatty acids, which are available for the synthesis of TG. Pioglitazone enhances lipoprotein lipase activity and insulin sensitivity by increasing the expression and differentiation of adiponectin resulting in reduced TG levels and increased serum HDL-C levels [15, 16]. This may provide another explanation for the improvement in insulin sensitivity despite weight gain by pioglitazone.

Synbiotics improves lipid profile in diabetic animals by producing SCFA, carbon disulfide and methyl acetate and can increase the lipolytic activity [17]. Based on previous *in vitro* and *in vivo* trials, probiotics accounted for serum cholesterol reduction by improving lipid profiles. Probiotics controls cholesterol metabolism by several ways: (1) They removes cholesterol by assimilation in the small intestine, (2) probiotics reduces absorption of cholesterol in the intestine which in turn reduces the serum cholesterol, and (3) probiotics incorporates the cholesterol into cell membranes. The current study results are in consistent with Liong *et al.* [18], stated that intake of synbiotic for 8 weeks resulted in a decreased serum TG, TC levels and increased HDL-C concentrations in hypercholesterolemic pigs. In Group 6, the administration of insulin, pioglitazone and synbiotic revealed a significant alteration in lipid profile to normal.

In the diabetic control group, the GPx activity, and the TBARS and protein carbonyls levels were significantly increased with a significant decrease in GSH level. These findings indicate ongoing free radical-induced oxidative damage in the living system by autoxidative glycosylation, hence depriving the antioxidant defenses. The antioxidant activity of pioglitazone is reported to be mediated by blocking the vicious cycle of reactive oxygen species production, enhancing the insulin sensitivity and arrest the proinflammatory signaling transduction [19, 20]. The probiotic *B. bifidum* present in synbiotic has defense mechanisms, exerts by modulating the mucosal immune system by blocking the proinflammatory cytokines, inhibit the attachment of pathogenic bacteria by producing antibacterial compounds and enhance the protective function of epithelial cells, ability to capture and make free radicals harmless and maintains homeostasis of digestive tract thereby reducing the oxidant levels and acts as antioxidants [21]. Treatment with insulin, pioglitazone and synbiotic in Group 6 resulted in the revival of antioxidant defenses toward normal, which confirms synergistic antioxidant potential of pioglitazone and synbiotic.

Conclusion

In summary, the present study demonstrated that combination of insulin, pioglitazone and synbiotic could significantly improve blood glucose concentration, improves lipid profile, and decrease oxidative stress in diabetic rats as compared to other treatments tested in this experiment, which was evident from the significant reversal of biochemical changes.

Authors' Contributions

This study is the major component of the work toward the PhD thesis of KK, under the guidance of the second author AGR. KK conducted the experiment and organized the manuscript, and AGR and KKR thoroughly revised the same. CSVSK, GB, JK assisted in housing and maintenance of rats, blood collection, organ collection, data analysis and interpretation. All authors read and approved the final manuscript.

Acknowledgments

The authors are thankful to the Associate Dean, College of Veterinary Science, Rajendranagar, Hyderabad for providing facilities and funds to carry out this experiment.

Competing Interests

The authors declare that they have no competing interests.

References

1. Wang, C., Guan, Y. and Yang, J. (2010) Cytokines in the progression of pancreatic β-cell dysfunction. *Int. J. Endocrinol.*, 2010: 1-10.

2. Shanmugam, K.R., Mallikarjuna, K. and Reddy, K.S. (2011) Effect of alcohol on blood glucose and antioxidant enzymes in the liver and kidney of diabetic rats. *Indian J. Pharmacol.*, 43: 330-335.

3. Biswas, A., Rabbani, S.I. and Devi, K. (2012) Influence of experimental heart failure and hyperlipidemia in rats. *Indian J. Pharmacol.*, 44: 333-339.

4. Pérez-Cobas, A.E., Moya, A., Gosalbes, M.J. and Latorre, A. (2015) Colonization resistance of the gut microbiota against *Clostridium difficile*. Antibiotics, 4: 337-357.

5. Canis, P.D., Possemiers, S., Van de Wiele, T., Guiot, Y., Everard, A., Rottier, O., Geurts, L., Naslain, D., Neyrinck, A. and Lambert, D.M. (2009) Changes in gut microbiota control inflammation in obese mice through a mechanism involving GLP-2-driven improvement of gut permeability. *Gut,* 58: 1091-1103.

6. Asemi, Z., Khorrami-Rad, A., Alizadeh, S.A., Shakeri, H. and Esmaillzadeh, A. (2014) Effects of synbiotic food consumption on metabolic status of diabetic patients: A double-blind randomized cross-over controlled clinical trial. *Clin. Nutr.*, 33(2): 198-203.

7. Patterson, J.W. and Lazarow, A. (1955) Determination of glutathione. *Methods Biochem. Anal.*, 2: 259-278.

8. Paglia, D.E. and Valentine, W.N. (1967) Studies on the quantitative and qualitative characterization of erythrocyte glutathione peroxidase. *J. Lab. Clin. Med.*, 70: 158-159.

9. Balasubramanian, K.A., Manohar, M. and Mathan, V.I. (1988) An unidentified inhibitor of lipid peroxidation in intestinal mucosa. *Biochem. Biophys.*, 962: 51-58.

10. Levine, R.L., Garland, D., Oliver, C.N., Amici, A., Climent, I., Lenz, A.G., Ahn, B.W., Shaltiel, S. and Stadtman, E.R. (1990) Determination of carbonyl content in oxidatively modified proteins. *Methods Enzymol.*, 186: 464-478.

11. Suthagar, E.S., Soudamani, S., Yuvaraj, S., Aruldhas, M.M. and Balasubramanian, K. (2009) Effects of streptozotocin-induced diabetes and insulin replacement on rat ventral prostate. *Biomed. Pharmacother.*, 63: 43-50.

12. Derosa, G. and Maffioli, P. (2012) Peroxisome proliferator activated receptor-γ (PPAR-γ) agonists on glycemic control, lipid profile and cardiovascular risk. *Curr. Mol. Pharmacol.*, 5: 272-281.

13. Bogacka, I., Xie, H., Bray, G.A., and Smith, S.R. (2004) The effect of pioglitazone on peroxisome proliferator-activated receptor-γ target genes related to lipid storage *in vivo. Diabetes Care*, 27: 1660-1667.

14. Roselino, M.N., Pauly-Silveira, N.D., Cavallini, D.C., Celiberto, L.S., Pinto, R.A., Vendramini, R.C. and Rossi, E.A. (2012) A potential synbiotic product improves the lipid profile of diabetic rats. *Lipids Health Dis.*, 11: 114.

15. Devesh, C., Kritika, M., Anroop, N., Kumar, S.P. and Sumeet, G. (2012) Spirulina reverses histomorphological changes in diabetic osteoporosis in pioglitazone treated rats. *J. Diabetes Metab.*, S1-006: 2-7.

16. Ozasa, H., Ayaori, M., Iizuka, M., Terao, Y., UtoKondo, H., Yakushiji, E. and Ikewaki, K. (2011) Pioglitazone enhances cholesterol efflux from macrophages by increasing ABCA1/ABCG1 expressions via PPARγ/LXRα pathway: Findings from *in vitro* and *ex vivo* studies. *Atherosclerosis*, 219: 141-150.

17. Vitali, B., Ndagijimana, M., Maccaferri, S., Biagi, E., Guerzoni, M.E. and Brigidi, P. (2012) An *in vitro* evaluation of the effect of probiotics and prebiotics on the metabolic profile of human microbiota. *Anaerobe*, 18: 386-391.

18. Liong, M.T., Dunshea, F.R. and Shah, N.P. (2007) Effects of a synbiotic containing *Lactobacillus acidophilus* ATCC

4962 on plasma lipid profiles and morphology of erythrocytes in hypercholesterolaemic pigs on high- and low-fat diets. *Br. J. Nutr.*, 98: 736-744.

19. Hsiao, P.J., Hsieh, T.J., Kuo, K.K., Hung, W.W., Tsai, K.B., Yang, C.H. and Shin, S.J. (2008) Pioglitazone retrieves hepatic antioxidant DNA repair in a mice model of high fat diet. *BMC Mol. Biol.*, 9(1): 82.

20. D'Souza, A., Fordjour, L., Ahmad, A., Cai, C., Kumar, D. and Valencia, G. (2010) Effects of probiotics, prebiotics, and synbiotics on messenger RNA expression of caveolin-1, NOS, and genes regulating oxidative stress in the terminal ileum of formula-fed neonatal rats. *Pediatr. Res.*, 67: 526-531.

21. Mandal, A., Patra, A., Mandal, S., Roy, S., Mahapatra, S.D., Mahapatra, T.D., Paul, T., Das, K., Mondal, K.C. and Nandi, D.K. (2015) Therapeutic potential of different commercially available synbiotic on acetaminophen-induced uremic rats. *Clin. Exp. Nephrol.*, 19(2): 168-177.

15

Serum muscle-derived enzymes response during show jumping competition in horse

Anna Assenza[1], Simona Marafioti[2], Fulvio Congiu[2], Claudia Giannetto[2], Francesco Fazio[2], Daniele Bruschetta[3] and Giuseppe Piccione[2]

1. Department of Cognitive Science, Education and Cultural Studies, University of Messina, Via Concezione n 6-8, 98122, Messina, Italy; 2. Department of Veterinary Sciences, University of Messina, Polo Universitario dell'Annunziata, 98168, Messina, Italy; 3. Department of Biomedical Sciences and Morpho-functional Imaging, University of Messina, Via Consolare Valeria 1, Messina, Italy.

Corresponding author: Giuseppe Piccione, e-mail: gpiccione@unime.it,
AA: aassenza@unime.it, SM: smarafioti@unime.it, FC: fcongiu@unime.it, CG: claudiagiannetto@alice.it,
FF: ffazio@unime.it, DB: daniele.bruschetta@unime.it

Abstract

Aim: The effect of two jumping competitions, performed in two consecutive weekends, on serum creatine phosphokinase (CPK), aspartate aminotransferase (AST), and lactate dehydrogenase (LDH), urea, creatinine (CREA) concentrations were evaluated in 12 healthy jumper horses.

Materials and Methods: Blood sampling was performed before the 1st day of competition (T_0), at the end of each show (J_1, J_2), on the day after the competition (T_1); the same sampling plan was followed during the second weekend (J_3, J_4 and T_2).

Results: One-way repeated measures analysis of variance showed an increase in CPK at J_1 and J_2 respect to T_0 and at J_3 and J_4 respect to all other time points ($p<0.05$). LDH activity showed an increase at J_2 respect to T_0, at J_3 respect to T_0, J_1, J_2 and at J_4 respect to all other time points ($p<0.05$). AST values increased at J_1 and J_2 respect to T_0 ($p<0.05$). A significant increase of CREA was found at J_3 respect to T_0, T_1 and J_1 and at J_4 respect to all other time points ($p<0.05$). A decrease in serum urea levels was found at J_1 respect to T_0, at J_2 and J_4 respect to T_0 and T_1; at T_2 respect to T_0 ($p<0.05$). A positive correlation between urea/CPK ($p=0.0042$, $r^2=0.030$), LDH/CPK ($p<0.0001$, $r^2=0.535$), CREA/LDH ($p<0.0001$, $r^2=0.263$), CREA/CPK ($p<0.0001$, $r^2=0.496$) was observed.

Conclusion: Our results suggest that 5 days recovery period between the two consecutive competition weekends is insufficient to allow muscle recovery and avoid potential additional stress. The findings obtained in this study improve the knowledge about metabolic changes occurring in athlete horse during the competition to identify muscle alterations following show jumping competitions.

Keywords: horse, muscle enzymes, physical exercise, show jumping competition.

Introduction

The performance of athletic horse is determined by many complicated interdependent biological and physiological processes. Similarity to other stressors, including delivery, transport and environmental conditions exercise need adequate response to re-establish homeostatic equilibrium [1]. Several cardiovascular and hematological adaptations are necessary to guarantee the correct supply of oxygen to active muscles during exercise. Physiological, hematological, and biochemical changes associated with exercise have been extensively analyzed in several types of horses such as thoroughbreds [2,3] eventers [4,5], show jumpers [6-9], and endurance horses [10,11].

One of the organs affected by exercise is the muscle, which suffers microdamage due to effort employed load [12]. Many researchers have compared muscular adaptations that occur after several training programs with different exercise intensities [13,14], others have examined the combined effect of intensity and duration of the exercise [15], or assessed adequate recovery after exercise.

Repeated workload leads the muscular apparatus to constant damage that can be assessed by laboratorial determination of some serum constituent such as urea and creatinine (CREA) and enzymes such as creatine phosphokinase (CPK), aspartate aminotransferase (AST), and lactate dehydrogenase (LDH) [16]. The activity of these enzymes has been studied by several researchers before and after exercise and can be used to detect muscle diseases [17], characterization of exercise intensity [11,18] and predicting possible complications that can arise from the exercise [19]. Despite the existing literature describing muscular adaptations to training in horses, little is still known about the durations and intensities of exercise that promote optimal response in skeletal muscles [20]. Considering the metabolic and clinical role of serum parameters above mentioned and considering the effect of physical exercise on them, studying changes in these muscle damage markers after exercise has become more important [21].

Therefore, the objective of this study was to evaluate the serum concentration of urea, CREA and the serum activities of CPK, AST and LDH of jumper horses before and after jumping competition.

Materials and Methods

Ethical approval

Protocols of animal husbandry and experimentation were reviewed and approved in accordance with the standards recommended by the Guide for the Care and Use of Laboratory Animals and Directive 2010/63/EU for animal experiments.

Animals

The study was carried out on 12 healthy and regularly trained Italian Saddle horses (7 geldings and 5 females, 9-12-year-old, mean body weight 500±20 kg). All horses were managed equally, housed in individual boxes under natural photoperiod (mean temperature 25±6°C, relative humidity 67±3%). The horses were fed standard rations, calculated to fulfill all the nutritional requirements according to National Institute of Agronomic Research specifications [22] constituted hay (first cut meadow hay, sun cured, late cut, and a mixture of cereals) oats and barley, 50% each.

The percentage composition of the mixture was dry matter 87% and moisture 13%. The dry matter contained 9.11% digestible protein, 13.05% crude protein, 20.7% crude fiber, and 3.42% crude lipid, as well as 0.80 Unitè Fouragire Cheval/kg. The ration was administered 3 times a day: 8:00 AM, 12:00 PM and 5:00 PM. Water was available *ad libitum*.

Show jumping course

Horses took part in jumping competitions held in two consecutive courses at distance of 5 days. Each completion session was preceded by 20 min warm-up consisting of walk, trot and gallop with six jumps (height: From 100 to 140 cm). During the 1st day of both weekends, horses competed with the following technical specifications: Total length - 550 m; obstacles height - 140 cm; total efforts 13 (7 verticals, 6 oxers, 1 triple combination). During the 2nd day of both weekend competitions, horses competed with the following technical specifications: Total length - 600 m; obstacles height - 145 cm; and mixed competition including efforts 15 (8 verticals, 7 oxers, 1 double combination, 1 triple combination).

All horses during the week between both competitions performed the following daily training schedule warm-up (10 min walk, 20 min trot, 10 min gallop) and show jumping course with 7 fences of 80±10 cm average height.

Blood sampling and analysis

Blood samples were collected by jugular venipuncture in vacutainer tubes with cloth activator for serum analyses (Terumo Co., Tokyo, Japan). Blood sampling was performed before the 1st day of competition (T_0), within 10 min from the end of each competition (J_1, J_2) and on the day after competition (T_1), same plan was followed during second weekend (J_3, J_4, and T_2). Immediately after collection, blood samples were placed in refrigerated bags and transported to the laboratory for the analysis. Tubes were centrifuged at 3000 rpm for 10 min and on obtained sera the concentration of CPK, LDH, AST, urea, CREA were determined by commercial available kit by means of an automated analyzer, Model 7070 (Hitachi Ltd., Tokyo).

The same operator assayed all samples in duplicate each time. Samples exhibited parallel displacement to the standard curve; the intra-assay and the inter-assay coefficients of variation were <7% and <9%, respectively, for all measured parameters.

Statistical analysis

The obtained data are expressed as mean ± standard deviation (SD) of the mean. Data were normally distributed (p>0.05, Kolmogorov–Smirnov test). One-way repeated measures analysis of variance (ANOVA) was applied to determine the statistically significant effect of exercise on all parameters. p<0.05 were considered statistically significant. Bonferroni's multiple comparison tests were applied for *post-hoc* comparison. A simple linear regression model was applied to evaluate the correlation between the studied parameters. A statistical analysis was performed using Stats package of R Core Team (2013) (R: A language and environment for statistical computing. R Foundation for Statistical Computing, Vienna, Austria. ISBN 3-900051-07-0, 2013, URL: http://www.R-project. org/).

Results

ANOVA showed an increase in CPK at J_1 and J_2 respect to T_0 and at J_3 and J_4 respect to all other time points. LDH activity showed an increase at J_2 respect to T_0, at J_3 respect to T_0, J_1, J_2 and at J_4 respect to all other time points. AST values increased at J_1 and J_2 respect to T_0. A significant increase of CREA was found at J_3 respect to T_0, T_1 and J_1 and at J_4 respect to all other time points. A decrease in serum urea levels was found at J_1 respect to T_0, at J_2 and J_4 respect to T_0 and T_1; at T_2 respect to T_0.

A positive correlation between CREA/LDH (p<0.0001, r^2=0.263), CREA/CPK (p<0.0001, r^2=0.496) urea/CPK (p=0.0042, r^2=0.030), LDH/CPK (p<0.0001, r^2=0.535), was observed (Figure-1).

Discussion

The obtained results showed that hematochemical modifications occur after exercise in jumper horses. With regard to the muscle enzymes, an increase

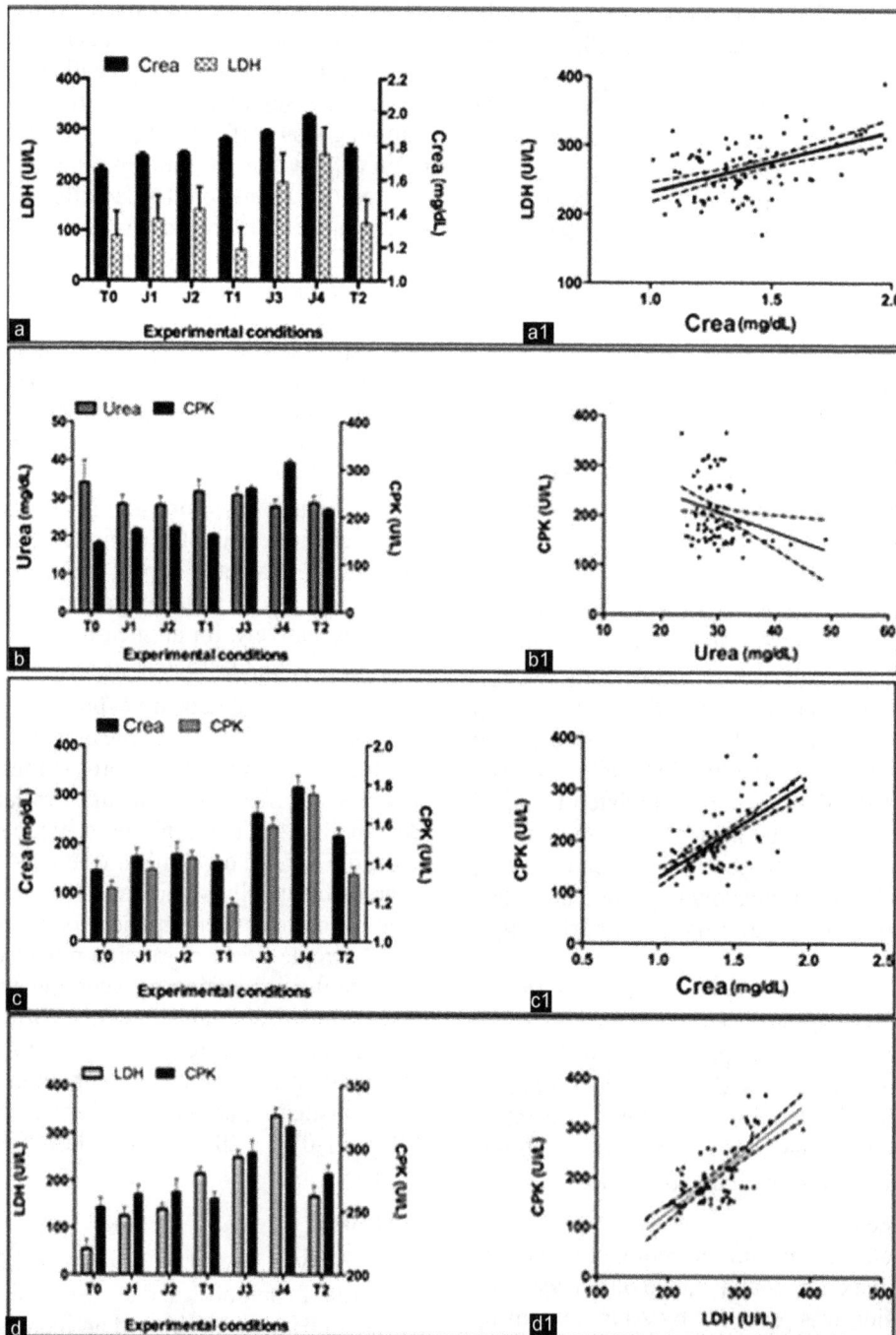

Figure-1: (a) Pattern of serum creatinine (CREA) and lactic dehydrogenase (LDH) observed during experimental period; (a1) Graphical representation of simple linear regression of LDH vs. CREA; (b) Pattern of CREA and creatine phosphokinase (CPK) observed during experimental period; (b1) Graphical representation of simple linear regression of CPK versus CREA, (c) Pattern of serum urea and CPK observed during experimental period; (c1) Graphical representation of simple linear regression of CPK versus urea; (d) Pattern of LDH and CPK observed during experimental period; (d1) graphical representation of simple linear regression of CPK versus LDH.

in the post-exercise activities of CPK, AST and LDH was fond compared to baseline values measured at T_0. According to our results, increase in serum CPK, AST, and LDH activities have been seen in response to exercise [23]. These increases are believed to relate either to overt damage or to a change in the muscle fiber membrane causing a transient increase in permeability [24]. However, physiological increases have been also shown to occur without any tissue

alteration [25]. The effects of physical effort on serum enzymatic activity may depend on the level of performance of the animal, and the intensity and duration of exercise [26].

A significant increase of CPK was observed after the competitions. The post-exercise increase of CPK levels could be attributed to the muscle metabolism and to the increasing energy requirements occurring during physical exercise [27]. It is well stated that the tissue CPK activity may augment energetic capacity and improve myofibril contraction responses through enhancing vascular tone and vasoconstrictor reserves [27]. At T_1, it showed slightly, but no significant decrease respect to J_1 and J_2, although remained highest, but no significantly, respect to T_0. This probably because blood sampling at T_1 occurred 24 h after the first weekend of competition and this is an insufficient time to determine a return to normal serum concentration. During the second weekend of competition, CPK assumed higher levels respect to the previous week and reached its peak levels in J_4. Its values remained significantly higher at T_2 respect to T_0 assuming that the shorter recovery period to the first competition (only 4 days) associated with another rise post-exercise, could increase the probability of muscle damage. CPK has relatively shorter half-life of 2 h [28]. Therefore, will become elevated sooner and return to normal range after an episode of muscle strain, unless the effort is so high as to delay its return to the baseline levels. For this reason, it is preferred to evaluate muscle enzyme for diagnosing and monitoring muscle recovery and considered a reliable marker of skeletal muscle injury [28]. LDH activity showed a significant increase at J_2 respect to T_0, probably due both to the increased effort respect to J_1 and to the increase of enzyme activity after 24 h post exercise (T_1). LDH have a longer half-life respect to CPK, in fact, it peaks 24 h after effort and could remain high for 48 h after exercise [11]. Therefore, since blood sampling at T_1 occurred 24 h after the last jumping round of the 1st week of completion, return to baseline levels could not be determined. Our study showed a greater increase in the levels of this enzyme at J_3 and J_4 revealing, as well as in CPK activity, a reduced capacity to recovery by effort probably due to the horses have performed competitions in two consecutive weekend.

AST activities may increase during exercise without observation of clinical signs or histological detection of changes in muscle cell structure [29]. In our study, AST values increased immediately after exercise, whereas they decreased at T_1 reaching levels measured at T_0.

In this study, a slightly but significant increase of CREA was found in J_3 and J_4. CREA is produced from the decomposition of creatine, a nitrogen compound used by muscle cells to store energy. The serum concentration of CREA varies according to creatine synthesis and the amount of muscle mass and exercise as reported by Nogueira et al. [30] in thoroughbred.

During the exercise phases and the recovery period, all animals showed a decrease in serum Urea levels respect to T_0. Urea is filtered by the glomerular capillaries, and it enters the renal tubule. Approximately half of urea is reabsorbed passively by diffusion, but the remainder is excreted in the urine. Lower urea levels suggest an increased glomerular filtration and an excretion in the urine or a diminished reabsorption in the tubules.

On the basis of our results, we can affirm that the higher levels of CPK and LDH in J_2 and J_4 (increased effort) respect to J_1 and J_3 confirmed that the effects of physical effort on serum activities of muscle enzymes is strictly linked with intensity and duration of exercise; the increased levels of CPK and LDH occurred during the second weekend of competition (J_3 and J_4) respect to the first, seem to indicate that the two jumping session were temporally too close and did not allow the horse adequate recovery.

Conclusion

Our results improved the knowledge about metabolic changes occurring in athlete horse during competition and underline that the physiological activity of enzymes, if not associated with the adequate recovery period, can increase the probability of muscle damage.

Authors' Contributions

AA and GP designed the study and supervised the research as major advisor. SM, FC and FF worked and collaborated in the lab work and compilation of the results as well as the manuscript. GC and DB provided valuable suggestions regarding the design of the experiment and analysis of the data collected during research. All authors read and approved the final manuscript.

Acknowledgments

The work presented in this manuscript was supported by the Department of Veterinary Science - University of Messina, Italy. The authors are thankful to all staff of the Equine Horse Center "La Pineta"- Italy.

Competing Interests

The authors declare that they have no competing interests.

References

1. Piccione, G., Rizzo, M., Arfuso, F., Giannetto, C., Di Pietro, S., Bazzano, M. and Quartuccio, M. (2015) Leukocyte modifications during the first month after foaling in mares and their newborn foals. *Polish J. Vet. Sci.*, 18(3): 621-625.

2. Fazio, F., Assenza, A., Tosto, F., Casella, S., Piccione, G. and Caola, G. (2011) Training and haematochemical profile in thoroughbreds and standard breds: A longitudinal study. *Livest. Sci.*, 141: 221-226.

3. Mukai, K., Takahashi, T., Eto, D., Ohmura, H., Tsubone, H. and Hiraga, A. (2007) Heart rates and blood lactate response in thoroughbreds horses during a race. *J. Equine Sci.*, 18: 153-160.

4. Muñoz, A., Riber, C., Santisteban, R., Rubio, M.D., Agüera, E.I. and Casteión, F.M. (1999) Cardiovascular and metabolic adaptations in horses competing in cross-country events. *J. Vet. Med. Sci.*, 69:13-20.

5. White, S.L. (1998) Fluid, electrolyte, and acid-base balances in three-day, combined-training horses. *Vet. Clin. North Am. Equine Pract.*, 14: 137-145.

6.   Assenza, A., Bergero, D., Congiu, F., Tosto, F., Giannetto, C. and Piccione, G. (2014) Evaluation of serum electrolytes and blood lactate concentration during repeated maximal exercise in horse. *J. Equine Vet. Sci.,* 34: 1175-1180.

7.   Piccione, G., Giannetto, C., Assenza, A., Fazio, F. and Caola, G. (2007) Serum electrolyte and protein modification during different workload in jumper horse. *Comp. Clin. Path.,* 16: 103-107.

8.   Piccione, G., Casella, S., Giannetto, C., Messina, V., Niutta, P.P. and Giudice, E. (2011) Effect of hydrocortisone on platelet aggregation in jumper horses. *Vet. Arch.,* 81: 153-162.

9.   Fazio, F., Casella, S., Assenza, A., Arfuso, F., Tosto, F. and Piccione, G. (2014) Blood biochemical changes in show jumpers during a simulated show jumping test. *Vet. Arch.,* 84: 143-152.

10. Muñoz, A., Cuesta, I., Riber, C., Gata, J., Trigo, P. and Castejon, F.M. (2006) Trot asymmetry in relation to physical performance and metabolism in equine endurance rides. *Equine Vet. J.,* 36: 50-54.

11. Teixeira-Neto, A.R., Ferraz, G.C., Moscardini, A.R.C., Balsamão, G.M., Souza, J.C.F. and Queiroz-Neto, A. (2008) Alterations in muscular enzymes of horses competing long-distance endurance rides under tropical climate. *Arq. Bras. Med. Vet. Zootec.,* 60: 543-549.

12. Brioschi Soares, O.A., de Freitas D'angelis, F.H., Feringer Jr, W.H., Bacciotti Nard, I.K., Trigo, P., Queiroz de Almeida, F., Tavares Miranda, A.C., Queiroz-Neto, A. and de Camargo Ferraz, G. (2013) Serum activity of creatine kinase and aminotransferase aspartate enzymes of horses submitted to muscle biopsy and incremental jump test. *Rev. Bras. Saúde Prod. Anim.,* 14: 299-307.

13. Eaton, M.D., Hodgson, D.R., Evans, D.L. and Rose, R.J. (1999) Effects of low- and moderate-intensity training on metabolic responses to exercise in thoroughbreds. *Equine Vet. J. Suppl.,* 30: 521-527.

14. Sinha, A.K., Ray, S.P. and Rose, R.J. (1993) Effect of constant load training on skeletal muscle histochemistry of thoroughbred horses. *Res. Vet. Sci.,* 54: 147-159.

15. Gansen, S., Lindner, A., Marx, S., Mosen, H. and Sallmann, H.P. (1999) Effects of conditioning horses with lactate-guided exercise on muscle glycogen content. *Equine Vet. J. Suppl.,* 30: 329-331.

16. Overgaard, K., Fredsted, A., Hyldal, A., Gissel, H. and Clausen, T. (2004) Effects of running distance and training on Ca^{2+} content and damage in human muscle. *Med. Sci. Sports Exerc.,* 36: 821-829.

17. Boffi, F.M., editor. (2007) Pathologies affecting the athletic performance. Muscle disorders. In: Equine Exercise Physiology. Blockwell, Buenos Aires. p145-151.

18. Ferraz, G.C., Soares, O.A.B., Foz, N.S.B., Pereira, M.C. and Queiroz-Neto, A. (2010) The workload and plasma ion concentration in a training match session of high-goal (elite) polo ponies. *Equine Vet. J.,* 42: 191-195.

19. Trigo, P., Castejon, F., Riber, C. and Muñoz, A. (2010) Use of biochemical parameters to predict metabolic elimination in endurance rides. *Equine Vet. J. Suppl.,* 38: 142-146.

20. Rivero, J.L.L., Ruz, A., Martí-Korff, S., Estepa, J.C., Aguilera-Tejero, E., Werkman, J., Sobotta, M. and Lindner, A. (2007) Effects of intensity and duration of exercise on muscular responses to training of thoroughbred racehorses. *J. Appl. Physiol.,* 102: 1871-1882.

21. Amir-Shaqaqi, M. (2006) Effects of a Period of Selected Plyometric Exercises on LDH, CK, and UREA Levels in Elite Female Soccer Players. Master's Thesis, Central Tehran Branch of IAU.

22. Martin-Rosset, W. (1990) Horse nutrition. INRA Editions. Versailles, France. p232.

23. Harris, P.A. (1998) Musculoskeletal disease. In: Reed, S.M., Bayly, W.M., editors. Equine Internal Medicine. Saunders, Philadelphia. p375-397.

24. Anderson, M.G. (1975) The influence of exercise on serum enzyme levels in the horse. *Equine Vet. J.,* 7: 160-165.

25. Valberg, S., Johnson, L., Lindholm, A. and Holmgren, N. (1993) Muscle histopathology and plasma aspartate aminotransferase, creatine kinase and myoglobin changes with exercise in horses with recurrent exertional rhabdomyolysis. *Equine Vet. J.,* 25: 11-16.

26. Bogdanis, G.C. (2012) Effects of physical activity and inactivity on muscle fatigue. *Front. Physiol.,* 3: 142.

27. Brewster, L.M., Mairuhu, G., Bindraban, N.R., Koopmans, R.P., Clark, J.F. and Van Montfrans, G.A. (2006) Creatine kinase activity is associated with blood pressure. *Circulation,* 114: 2034-2039.

28. Octura, J.E.R., Lee, K.J., Cho, H.W., Vega, R.S.A., Choi, J.Y., Park, J.W., Shin, T.S., Cho, S.K., Kim, B.W. and Cho, B.W. (2014) Elevation of blood creatine kinase and selected blood parameters after exercise in thoroughbred racehorses (*Equus caballus* L.). *J. Res. Agric. Anim. Sci.,* 2: 7-13.

29. Câmara, E., Silva, I.A., Dias, R.V.C. and Soto-Blanco, B. (2007) Determination of serum activities of creatine kinase, lactate dehydrogenase, and aspartate aminotransferase in horses of different activities classes. *Arq. Bras. Med. Vet. Zootec.,* 59: 250-252.

30. Nogueira, G.P., Barnabe, R.C., Bedran-De-Castro, J.C., Moreira, A.F., Fernandes, W.R., Mirandola, R.M.S. and Howard, D.L. (2002) Serum cortisol, lactate and creatinine concentrations in Thoroughbred fillies of different ages and states of training. *Braz. J. Vet. Res. Anim. Sci.,* 39: 54-57.

16

Economic effects of foot and mouth disease outbreaks along the cattle marketing chain in Uganda

Sylvia Angubua Baluka

Department of Biosecurity, Ecosystem & Veterinary Public Health, College of Veterinary Medicine, Animal Resources & Biosecurity, Makerere University, Kampala, Uganda.
Corresponding author: Sylvia Angubua Baluka, e-mail: sbaluka3@gmail.com

Abstract

Aim: Disease outbreaks increase the cost of animal production; reduce milk and beef yield, cattle sales, farmers' incomes, and enterprise profitability. The study assessed the economic effects of foot and mouth disease (FMD) outbreaks along the cattle marketing chain in selected study districts in Uganda.

Materials and Methods: The study combined qualitative and quantitative study designs. Respondents were selected proportionally using simple random sampling from the sampling frame comprising of 224, 173, 291, and 185 farmers for Nakasongola, Nakaseke, Isingiro, and Rakai, respectively. Key informants were selected purposively. Data analysis combined descriptive, modeling, and regression analysis. Data on the socio-economic characteristics and how they influenced FMD outbreaks, cattle markets revenue losses, and the economic cost of the outbreaks were analyzed using descriptive measures including percentages, means, and frequencies.

Results: Farmers with small and medium herds incurred higher control costs, whereas large herds experienced the highest milk losses. Total income earned by the actors per month at the processing level reduced by 23%. In Isingiro, bulls and cows were salvage sold at 83% and 88% less market value, i.e., a loss of $196.1 and $1,552.9 in small and medium herds, respectively.

Conclusion: All actors along the cattle marketing chain incur losses during FMD outbreaks, but smallholder farmers are most affected. Control and prevention of FMD should remain the responsibility of the government if Uganda is to achieve a disease-free status that is a prerequisite for free movement and operation of cattle markets throughout the year which will boost cattle marketing.

Keywords: chain, cost, economics, financial losses, market, outbreak.

Introduction

Uganda's well-being is inextricably tied to livestock with 70% of households owning cattle, goats, sheep, pigs, or chicken. About 22% and 60% of households nationally and in the cattle corridor, respectively, derive their livelihood from livestock [1,2]. Animal diseases are a major constraint to livestock production and trade in Uganda [3]. The presence of infectious diseases such as foot and mouth disease (FMD) limits Uganda's ability to access major export markets, and her performance in the global export trade in livestock and livestock products is negligible due to FMD [4]. Frequent FMD outbreaks and subsequent bans on cattle and cattle products movement to and from the affected areas during quarantine period cripples cattle marketing [3,5]. Furthermore, livestock diseases impose heavy costs on farmers and reduce incentives to invest in higher yielding cross breeds or exotic animals that are more susceptible to tropical diseases [2].

FMD causes serious production losses, is highly contagious, transmitted through multiple routes and hosts which makes it one of the most important diseases affecting trade in livestock [6-8]. Animal diseases affect the amount as well as the timing and certainty of income from livestock enterprises and undermine the livestock sector potential, compromise food security, affect livelihoods by reducing milk yield and body weight while increasing losses due to disease control costs and mortalities [9-11]. These diseases reduce the level of sales for cattle and cattle products [12], perceived or actual output quality, input utilization efficiency [13], necessitate international trade restrictions thus reducing the benefits derived by mankind from livestock farming [14,15], and cause losses of up to 30% of the annual livestock output in developing countries [16].

Despite 75% of the world's cattle living in low- and middle-income countries, livestock product exports from these countries account for less than 15% of the global value [17] with exception of Brazil that is ranked among the largest beef producers and exporters globally [18]. This paradox is partly explained by the presence of transboundary animal diseases (TADs) such as FMD that restrict livestock trade [9,19] and often precede uncontrolled livestock movements typical of grazing systems in these countries [20,21].

Controlling production costs are important in modern livestock farming. Improving animal health and fertility can play a major role in achieving efficient and economically rewarding production [22,23]. Policy makers and livestock industry stakeholders need means of assessing a disease's economic impacts when evaluating prevention and mitigation measures [24]. This study assessed the economic costs incurred by the various actors along the cattle marketing chain during FMD outbreaks in selected study districts.

Materials and Methods

Ethical approval

The research proposal and data collection instruments that led to this manuscript were vetted and approved by the College of Veterinary Medicine, Animal Resources and Biosecurity, Makerere University Research Ethics Committee.

Study design

The study combined qualitative and quantitative study designs. Desk review of disease outbreak reports in Ministry of Agriculture Animal Industry and Fisheries archives was done. The study was phased into reconnaissance visit that involved site selection and participatory discussions, semi-structured interviews with key stakeholders (extension staff, policy makers, and local leaders), survey using a structured questionnaire and case studies. The qualitative design employed focus group discussions (FGDs) and key informant interviews (KIs).

The study population, study design, and sample size determination

Livestock markets from the sub-counties most affected by the previous FMD outbreaks were identified, and they provided a nucleus for selecting study sites. Two livestock markets per district were selected for the study, which involved three stratified populations: Farmers, livestock traders/transporters, and processors. The herd was the unit of study at the farmers' level, and it was most appropriate given the epidemiology and morbidity of FMD within infected herds.

The catchment areas (parishes) that supplied livestock to the selected livestock markets were identified, and sampling frames were constructed to include farmers from all the listed parishes with the help of extension veterinarians and farmers' association leaders. Sample sizes from each stratum were obtained using proportional sampling. The sampling frames comprised 224, 173, 291, and 185 farmers for Nakasongola, Nakaseke, Isingiro, and Rakai districts, respectively. The study farms from each district were selected from the sampling frame using simple random sampling. Veterinary extension staff, local leaders, and farmers for the KIs and FGDs were selected purposively. Traders were considered as an aggregate rather than by district since they operate in several districts and a total of 45 cattle traders were interviewed.

FMD case studies were done in 17 herds that had experienced FMD outbreaks in Mbaare, Isingiro; 3, 9,

and 5 herds were selected to represent small, medium, and large herds. Small, medium, and large herds refer to herd sizes of 10-50, 51-150, and 151-350 heads of cattle, respectively.

The main questions asked during FGDs

The main questions asked during FGDs with cattle farmers addressed the major livelihood activities, type of cattle production system used, cattle marketing channels and mode of transport used, and impact of FMD on cattle prices and household incomes.

The main questions asked during the FGDs with cattle traders included the following: How often do you buy cattle for sale? Where do you buy cattle from and where do you resale them? Where do you obtain information on markets and cattle prices from? Have you ever sold cattle outside Uganda's borders, i.e., to other neighboring countries? At what price did you buy/sell cattle before, during and after the FMD outbreak? How many cattle did you buy/sell before, during, and after the FMD outbreak? Were you able to get alternative suppliers of cattle during FMD outbreak? Which extra costs did you incur during the FMD outbreak?

The main questions asked during the FGDs with cattle processors included; how often do you buy/ slaughter cattle? Where do you normally buy your slaughter cattle from? How many people do you employ in your cattle slaughter/butchery business? Where do you obtain information on cattle markets and prices from? How do you transport your purchased cattle from the cattle markets to the holding farm/slaughter place? How was your cattle slaughter business affected during the last FMD outbreak?

The main questions asked during the key KIs with Veterinary Extension staff at the districts, i.e. DVOs included how long they had served in the current employment in the study district, the major constraints/challenges affecting livestock farming in the district, whether they had experienced outbreaks in their district in the period under study.

The main questions asked during the KIs with policy makers and regulators from the ministry included; the laws and regulations regarding prevention and control of TADs, number of outbreaks and cases reported in the area in the period under study, policies, and institutional arrangements for control of FMD.

Structured questionnaire interviews

Structured questionnaire interviewing was the most appropriate technique for gathering data to quantify the economic effects of FMD at the production and marketing levels because it gives the researcher control over the process, achieves high response rates, and ensures complete information.

The main questions asked during the structured questionnaire interviews with farmers

The farmers' structured questionnaire survey captured information on household demographics such as sex, age, education level, and experience in years in livestock rearing for the household head, reasons for keeping cattle, household assets and income sources, land ownership tenure or user rights, sources of market information, major channels used for selling cattle, major mode of transportation of cattle to the market, major channels for sales and purchases of cattle, source of breeding stock, vaccination schedules against FMD, husbandry practices in regards to feeding and watering, and major inputs into cattle production, costs associated with FMD control and treatment, constraints to cattle production and marketing and overall impact of FMD on farmers.

The main questions asked during the structured questionnaire interviews with cattle traders

The traders' structured questionnaire survey captured information on demographics such as sex, age, educational level, years in cattle trading business, major livelihood activity and income source, cattle commodity traded, sources, and amount of capital, scale of operations, percentage contribution of cattle trade toward their household income, number of workers employed in their cattle trading business, how much they pay the workers per month or in kind, availability of cattle holding grounds in their area of operation, mode of transportation of cattle, whether they use brokers or middlemen, quality attributes sought for when purchasing cattle, percentage of cattle purchases by different channels, constraints in livestock marketing, access to cattle marketing facilities, source of marketing information, volume of cattle sold per week, impact of FMD on cattle and beef prices during outbreaks, major opportunities and constraints in cattle trading.

The main questions asked during the structured questionnaire interviews with cattle processors/slaughter facility operators captured information on major livelihood activity, years in cattle processing business, whether they have received any specialized training in cattle processing, major income sources and percentage contribution per month, number of workers employed, how much they pay the workers in cash or kind per month, whether they belong to any association or cooperative for processors, legal status of their business, quality attributes sought for when purchasing beef, common terms of payment in their trade, constraints faced in their business, source of market information, how the FMD outbreak affected cattle and beef prices. Data on slaughter capacity, number of livestock species slaughtered in the facility, number of days the slaughter facility operates and changes in slaughter volumes during outbreaks were also captured.

Determination of market revenue earned from livestock markets

Market revenue analysis considered bad and good cattle marketing seasons. The bad season falls within the dry season when cattle move long distances

in search for pastures and water, they lose weight and are generally in poor body condition, the total cattle turnover in markets and prices are low. The good season occurs during the rainy season when cattle have enough pasture and water; they are in good body condition, total cattle turnover in markets and prices are high. The good season also includes festive seasons such as Christmas, Easter, and Eid. The total annual market revenue losses were assumed equal to total income earned from cattle during good season months + total income earned from cattle sales during the bad season months.

Where by:

Annual total income earned from cattle during good season months=number of months in a year, in which cattle were sold during good season*price levied per head of cattle*average number of cattle sold per market day. Annual total income earned from cattle during bad season months=number of months in the year, in which cattle are sold during bad season*price levied per head of cattle*average number of cattle sold per market day. Estimation of cattle market revenue losses was based on the assumption that if the outbreak lasted 14 months, the quarantine period was 6 months; 2 months fell within the good season and 4 months fell within the bad season. Moreover, if an outbreak lasted for 6 months or more then the quarantine period lasted for 1-year or longer. The cattle prices levied per head of cattle were made comparable to price values charged during 2010 by compounding the prices charged in the previous years (2006-2009) using the formula:

$$P = P_{i(1+r)}{}^n$$

Where,

P=Discounted price in previous year earlier than 2010

P_i=Price during previous year earlier than 2010

n=number of years before 2010

r=discounting rate of 7%.

The market losses in the two district categories (inland and border districts) and between districts within the same district category were estimated. The significant difference in revenue was determined using a Chi-square test. The market revenues were determined under the following scenarios:

- Revenue earned when there was no FMD outbreak
- Revenue earned during FMD outbreaks
- Income lost during FMD outbreaks.

Determination of household incomes

Household incomes were determined in a four step process:

- Identifying and listing all the major inputs into the cattle enterprises. These included farm infrastructures such as fence maintenance, hired labor, water, tick control costs, vaccination costs, treatment costs, mineral salts, and supplements.
- Obtaining the unit cost of each input and then determining the average annual household

expenditures on the various inputs into a given cattle enterprise.

- Identifying and listing all the various outputs from a given cattle enterprise. The major outputs included milk, manure (cow dung that is sold in most study districts apart from Nakasongola), and sale of live cattle.

- The last step involved quantifying how much of the outputs were produced per household per week, month and then computed the average household income earned annually from the cattle enterprise.

Gross margin analysis (GMA)

GMA was performed by a spreadsheet model developed using Microsoft Excel Version 5.0, Microsoft Corporation, USA, on households when there were no FMD outbreaks using [25] procedure. GM was taken as the gross income of an enterprise less variable costs. Total livestock income or output was taken as a sum of income from the sale of live animals, milk, and manure. Draft power was not important in the study areas and was, therefore, excluded from the analysis. GM can be represented by the equation: $GM = \sum (y_i \times py_i) - \sum (X_i \times PX_i)$

Where,

$\sum (yi \times pyi)$ = Gross income,
Y_i = Quantities of products,
Py_i = Respective prices of the products,
$\sum (X_i \times PX_i)$ = Total variable costs,
X_i = Quantities of costs,
Px_i = Respective prices of variable inputs.

Determination of economic cost of FMD outbreaks in the case study herds

The FMD economic cost comprised of the control costs (vaccination and treatment of secondary infections in affected cattle herds), losses due to weight loss, abortion, losses in milk production, reduced manure production, salvage sales during the outbreak and mortality. The economic cost of FMD outbreaks in the case study herds were calculated as follows:

Milk yield losses for rainy and dry seasons = Average herd size × % lactating cows × milk yield × % milk reduction.

Herd-specific abortions losses = Average herd size × % Cows ×Average number of calves per year × % calf reduction.

Age-specific mortality losses for bulls, cows, heifers, and calves=Age-specific prices × Herd size × % Composition × % dead.

Age-specific weight losses for bulls, cows, heifers, and calves = Herd size × % Bulls × Average weight of bulls × % weight reduction.

Treatment costs for FMD=Average herd size × % infected × Average cost of treatment per head.

Vaccination costs for FMD = Average herd size × Average cost of vaccination per head × Number of vaccinations per year.

Age-specific salvage sale losses were calculated by considering cattle prices before, during, and after the last FMD outbreak.

Age-specific salvage sale losses for bulls, cows, heifers, and calves (female and male) = Age-specific prices × Herd size × % Composition × % Price reduction.

Data analysis

The study used qualitative data, which were captured using FGDs, semi-structured questionnaire; KIs and quantitative data captured using the structured questionnaire. Qualitative data were analyzed by summarizing content according to the major themes. Quantitative data were entered using MS Excel and analyzed using STATA. Data from case studies were analyzed using regression analysis. Data analysis combined descriptive and regression analysis with inferential statistics to compare market revenue losses and economic costs during FMD outbreaks.

Results

Financial analysis of cattle enterprises in the study districts

The major inputs into the cattle enterprises included labor, treatment or veterinary drugs, acaricides (tick control chemicals), mineral salts, vaccination, fencing, and farm maintenance. While the major outputs from cattle enterprises were milk, live cattle sales, and manure. The average household daily milk production including the amount consumed, sold and given to herdsmen as a form of payment for their labor during the rainy and dry seasons and the prices per study district were as shown in Table-1. In all the study districts, milk yield was significantly different between the dry and wet seasons. The variance was more prominent in Nakasongola compared to the rest of the study districts. Prices increased and fell in the dry and wet seasons, respectively, in all the districts, but the variance was more prominent in Rakai where the prices increased by nearly 50% (Table-1).

Nakaseke earned higher revenues from milk annually compared to the rest of the study districts. Ironically, all the study districts earned more revenues from milk during the dry season than in the wet season (Table-2).

During the normal marketing periods (without outbreaks), bulls and cows fetched higher prices than other cattle types in all the study districts. Notably, the prices for bulls and cows are much higher in Nakaseke than in the other study districts (Table-3). Farmers in all the four study districts mainly sell cows (culled animals) as compared to the other age groups, which explains the generally low off-take rate (Table-4).

On average, households in Nakaseke earned more revenue from cattle sales than households in other study districts (Table-5). Nakaseke had a higher off-take rate and earned more income from cattle sales compared to the rest of the study districts (Table-6).

Table-1: Average household daily milk production, consumption, and sales; and prices during the wet and dry seasons in the study districts.

Item	Season	Nakasongola	Nakaseke	Isingiro	Rakai
Daily milk yield (liters)	Wet	17.5	51.6	23.9	12.0
	Dry	6.0	25.5	11.3	6.6
Daily milk consumption	Wet	4.5	9.5	12.6	9.2
	Dry	2.3	8.6	7.5	5.0
Daily milk sales	Wet	13.0	42.0	11.4	3.0
	Dry	3.9	16.8	3.7	1.7
Milk payment to herdsmen in-kind	Wet	3.0	4.7	5.3	2.5
	Dry	1.4	2.1	2.9	1.0
Prices/liter (UGX)	Wet	326.8	270.0	320.0	492.9
	Dry	420.1	380.3	421.5	632.1

Table-2: Average annual total revenue from milk in US dollars per household in the study districts.

Outputs	Season	Nakasongola	Nakaseke	Isingiro	Rakai
Milk sales	Wet	450	1201	386	201
	Dry	174	677	165	114
Ghee sales		548	98	130	193
Home consumption	Wet	156	272	427	480
	Dry	102	346	335	335
Milk payment to herdsmen in-kind	Wet	104	209	180	131
	Dry	62	85	129	67
Total output	Wet	1258	1780	1123	1004
	Dry	338	1107	629	515
Average total output		798	1443	876	760

Table-3: Normal average age-specific prices of cattle (US dollars) in the study districts.

Category	Nakasongola	Nakaseke	Isingiro	Rakai
Female calves	77	66	52	121
Male calves	77	66	52	59
Steers	132	206	59	127
Heifers	162	235	147	127
Cows	265	309	221	217
Bulls	438	577	309	309

Table-4: Percentage age-specific off-take sale composition per district between January 2010 and January 2011 as revealed by sub-county livestock markets records.

Category	Rakai	Isingiro	Nakasongola	Nakaseke
Female calves	14.8	10.8	8.4	2.4
Male calves	21.6	19.0	5.3	6.2
Steers	3.4	9.0	9.9	4.1
Heifers	23.5	12.5	23.2	9.8
Cows	35.7	46.0	48.2	72.8
Bulls	0.9	2.6	5.0	4.7

Milk yield loss during FMD outbreaks affected households in all the study districts, and it resulted into loss of income from milk and live cattle sales (Table-7). There was a significant difference in income lost due to a decrease in milk and live cattle sales. The loss of income due to milk loss and live cattle sales was more significant in Nakasongola compared to Rakai (Table-8).

The most significant difference between farmers' expenditure on drugs, vaccines, and labor during FMD outbreaks was observed in Nakasongola as opposed to Rakai (Table-9). Another major effect of FMD on the

farmers during outbreaks was via abortion. Foot and mouth disease outbreaks were associated with abortions in all the study districts; (84.7%) for Isingiro, 100% for Nakasongola and Nakaseke, and 76.7% for Rakai.

FMD control cost per head of cattle was highest in the small herds ($19), more than thrice and eight times for medium and large herds, respectively. Mortality losses in small and medium case study herds were $429 and $214, respectively, and there was no mortality in large herds. The salvage losses in small and medium case study herds were $143 and $113, respectively, and there were no salvage losses in large herds, i.e. large herds did not sell any cattle at salvage prices during outbreaks and quarantine (Table-10).

The economic loss due to the reduction of milk production during FMD outbreak and losses due to the absence of milk sales during the quarantine period were as shown in Table-11. Average milk yield per cow was 0.9±0.45 and 2.1±0.3 during dry and wet season, respectively, with each liter of milk costing $0.12 and $0.09, respectively. During FMD outbreaks, there was 42% drop in milk yield in infected cattle over a period of 12 weeks. 12% of the milk produced which is usually sold was not sold during this period. During FMD quarantine periods, milk production gradually resumes in recovered cattle; however, only 12% of the milk was sold (Table-11).

Mortality loss, salvage sale loss, and milk loss accounted for the greatest percentage of the total economic cost due to FMD in small, medium, and large

Table-5: Total cattle populations, number of cattle sold, revenue earned (US dollars) from cattle sales, and number of households that sold cattle per district.

District	Total cattle population	Total number of cattle sold	Total revenue earned from cattle sales	Number of households that sold cattle per district
Isingiro	396,700	918	136,618	330
Rakai	279,394	582	84,332	205
Nakasongola	222,185	604	127,143	242
Nakaseke	160,737	1717	496,088	246

Table-6: The percentage of the cattle herd sold and average annual household income in US dollars earned from cattle sales per district.

District	% of cattle herds sold	Average annual household income from cattle sales
Isingiro	0.23	414
Rakai	0.28	411
Nakasongola	0.27	525
Nakaseke	1.07	2017

herds, respectively, in case study herds in Isingiro (Table-12).

Large herds spent more on vaccination than the small and medium herds (Table-13).

The potential total number of cattle that can be sold in the study markets annually and the representative total off-take per district when there was no FMD outbreak were as shown in Table-14.

The inland districts (Nakaseke and Nakasongola) had higher off-take rates than the international border districts (Rakai and Isingiro) as shown in Table-14. The inland districts would earn very highly significant income (p<0.001); Nakaseke and Nakasongola had the potential to earn 38.6% and 34.1% of the grand total earned by all study districts, respectively, as compared to districts along international borders. The total cattle markets revenue loss during FMD outbreaks from 2006 to 2010 amounted to $340543. The international border districts lost less income (p<0.001, $122514, 47.2%) of the grand total than the inland districts ($137371, 52.9%) during FMD outbreaks in the 5-year period under study.

The total income earned by processing actors per head of cattle during the outbreak and non-outbreak periods in Nakasongola district is presented in Table-15. The total income earned by the actors per month at the processing level reduced by 23% during outbreaks (Table-15).

Discussion

Milk yield loss during FMD outbreaks affected farming households in all the study districts, and it resulted into loss of income due to a decrease in milk sales. However, FMD outbreaks affected households in the study districts differently. For instance, loss of income due to loss of milk and live cattle sales was more significant in Nakasongola than in Rakai.

The economic cost per head of cattle was highest in the small herds followed by the medium herds and was lowest in the large herds. The greatest percentage of the economic cost due to FMD arose from milk losses in large herds compared to the economic costs in small and medium herds that were mainly due to market blockage caused by continued persistence of the disease in the affected cattle farming areas.

Vaccination comprised a major control cost although FMD remains endemic in the study area. An optimal strategy for FMD control in Uganda is yet to emerge, and it will only be possible if the unique circumstances such as production systems, livestock movements to the market are considered as recommended [26]. Thus, FMD disproportionately affects the smallholders and probably the poorer households who may not afford the cost of prevention and control of the disease. In calf cows aborted as a result of FMD, abortions affect the herd structure and undermine the farmers' economic objective of one calf per cow per year [27]. FMD related age-specific mortality as perceived by farmers was generally low, and calves were most affected which agrees with [20]. FMD outbreaks had food security effects on the farmers by causing starvation which is in agreement with previous studies [28,29].

Processors experienced physical loss of meat products and negative demand shifts which greatly reduced the price of beef and profitability, and these findings are in tandem with [23]. In Nakaseke, under normal circumstances processors earned net monthly income of about $14 after paying off all the operational costs, but this income was lost during the outbreaks. Processors found themselves out of employment, i.e. slaughters reduced from 5 heads of cattle before FMD outbreak to 1/day.

All the study districts highly significantly (p<0.001) suffered from starvation due milk loss during outbreaks which agree with [29] who reported that households and communities that depend more or solely on livestock for their livelihoods suffer more during FMD outbreaks since livestock provide a safety net for farmers throughout the developing world [30]. However, the current findings defer in that districts that were less dependent on livestock for their livelihoods suffered from starvation more than Nakaseke that had a higher sole dependency probably because Nakaseke had the lowest prevalence for FMD.

Table-7: Effects of milk yield loss (percentage) on households during FMD outbreaks.

Effects of milk yield losses on the household	Nakasongola	Nakaseke	Isingiro	Rakai
Starvation due to loss of milk for food	26.8	8.7	30.7	33.9
Loss of income from milk and live cattle sales	69.5	58.4	48.6	25.6
Increased household expenditure on drugs, vaccines, and labor	14.1	31.9	20.7	40.5

FMD=Foot and mouth disease

Table-8: Loss of income due to milk loss and live cattle sales.

Districts compared	χ^2 value	Level of significance difference
Nakasongola versus Rakai	38.4	p<0.001
Nakasongola versus Isingiro	5.6	p<0.01
Nakaseke versus Isingiro	2.7	p>0.05
Rakai versus Nakaseke	22.5	p<0.01
Rakai versus Isingiro	11.7	p<0.01

Table-9: Household expenditure on drugs, vaccines, and labor during FMD outbreaks.

Districts compared	χ^2 value	Level of significance difference
Nakasongola versus Nakaseke	8.14	p<0.01
Nakasongola versus Isingiro	1.36	p>0.05
Nakasongola versus Rakai	17	p<0.001
Rakai versus Nakaseke	1.8	p>0.05

FMD=Foot and mouth disease

Table-10: FMD control costs in case study herds in Isingiro district.

Control item	Herd category	Small	Medium	Large
Treatment	Bulls	57	29	0
	Cows	86	357	143
	Heifers	29	29	214
	Steers	0	0	0
	Calves	43	43	114
	Total	214	457	471
Vaccination costs		4.3	23	74
Veterinary costs		6	6	6
Total FMD control costs		224	487	551
FMD control cost per head of cattle		19	6	2

FMD=Foot and mouth disease

FMD outbreaks caused financial losses at the farmer and regional levels within inland and border districts as well as at the national level. FMD outbreaks caused even more impact on cattle sector performance due to losses incurred from reduced productivity, treatment, and control costs besides the trade bans [31]. In agreement with other studies, efficiency was undermined, and all actors in the cattle-beef marketing chain lost significant income streams during the outbreaks [32]. At the processing level, various actors lost income amounting to 77% which means that during the outbreaks the actors only earn 23%, which severely affects their livelihoods, food security, and ability to meet basic needs in their households [8,7].

FMD outbreaks affected farmers and beef marketing by lowering cattle and meat prices with a resultant loss of income which agrees with earlier studies [33,34]. Cattle traders were affected during the FMD outbreaks because quarantine period made it difficult for them to obtain stock from the affected areas and at the same time they faced difficulty in finding alternative suppliers thus they were rendered jobless. Consequently, it was difficult for the processors to obtain slaughter animals during the same period.

The government of Uganda should retain responsibility for controlling and preventing FMD since this disease affects the poor most who cannot afford to control or prevent the disease without government support. The magnitude of financial losses estimated justifies investments in prevention and control of FMD at all levels of the cattle marketing chain.

Conclusion

All actors along the cattle marketing chain incur losses during FMD outbreaks, but smallholder farmers are most affected. Control and prevention of FMD should remain the responsibility of the government if Uganda is to achieve a disease-free status that is a prerequisite for free movement and operation of cattle markets throughout the year which will boost cattle marketing.

Authors' Contributions

The author was the principal investigator and she designed the study, prepared the data collection instruments and collected the data with the help of research assistants, analyzed the data and wrote the manuscript that was submitted for this publication.

Acknowledgments

The author acknowledges Makerere University Council, Carnegie Corporation of New York Next Generation of Academics Program, and the International Livestock Research Institute – Germany Academic Exchange Program (ILRI – DAAD) In-Country/In-Region Fellowships for

Table-11: Milk production losses in US dollars due to lack of milk sales during FMD outbreaks in case study herds.

Herd size category	Loss due to reduction of milk production during FMD outbreak	Loss due to absence of sales during FMD outbreak	Milk sale loss caused due to FMD quarantine	Total milk loss due to FMD
Small herds	42	11	213	267
Medium herds	144	43	441	629
Large herds	613	183	1873	2670
Average	266	80	814	1160
% composition of type of milk loss to total milk economic loss	23	6.9	70.1	

FMD=Foot and mouth disease

Table-12: The percentage of each economic cost to total FMD cost in Isingiro district.

Economic loss	Small	Medium	Large
Mortality loss	40	9	0
Salvage sale loss	13	46	0
Milk loss	25	26	83
Treatment	20	19	15
Vaccination	0	1	2
Veterinary costs	1	0	0

FMD=Foot and mouth disease

Table-13: Average vaccination costs in US dollars against FMD for all herd categories.

Age category	Small	Medium	Large
Bulls	1	2	6
Cows	5	12	25
Heifers	3	7	6
Steers	0.3	3	1.2
Calves	2	7	5.3
Total	10	30	43

FMD=Foot and mouth disease

Table-14: Annual potential volume of cattle that can be sold per market and percentage off-take from two markets per district.

District	Market	Number of cattle sold yearly	% off-take of the total district herd
Nakasongola	Wabinyoyi	4500	10.7
Nakaseke	Nakitoma	19200	
	Subtotal	23700	
Rakai	Ngoma	19200	19.4
	Kinyogoga	12000	
	Subtotal	31200	
	Kibanda	7200	5.2
	Kakuuto	7,320	
	Subtotal	14520	
Isingiro	Bugango	8880	3.6
	Rwenseke	5400	
	Subtotal	14280	

Table-15: Total income earned (US dollars) by processing actors per head of cattle during outbreaks and non-outbreak periods in Nakasongola district.

Actor	Income earned weekly without outbreak	Income earned monthly without outbreak	Income earned weekly during outbreak	Income earned monthly during outbreak
Weighing scale owner	30	120	1	24
Local government	30	120	1	24
Veterinary inspectors	30	120	1	24
Public health inspector	30	120	1	24
Slaughter man/moslem	30	120	1	24
Other operational costs	86	343	1	23
Butchery workers	51	206	0.4	41
Processors	2700	10800	26	2571
Total income	2987	11949	689	2755

funding the research that the led to this publication. The author also acknowledges the support of the research assistants throughout the study and all the respondents for their cooperation and participation in the study.

Competing Interests

The authors declare that they have no competing interests.

References

1. Ministry of Agriculture Animal Industry and Fisheries, Uganda. (2005) National Livestock Productivity Improvement Project. Baseline Survey Report. A Benchmark for Measuring Project Impact.
2. Ministry of Agriculture Animal Industry and Fisheries, Uganda, Uganda Bureau of Statistics, Food and Agriculture Organization of the United Nations, International Livestock Research Institute and World Resources Institute. (2010) Mapping A Better Future: Spatial Analysis and Pro-Poor Livestock Strategies in Uganda. World Resources Institute, Washington, DC, Kampala.
3. King, A. (2002) Joint Donor Agencies Study on the Performance of Growth Prospects for Strategic Exports in Uganda. A Case Study of Livestock, Hides and Skins and Leather Products. Delegation of the European Commission.
4. Moyini, Y., Masiga, M. and Nabatanzi, M. (2005) Improving Market Access For Dry lands Commodities, United Nations Development Programme Uganda Country Office Report.
5. Balinda, S.N., Belsham, G.J., Masembe, C., Sangula, A.K., Siegismund, H.R. and Muwanika, W.B. (2010) Molecular characterization of SAT2 food and mouth disease virus from post-outbreak slaughtered animals. Implications for disease control in Uganda. *Epid. Infect. Dis.*, 138(8): 1204-1210.
6. Paton, D.J., Keith, J.S. and Charleston, B. (2009) Options for control of foot and mouth disease: Knowledge, capability and policy. *Philos. Trans. R. Soc.*, 364: 2643-2655.
7. Di Nardo, A., Knowles, N.J. and Paton, D.J. (2011) Combining livestock trade patterns with phylogenetics to help understand the spread of foot and mouth disease sub-Saharan Africa, the Middle East and South East Asia. *Rev. Sci. Tech. Off. Int. Epiz.*, 30(1): 63-85.
8. Picardo, A., Speybroeck, N., Kivaria, F., Mosha, R.M., Sumaye, R.D., Casal, J. and Berkvens, D. (2011) Foot-and-mouth disease in Tanzania from 2001 to 2006. Transbound. *Emerg. Dis.*, 58(1): 44-52.
9. Vosloo, W., Bastos, A.D., Sangaro, O., Hargreaves, S.K. and Thomson, G.R. (2002) Review of the status and control of food and mouth disease in sub-Saharan Africa. *Rev. Sci. Tech.*, 21(3): 437-449.
10. Upton, M. (2006) A Framework for Identifying Market and Trade Impacts of HPAI and its Control. A Paper Presented at Symposium on the Market and Trade Dimension on Avian Influenza. Rome, Italy. 14 November; 2006.
11. Rich, K.M. and Wanyoike, F. (2011) An assessment of the regional and national socio-economic impacts of the 2007 rift valley fever outbreak in Kenya. *Am. J. Trop. Med. Hyg.*, 83 Suppl 2: 52-57.
12. Bennet, R. (2003) The 'direct costs of livestock diseases: The development of a system of models for the analysis of thirty endemic livestock diseases in Great Britain. *J. Agric. Econ.* 54(1): 55-71.
13. Fevre, E.M., Bronsvoort, B.M., Hamilton, K.A. and Cleveland, S. (2006) Animal movements and the spread of infectious diseases. *Trends Microbiol.*, 14(3): 125-31.
14. African Union Inter African Bureau of Animal Resources. (2010) Framework for Mainstreaming Livestock in the CAADP Pillars. African Union Inter African Bureau of Animal Resources, Nairobi.
15. Webber, C.M. and Labaste, P. (2010) Building Competitiveness in Africa's Agriculture. A Guide to Value Chain Concepts and Applications. The International Bank for Reconstruction and Development/The World Bank, New York, USA.
16. Tambi, N.E., Maina, W.O. and Ndi, C. (2006) An estimation of the economic impact of contagious bovine pleuropneumonia in Africa. *Rev. Sci. Tech. Off. Int. Epiz.*, 25(3): 999-1012.
17. Heath, S.E. (2006) Challenges and options for animal and public health services in the next two decades. *Rev. Sci. Tech.*, 25(1): 403-419.
18. Somwaru, A. and Valdes, C. (2004) Brazil's Beef Production and its Efficiency: A Comparative Study of Scale Economies. GTAP Seventh Annual Conference on Global Economic Analysis. Trade, Poverty and the Environment. June 17-19, 2004. The World Bank, Washington, DC, United States.
19. Heath, S.E. (2008) The impact of epizootics on livelihoods. *J. Appl. Anim. Welf. Sci.*, 11(2): 98-111.
20. Rufael, T., Catley, A., Bogale, A., Sahle, M. and Shiferaw, Y. (2008) Foot and mouth disease in the Borana pastoral system, Southern Ethiopia and implications for livelihoods and international trade. *Trop. Anim. Health Prod.*, 40(1): 29-38.
21. Meckonen, H., Beyene, D., Rufael, T., Fevisa, A. and Abunna, F. (2011) Study on the prevalence of foot and mouth disease in the Borana and Guji zones, Southern Ethiopia. *Vet. World*, 4(7): 293-296.
22. Dijkhuizen, A., Huirne, R.B.M. and Jalvingh, A.W. (1995) Economic analysis of animal diseases and their control. *Prev. Vet. Med.*, 25: 135-149.
23. Perry, B.D., Nin Pratt, A., Sones, K. and Stevens, C. (2005) An Appropriate Level of Risk. Balancing the Need for Safe Livestock Products with Fair Market Access for the Poor. Food and Agriculture Organization of the United Nations (FAO), PPLPI Working Paper Number 23. July 13; 2005.
24. Pritchett, J., Thilmany, D. and Johnson, K. (2005) Animal disease economic impacts: A survey of literature and typology of research approaches. *Int. Food Agribus. Manag. Rev.*, 8(1): 23-45.
25. Ocaido, M., Muwazi, R.T. and Opuda, J.A. (2009) Disease incidence in ranch and pastoral livestock herds around Lake Mburo National Park, in South Western Uganda. *Trop. Anim. Health Prod.*, 41: 1299-1308.
26. Traulsen, I., Rave, G., Teuffert, J. and Krieter, J. (2011) Consideration of different outbreak conditions in the evaluation of preventive culling and emergency vaccination to control foot and mouth disease epidemics. *Res. Vet. Sci.*, 91(2): 219-224.
27. Rushton, J. (2009) The Economics of Animal Health and Production. CAB International, Oxford.
28. Mazengia, H., Taye, M., Negussie, H., Alemu, S. and Tassew, A. (2010) Incidence of foot and mouth disease and its effect on milk yield in dairy cattle at Andassa dairy farm, North West Ethiopia. *Agric. Biol. J. North Am.*, 1(5): 969-973.
29. Rutagwenda, T. (2003) The implications and consequences of foot and mouth disease outbreak on food security and household incomes in selected districts in Uganda. A report to Food and Agriculture Organization, TCP/UGA/O168 (E) 1 May 2003.
30. Forman, S.F., Belton, G., Evans, D., Francois, B., Murray, J.L., Sheesley, G., Vandersmissen, D.A. and Yoshimura, S. (2009) Moving towards the global control of foot and mouth disease: An opportunity for donors. Health programmes in developing countries. FAO Expert Consultation, Rome. *Rev. Sci. Tech. Off. Int. Epiz.*, 28(3):883-896.
31. Zhang, L., Zhang, J., Chen, H., Zhou, J., Ma, L., Yao-Zhong,

D. and Yong-sheng, L. (2011) Research in advance for FMD novel vaccines. *Virol. J.,* 8: 268.

32. Koopman, R.B. and Laney, K. (2012) Brazil: Competitive Factors in Brazil affecting US and Brazilian Agricultural Sales in Selected Third Country Markets. US International Trade Commission. Publication 4310 April; 2012.

33. Perry, B.D. and Grace, D. (2009) The impacts of livestock diseases and their control on growth and development processes that are pro-poor. *Philos. Trans. R. Soc.,* 364: 2643-2655.

34. Rich, K.M. and Perry, B.D. (2011) The economic and poverty impacts of animal diseases in developing countries: New roles, new demands for economics and epidemiology. *Rev. Sci. Tech. Off. Int. Epiz.,* 101(3-4): 133-147.

17

Influence of combinations of fenugreek, garlic, and black pepper powder on production traits of the broilers

A. Kirubakaran[1], M. Moorthy[2], R. Chitra[3] and G. Prabakar[2]

1. Veterinary University Training and Research Centre, Erode - 638 004, Tamil Nadu, India; 2. Department of Poultry Science, Veterinary College and Research Institute, Namakkal - 637 002, Tamil Nadu, India; 3. Department of Animal Husbandry Statistics and Computer Applications, Veterinary College and Research Institute, Namakkal - 637 002, Tamil Nadu, India.
Corresponding author: A. Kirubakaran, e-mail: kirubavet@yahoo.co.in,
MM: m.moorthy@tanuvas.org.in, RC: chitra@tanuvas.org.in, GP: prabavet@gmail.com

Abstract

Aim: To study the effects of combinations of fenugreek (*Trigonella foenum-graecum* L.), garlic (*Allium sativum*), and black pepper (*Piper nigrum*) powder supplementation on production traits of broiler chickens.

Materials and Methods: A total of 288 commercial broiler chicks were randomly assigned to 1-9 groups with 4 replicates each. An experiment was conducted in broilers with different feed formulations; control feed, with no added fenugreek, garlic, and black pepper powder; and 8 treatment groups receiving feed supplemented with different combinations of fenugreek, garlic, and black pepper powder. The individual broilers' body weight and feed consumption were recorded and calculate the body weight gain and feed conversion ratio (FCR).

Results: Broiler's weight gain and FCR were significantly higher in groups receiving feed supplemented with garlic and black pepper powder combinations (p<0.01). Cumulative feed consumption was significantly higher in groups receiving feed supplemented with garlic and black pepper powder combinations (p<0.01).

Conclusion: The combination of garlic and black pepper powder supplemented broiler feed fed groups showed higher production performance. The 5 g/kg garlic powder+1 g/kg black pepper powder and 10 g/kg garlic powder+2 g/kg black pepper powder significantly improved the weight gain and FCR.

Keywords: black pepper, body weight, feed conversion ratio, fenugreek, garlic.

Introduction

Antibiotics are used to control the disease and infection effect in the poultry industry. The commercial broilers are genetic engineering birds, and it can attain maximum body weight (above 2 kg) during its short growing time interval of 35 days. The commercial broilers faced much stress during its growing period, due to attain maximum body weight in shorter duration interval. The poultry nutritionists are added stress relieving medicines to feed to trying to ease stress from broilers and improve the body weight. Large number of laboratory derived antistress and growth promoting medicines are available in the field to improve its performance. However, the use of chemical products, especially hormones and antibiotics, may cause adverse side effects. Attempts to use the natural resources such as medicinal plants could be widely accepted as feed additives to improve the efficiency of feed utilization and productive performance in poultry.

Antibiotic have a certain period as a pulling out time. If the antibiotics are not reserved from the broiler diet before catching the birds for slaughter, it will lead to a problem, like deposition of antibiotic residues in commercial broiler meats and also delivered the antibiotic residues to the consumers through this meat consumption. Poultry nutritionists are trying to rectify this problem through supplementation of phytoadditives, which contain antibiotic and antibacterial properties. The majority of medicinal plants do not have the residual effects [1].

Fenugreek, garlic, and black pepper plants contain beneficial phytoadditives in its parts. Their phytochemical efficiency was also analyzed by many researchers, and there was a great need to judge its efficacy and economic feasibility on the basis of different dosage levels in the broiler diet. The broilers' body weight was significantly (p<0.01) increased in fenugreek seed powder (0, 10, 20, and 40 g/kg) fed groups compared to control (1382, 2587, 2328, and 2192.5 g/bird) and observed significantly (p<0.01) decreased feed consumption and significant (p<0.01) improvement in feed conversion ratio between the groups [2]. The some researchers were reported the addition of fenugreek powder and extract to diet has improved the body weight gain in broilers [3,4]. The 42 days trial by feeding garlic powder at the rate of 0, 2 and, 4 g/kg in commercial broiler diet and found no significant effects on body weight and weight gain, no difference in feed consumption and feed efficiency during the experimental period [5]. The addition of garlic to the diet has improved the production performance of broiler [6-8]. The black pepper powder was added at the rate of 0, 5, 7.5, and 10 g/kg in broiler diet and noted significant ($p<0.05$) difference in body weight (1855, 1990, 2025, and 2144 g/bird), body weight gain (1810, 1945, 1980, and 2099 g/bird), increased feed consumption (3620, 3793, 3841, and 4030 g/bird), and positive significant ($p<0.05$) effect on feed conversion ratio (2.00, 1.95, 1.94, and 1.92) at 42 days of age [9]. Some researchers were found no difference in feed intake in broiler fed with black pepper for a period of 5-week [10,11].

The individual phytoadditives are used as an antibiotic replacer in poultry field. In these circumstances, combinations of fenugreek (*Trigonella foenum-graecum* L.), garlic (*Allium sativum*), and black pepper (*Piper nigrum*) are added to broiler in these trials and evaluated its efficacy.

Materials and Methods

Ethical approval

The biological trial was carried out at the Poultry Farm Complex and the Department of Poultry Science, Veterinary College and Research Institute (Namakkal, India) after permission of Institutional Animal Ethics Committee.

Experimental design and dietary treatments:

A total of 288 commercial broiler chicks at day old age, belonging to the same hatch and of uniform body size, were randomly assigned to 9 dietary treatments. Four replicates were randomly assigned to each of the 9 dietary treatments. Eight chicks were allotted to each of the replicates. The broilers are vaccinated with live B1 and Lasota strain on the end of 1st week

and end of 3rd week. The experimental designs are showed in Table-1.

Samples of fenugreek, garlic, and black pepper used in the experimental feeds were assayed in duplicate [12]. The experimental diet was formulated according to the standards prescribed in Bureau of Indian Standards [13]. The locally available fenugreek, garlic, and black pepper were purchased and powdered and incorporated into standard broiler diet to form different experimental diets. The phytoadditives, fenugreek, garlic, and black pepper combinations are added as feed supplements and act as antibiotic alternatives.

The total phenolic content of fenugreek powder was estimated and expressed as mg/l gallic acid equivalent of phenols [14]. Total flavonoid content of fenugreek powder was determined and expressed as mg/l quercetin equivalents of flavonoid [15]. The tannin content of fenugreek was determined and calculated as mg/l tannic acid equivalents of tannin [16]. Total phenolic content of garlic powder was determined in the garlic using the Folin-Ciocalteu method [14]. The total flavonoid content of garlic powder was determined expressed as micrograms of rutin equivalents per gram dry weight [17]. Total phenols and flavonoids contents in the black pepper powder extracts were also analyzed by UV spectroscopy [18,19].

Sample collection and analysis
Production traits

The body weight of the individual experimental bird was recorded on initial and weekly to 1-g accuracy from 1 to 6 weeks of age to determine the body weight gain. Replicate-wise feed intake and mortality (if any) were recorded to calculate the feed efficiency.

Statistical analysis

Data on the 9 dietary treatments were analyzed statistically by one-way ANOVA to determine whether a significant difference existed between the 9 different diets. Significance was tested by a *post-hoc* analysis method.

Table-1: Experimental design.

Treatment groups	Particulars	Number of replicates	Number of birds/replicate	Total
T_1	Control−standard broiler diet	4	8	32
T_2	Control+5 g fenugreek powder/kg of diet+5 g garlic powder/kg of diet	4	8	32
T_3	Control+10 g fenugreek powder/kg of diet+10 g garlic powder/kg of diet	4	8	32
T_4	Control+5 g fenugreek powder/kg of diet+ 1 g black pepper powder/kg of diet	4	8	32
T_5	Control+10 g fenugreek powder/kg of diet+ 2 g black pepper powder/kg of diet	4	8	32
T_6	Control+5 g garlic powder/kg of diet+1 g black pepper powder/kg of diet	4	8	32
T_7	Control+10 g garlic powder/kg of diet+2 g black pepper powder/kg of diet	4	8	32
T_8	Control+5 g fenugreek powder/kg of diet+5 g garlic powder/kg of diet+ 1 g black pepper powder/kg of diet	4	8	32
T_9	Control+10 g fenugreek powder/kg of diet+10 g garlic powder/kg of diet+2 g black pepper powder/kg of diet	4	8	32
Total				288

Table-2: Proximate composition (% DM basis) of fenugreek, garlic, and black pepper.

Nutrients	Fenugreek	Garlic	Black pepper
Moisture	7.18	6.10	11.23
Crude protein	28.58	15.93	11.55
Ether extract	7.55	1.30	7.93
Crude fiber	6.27	10.12	12.32
Total ash	2.39	7.31	3.93
Gross energy (kcal/kg)	4500	3797	4015
Metabolizable energy* (kcal/kg)	3877	1490	2550
Phytochemical concentration			
Phenol	110 mg/l	42 mg GAE/ 100 g	1.728 mg/g
Flavonoid	410 mg/l	0.39 mg rutin DW/g FW	1.087 mg/g
Tannin	100 mg/l	-	-

*Calculated values. DM=Dry matter, DW=Dry weight, GAE=Gallic acid equivalent

Results

The proximate composition (% dry matter basis) and phytochemical concentration of fenugreek, garlic, and black pepper are presented in Table-2.

Production traits

Comparisons for production traits, body weight, body weight gain, feed consumption, and feed conversion ratio are shown in Tables-3-6.

Discussion

Body weight and weight gain

The analysis of variance of data on mean body weight (g) and body weight gain of broilers revealed significant ($p<0.01$) difference from 1 to 6 weeks of age between treatment groups due to dietary supplementation of fenugreek, garlic, and black pepper combinations (Tables- 3 and 4). Fenugreek and garlic combinations (T_2 and T_3) revealed numerically higher body weight and weight gain than the control group at 6 weeks of age. This might be due to the presence of phytochemical, namely, allicin in garlic powder which improved digestibility and eradicates the pathogenic microbes in the intestine [20]. Fenugreek and black pepper combination fed group (T_4 and T_5) showed numerically higher body weight when compared to control group at 6 weeks of age. The higher body weight might be due to the active principle-piperine present in black pepper which has a digestive stimulatory effect. The higher body weight was observed in T_4 than T_5. The high proportion (40%) of soluble fiber in the fenugreek seed which forms a gelatinous structure, which might slow down the digestion and absorption of feed from the intestine and create a sense of fullness in the abdomen and thus suppressed appetite and resulted in more weight loss in T_5 than T_4 [21].

In garlic and black pepper combination (T_6 and T_7), fed broilers showed a significantly ($p<0.01$) higher body weight when compared to control. This might be due to the synergistic action of garlic phytochemical – allicin and black pepper phytochemical – piperine, which give better results in T_6 and T_7. Some researchers were observed significantly higher body weight and weight gain in broilers fed with individual black pepper only at 6 weeks of age [22-28]. The addition of garlic to broiler diet had increased the salivary flow rate and gastric juice secretion which resulted in improved digestibility and higher body weight [29].

The fenugreek, garlic, and black pepper combination group (T_8 and T_9) revealed lower body weight than T_6 and T_7. This might be due to the presence of fenugreek powder in diet T_8 and T_9.

Feed consumption

The statistical analysis revealed significant ($p<0.01$) difference between treatment groups in mean feed consumption and feed conversion ratio (Tables-5 and 6) at the end of every week due to dietary supplementation of fenugreek, garlic, and black pepper combinations. The mean cumulative feed consumption was significantly ($p<0.01$) higher in T_6 and T_7 group (3185.53 and 3236.37 g) when compared to control at 6 weeks of age. Similarly, significantly ($p<0.01$) superior feed conversion ratio was observed in T_6 and T_7 (1.59 and 1.58) when compared to control at the end of the experiment. This might be due to the positive synergism between active principles of garlic and black pepper, which resulted in better feed conversion ratio in T_6 and T_7 at 6 weeks of age.

Conclusion

This study clarified that the birds fed rations supplemented with garlic and black pepper combinations utilized their feed more efficiently resulting in higher body weight and also combinations of 5 g garlic+1 g black pepper and 10 g garlic+2 g black pepper powder had resulted in better feed consumption and feed conversion ratio in broilers.

Authors' Contributions

This study is the part of Ph.D. thesis of the first author AK, who carried out the research under the guidance of Professor MM. RC and GP helped during the trial. The article was drafted by AK. The revision was made by MM, RC and GP.

All authors have read and approved the final version of the manuscript.

Acknowledgments

The authors are highly thankful to Tamil Nadu Veterinary and Animal Sciences University, for providing necessary funds to carry out the work.

Competing Interests

The authors declare that they have no competing interests.

Table-3: Mean±SE body weight (g) of broilers fed with different combinations of fenugreek, garlic, and black pepper.

Weeks	T_1	T_2	T_3	T_4	T_5	T_6	T_7	T_8	T_9	p value
Hatch weight	48.56 ± 0.63	48.02 ± 0.57	47.02 ± 0.54	48.94 ± 0.67	47.75 ± 0.60	48.06 ± 0.65	48.10 ± 0.47	48.07 ± 0.60	48.12 ± 0.67	0.6562
1st week	$118.56^{D}\pm2.64$	$120.06^{D}\pm1.98$	$119.00^{D}\pm2.04$	$125.09^{CD}\pm2.04$	$121.09^{D}\pm1.43$	$144.03^{A}\pm1.81$	$149.40^{A}\pm1.68$	$130.00^{BC}\pm1.78$	$135.00^{B}\pm1.39$	<0.0001
2nd week	$282.96^{E}\pm6.49$	$300.90^{DEF}\pm5.18$	$290.59^{EF}\pm4.89$	$310.84^{CDE}\pm3.27$	$305.15^{DE}\pm3.85$	$350.00^{AB}\pm3.27$	$360.00^{A}\pm5.22$	$320.03^{CD}\pm3.56$	$330.12^{BC}\pm2.90$	<0.0001
3rd week	$560.75^{C}\pm13.37$	$575.06^{BC}\pm10.47$	$570.65^{BC}\pm10.30$	$618.03^{ABC}\pm11.30$	$603.18^{ABC}\pm13.65$	$650.03^{A}\pm13.65$	$660.00^{A}\pm12.78$	$625.50^{AB}\pm19.30$	$635.28^{A}\pm17.66$	0.0001
4th week	$880.81^{D}\pm21.75$	$900.90^{BCD}\pm13.85$	$890.00^{CD}\pm19.51$	$931.78^{ABCD}\pm17.54$	$924.15^{ABCD}\pm14.13$	$972.90^{A}\pm12.26$	$980.00^{A}\pm7.27$	$950.71^{ABC}\pm13.82$	$967.25^{AB}\pm14.98$	0.0001
5th week	$1295.93^{C}\pm16.90$	$1300.00^{BCD}\pm39.83$	$1295.18^{C}\pm23.07$	$1410.15^{ABC}\pm17.50$	$1369.84^{BC}\pm20.90$	$1450.62^{AB}\pm30.83$	$1490.62^{A}\pm11.54$	$1425.46^{AB}\pm21.33$	$1437.65^{AB}\pm19.36$	<0.0001
6th week	$1785.34^{D}\pm40.2$	$1801.37^{D}\pm28.88$	$1798.84^{D}\pm41.40$	$1905.09^{CD}\pm26.77$	$1896.84^{CD}\pm14.88$	$2053.12^{A}\pm14.88$	$2090.62^{A}\pm17.01$	$1915.28^{CD}\pm33.91$	$1946.25^{BC}\pm24.70$	<0.0001

Values given in each cell is the mean of 32 observations. $^{A\text{-}F}$Means within a row bearing different superscripts differ significantly (p<0.01). SE=Standard error

Table-4: Mean±SE body weight gain (g) of broilers fed with different combinations of fenugreek, garlic, and black pepper.

Weeks	T_1	T_2	T_3	T_4	T_5	T_6	T_7	T_8	T_9	p value
1st week	$69.99^{E}\pm2.70$	$72.04^{E}\pm2.09$	$71.97^{E}\pm1.93$	$76.15^{DE}\pm2.88$	$73.34^{DE}\pm1.66$	$95.96^{AB}\pm1.91$	$101.30^{A}\pm1.63$	$81.92^{CD}\pm1.98$	$86.87^{BC}\pm1.53$	<0.0001
2nd week	$234.40^{F}\pm6.38$	$252.88^{DEF}\pm5.15$	$242.90^{EF}\pm4.97$	$261.90^{CDE}\pm7.31$	$257.40^{DEF}\pm3.94$	$301.93^{AB}\pm3.27$	$311.90^{A}\pm5.28$	$271.95^{CD}\pm3.84$	$281.99^{BC}\pm2.99$	<0.0001
3rd week	$512.18^{D}\pm13.38$	$527.04^{BCD}\pm10.48$	$522.97^{CD}\pm10.30$	$569.08^{ABCD}\pm11.41$	$555.43^{ABCD}\pm10.46$	$601.96^{A}\pm13.70$	$611.90^{A}\pm12.79$	$577.42^{ABC}\pm19.41$	$587.15^{AB}\pm17.73$	0.0001
4th week	$832.24^{D}\pm21.80$	$852.88^{BCD}\pm13.97$	$842.31^{CD}\pm19.44$	$882.83^{ABCD}\pm17.71$	$876.96^{ABCD}\pm14.18$	$924.84^{A}\pm12.32$	$931.90^{A}\pm7.40$	$902.64^{ABC}\pm13.92$	$919.12^{AB}\pm14.93$	0.0005
5th week	$1247.37^{C}\pm16.91$	$1251.97^{C}\pm39.76$	$1247.50^{C}\pm23.00$	$1361.21^{ABC}\pm37.89$	$1322.65^{BC}\pm21.18$	$1402.55^{AB}\pm30.76$	$1442.52^{A}\pm11.42$	$1377.39^{AB}\pm21.48$	$1389.52^{AB}\pm19.13$	<0.0001
6th week	$1736.27^{D}\pm40.14$	$1753.35^{D}\pm28.97$	$1751.15^{D}\pm41.40$	$1856.15^{CD}\pm28.37$	$1849.65^{CD}\pm26.96$	$2005.05^{AB}\pm15.03$	$2042.52^{A}\pm17.09$	$1867.20^{CD}\pm34.01$	$1898.12^{BC}\pm24.52$	<0.0001

Value given in each cell is the mean of 32 observations. $^{A\text{-}F}$Means within a row bearing different superscripts differ significantly (p<0.01). SE=Standard error

Table-5: Mean±SE cumulative feed consumption (g) of broilers fed with different combinations of fenugreek, garlic, and black pepper.

Weeks	T_1	T_2	T_3	T_4	T_5	T_6	T_7	T_8	T_9	p value
1st week	93.21 ± 2.30	$79.50^{E}\pm0.08$	$78.00^{E}\pm0.76$	$84.75^{D}\pm0.34$	$79.46^{E}\pm0.92$	$101.96^{B}\pm0.33$	$110.00^{A}\pm1.68$	$91.50^{E}\pm0.68$	$95.81^{E}\pm0.89$	<0.0001
2nd week	$336.96^{BC}\pm2.77$	$294.50^{FG}\pm8.74$	$280.00^{G}\pm2.20$	$303.75^{EF}\pm0.91$	$298.21^{F}\pm3.98$	$349.71^{AB}\pm0.87$	$360.37^{A}\pm5.07$	$319.06^{DE}\pm2.41$	$328.31^{CD}\pm0.60$	<0.0001
3rd week	$770.40^{A}\pm9.74$	$672.00^{E}\pm8.55$	$660.00^{E}\pm6.67$	$724.96^{CD}\pm6.76$	$706.81^{D}\pm4.35$	$765.21^{AB}\pm1.18$	$768.50^{A}\pm5.91$	$740.31^{BC}\pm1.90$	$748.00^{ABC}\pm5.79$	<0.0001
4th week	$1329.14^{A}\pm14.93$	$1176.71^{DE}\pm12.08$	$1160.00^{E}\pm9.05$	$1215.96^{CD}\pm7.95$	$1211.18^{CD}\pm6.64$	$1275.84^{A}\pm4.71$	$1275.81^{BC}\pm3.82$	$1250.31^{BC}\pm1.90$	$1270.90^{B}\pm11.95$	<0.0001
5th week	$2226.33^{A}\pm14.62$	$2040.78^{C}\pm10.54$	$2039.06^{C}\pm9.98$	$2070.34^{C}\pm12.43$	$2065.56^{C}\pm13.43$	$2091.78^{BC}\pm9.86$	$2136.37^{B}\pm7.63$	$2090.37^{BC}\pm7.63$	$2086.21^{BC}\pm18.70$	<0.0001
6th week	$3076.33^{B}\pm22.16$	$2960.15^{D}\pm12.64$	$2950.00^{D}\pm13.20$	$2979.71^{D}\pm18.27$	$2970.09^{D}\pm13.11$	$3185.53^{A}\pm9.04$	$3236.37^{A}\pm7.65$	$2989.43^{CD}\pm8.28$	$3024.18^{C}\pm18.57$	<0.0001

Values given in each cell is the mean of four observations. $^{A\text{-}F}$Means within a row bearing different superscripts differ significantly (p<0.01). SE=Standard error

Table-6: Mean±SE cumulative feed conversion ratio of broilers fed with different combinations of fenugreek, garlic, and black pepper.

Weeks	T_1	T_2	T_3	T_4	T_5	T_6	T_7	T_8	T_9	p value
1st week	$1.35^{B}\pm0.05$	$1.13^{A}\pm0.04$	$1.11^{A}\pm0.03$	$1.16^{A}\pm0.04$	$1.10^{A}\pm0.03$	$1.07^{A}\pm0.02$	$1.09^{A}\pm0.03$	$1.13^{A}\pm0.02$	$1.11^{A}\pm0.02$	0.0003
2nd week	$1.44^{B}\pm0.05$	$1.18^{A}\pm0.04$	$1.16^{A}\pm0.02$	$1.19^{A}\pm0.04$	$1.16^{A}\pm0.02$	$1.16^{A}\pm0.01$	$1.16^{A}\pm0.02$	$1.18^{A}\pm0.01$	$1.16^{A}\pm0.01$	<0.0001
3rd week	$1.53^{B}\pm0.04$	$1.29^{A}\pm0.03$	$1.28^{A}\pm0.03$	$1.29^{A}\pm0.03$	$1.28^{A}\pm0.03$	$1.29^{A}\pm0.03$	$1.27^{A}\pm0.03$	$1.30^{A}\pm0.05$	$1.31^{A}\pm0.04$	0.0037
4th week	$1.60^{B}\pm0.04$	$1.39^{A}\pm0.03$	$1.40^{A}\pm0.04$	$1.39^{A}\pm0.04$	$1.39^{A}\pm0.04$	$1.38^{A}\pm0.03$	$1.30^{A}\pm0.01$	$1.39^{A}\pm0.02$	$1.39^{A}\pm0.02$	0.0002
5th week	$1.79^{D}\pm0.03$	$1.68^{CD}\pm0.05$	$1.65^{BCD}\pm0.03$	$1.56^{ABC}\pm0.04$	$1.57^{ABC}\pm0.03$	$1.51^{AB}\pm0.03$	$1.48^{A}\pm0.01$	$1.53^{ABC}\pm0.02$	$1.51^{AB}\pm0.02$	<0.0001
6th week	$1.80^{B}\pm0.04$	$1.70^{AB}\pm0.03$	$1.71^{AB}\pm0.04$	$1.61^{A}\pm0.03$	$1.62^{A}\pm0.03$	$1.59^{A}\pm0.01$	$1.58^{A}\pm0.01$	$1.61^{A}\pm0.01$	$1.60^{A}\pm0.02$	0.0010

Value given in each cell is the mean of four observations. $^{A\text{-}D}$Means within a row bearing different superscripts differ significantly (p<0.01). SE=Standard error

References

1. Tipu, M.A., Akhtar, M.S., Anjum, M.I. and Raja, M.L. (2006) New dimension of medicinal plants as animal feed. *Pak. Vet. J.*, 26: 144-148.

2. Mamoun, T., Mukhtar, M.A. and Tabidi, M.H. (2014) Effect of fenugreek seed powder on the performance, carcass characteristics and some blood serum attributes. *Adv. Res. Agric. Vet. Sci.*, 1(1): 6-11.

3. Duru, M., Erdogan, Z., Duru, A., Kuçukgul, A., Duzguner, V., Kaya, D.A. and Sahin, A. (2013) Effect of seed powder of an herbal legume fenugreek (*Trigonella foenum-graceum* L.) on growth performance, body components, digestive parts, and blood parameters of broiler chicks. *J. Zool.*, 45(4): 1007-1014.

4. Safaei, A., Rahanjam, S.M. and Gharajanlu, M. (2013) Effect of foenum-graecum on immune response and some blood parameters of broilers. *Sch. J. Agric. Sci.*, 3(4): 117-120.

5. Issa, K.J. and Omar, J.M.A. (2012) Effect of garlic powder on performance and lipid profile of broilers. *Open J. Anim. Sci.*, 2(2): 62-68.

6. Oladele, O.A., Emikpe, B.O. and Bakare, H. (2012) Effect of dietary Garlic (*Allium sativum* Linn.) supplementation on body weight and gut morphometry of commercial broilers. *Int. J. Morphol.*, 30(1): 238-240.

7. Suriya, R., Zulkifli, I. and Alimon, A.R. (2012) The effect of dietary inclusion of herbs as growth promoter in broiler chickens. *J. Anim. Vet. Adv.*, 11(3): 346-350.

8. Elagib, H.A.A., El-Amin, W.I.A., Elamin, K.M. and Malik, H.E.E. (2013) Effect of dietary garlic (*Allium sativum*) supplementation as feed additive on broiler performance and blood profile. *Anim. Sci. Adv.*, 3(2): 58-64.

9. Tazi, S.M.E., Mukhtar, M.A., Mohamed, K.A. and Tabidi, M.H. (2014) Effect of using black pepper as natural feed additive on performance and carcass quality of broiler chicks. *J. Pharm. Res. Anal.*, 4(2): 108-113.

10. Ademola, S.G. (2004) Growth, hematological and biochemical studies on garlic and ginger-fed broiler chicken. *Moor J. Agric. Res.*, 5(2): 122-128.

11. Doley, S., Gupta, J.J. and Reddy, P.B. (2009) Effect of supplementation of ginger, garlic and turmeric in broiler chicken. *Indian Vet. J.*, 86: 644-645.

12. A.O.A.C. (1995) Official Methods of Analysis. 16th ed. Association of Official Analytical Chemists, Arlington, Virgina, USA.

13. B.I.S. (1992) Nutrient Requirement for Poultry. Bureau of Indian Standards, I.S., New Delhi.

14. Wolfe, K., Wu, X. and Liu, R.H. (2003) Antioxidant activity of apple peels. *J. Agric. Food Chem.*, 51: 609-614.

15. Singleton, V. and Rossi, J.A. (1965) Colorimetry of total phenolics with phosphomolybdic - Phosphotungstic acid reagents. *Am. J. Enol. Viticult.*, 16(3): 144-158.

16. Shivakumar, B.S., Ramaiah, M., Hema, M.R., Vijay Kumar, M. and Vaidya, V.P. (2012) Quantitative determination of total content of phenol, flavonoid and tannin in leaf extract of *Barlaria Buxifolia* Linn. *Am. J. PharmTech. Res.*, 2(5): 418-422.

17. Sellappan, S. and Akoh, C.C. (2002) Flavonoids and antioxidant capacity of Georgia grown Vidalia onions. *J. Agric. Food Chem.*, 50(19): 5338-5342.

18. McDonald, S., Prenzler, P.D., Antolovich, M. and Robards, K. (2001) Phenolic content and antioxidant activity of olive extracts. *Food Chem.*, 73: 73-84.

19. Chang, C.C., Yang, M.H., Wen, H.M. and Chern, J.C. (2002) Estimation of total flavonoid content in propolis by two complementary colorimetric methods. *J. Food Drug Anal.*, 10: 78-182.

20. Meraj, I.C.A. (1998) Effect of garlic and neem leaves supplementation on the performance of broiler chickens. M.Sc., Thesis, Department of Poultry Sciences, University of Agriculture, Faisalabad, Pakisthan.

21. Geetha, M., Suneel, K.R., Krupanidhi, A.M., Muralikrishna, K.S., Avin, A.P. and Prashanth, P. (2011) Effect of fenugreek on total body and organ weights: A study on mice. *Pharm. Online*, 3: 747-752.

22. Mansoub, N.H. (2011) Comparison of using different level of black pepper with probiotic on performance and serum composition of broiler chickens. *J. Basic Appl. Sci. Res.*, 1(11): 2425-2428.

23. Akbarian, A., Golian, A., Kermanshahi, H., Gilani, A. and Moradi, S. (2012) Influence of turmeric rhizome and black pepper on blood constituents and performance of broiler chickens. *J. Biotechnol.*, 11(34): 8606-8611.

24. Shahverdi, A., Kheiri, F., Faghani, M., Rahimian, Y. and Rafiee, A. (2013) The effect of use red pepper (*Capsicum annum* L.) and black pepper (*Piper nigrum* L.) on performance and hematological parameters of broiler chicks. *Eur. J. Zoo Res.*, 2(6): 44-48.

25. Ghaedi, H., Nasr, J., Kheiri, F., Miri, Y. and Rahimian, Y. (2013) Effect of use virginiamycin as probiotic, black pepper extract as phytogenic feed additive on performance of broiler chicks. *Sch. J. Agric. Sci.*, 3(12): 521-525.

26. Al-Kassie, G.A.M., Mamdooh, A.M.A. and Saba, J.A. (2011) Use of black pepper (*Piper nigrum*) as feed additive in broilers diet. *Res Opin Anim. Vet. Sci.*, 1(3): 169-173.

27. Valiollahi, M.R., Rahimian, Y., Miri, Y. and Rafiee, A. (2013) Effect use ginger (*Zingiber officinale*), black pepper (*Piper Nigrum L*) powders on performance, some blood parameters and antibody titer against new castle vaccine on broiler chicks. *Sch. J. Agric. Sci.*, 3(12): 535-540.

28. Elkhair, R.A., Ahmed, H.A. and Selim, S. (2014) Effects of black pepper (*Piper nigrum*), turmeric powder (*Curcuma longa*) and coriander seeds (*Coriandrum sativum*) and their combinations as feed additives on growth performance, carcass traits, some blood parameters and humoral immune response of broiler chickens. *Asian Aust. J. Anim. Sci.*, 27(6): 847-854.

29. Raeesi, M., Aliabad, S.A.H., Roofchaee, A., Shahneh, A.Z. and Pirali, S. (2010) Effect of periodically use of garlic (*Allium sativum*) powder on performance and carcass characteristics in broiler chickens. *World Acad. Sci. Eng. Technol.*, 68: 1213-1219.

18

Analysis of viral protein-2 encoding gene of avian encephalomyelitis virus from field specimens in Central Java region, Indonesia

Aris Haryanto[1], Ratna Ermawati[1], Vera Wati[2], Sri Handayani Irianingsih[3] and Nastiti Wijayanti[4]

1. Department of Biochemistry, Faculty of Veterinary Medicine, Universitas Gadjah Mada, Yogyakarta, Indonesia;
2. Division of Biotechnology, Animal Disease Investigation Center Wates, Daerah Istimewa Yogyakarta Province, Indonesia; 3. Division of Virology, Animal Disease Investigation Center Wates, Daerah Istimewa Yogyakarta Province, Indonesia; 4. Department of Animal Physiology, Faculty of Biology, Universitas Gadjah Mada, Yogyakarta, Indonesia.
Corresponding author: Aris Haryanto, e-mail: arisharyanto@yahoo.com, arisharyanto@ugm.ac.id, RE: ratna. ermawati@yahoo.com, VW: verawatisutopo@gmail.com, SHI: handa_nie@yahoo.com, NW: nastitiw@yahoo.com

Abstract

Aim: Avian encephalomyelitis (AE) is a viral disease which can infect various types of poultry, especially chicken. In Indonesia, the incidence of AE infection in chicken has been reported since 2009, the AE incidence tends to increase from year to year. The objective of this study was to analyze viral protein 2 (VP-2) encoding gene of AE virus (AEV) from various species of birds in field specimen by reverse transcription polymerase chain reaction (RT-PCR) amplification using specific nucleotides primer for confirmation of AE diagnosis.

Materials and Methods: A total of 13 AEV samples are isolated from various species of poultry which are serologically diagnosed infected by AEV from some areas in central Java, Indonesia. Research stage consists of virus samples collection from field specimens, extraction of AEV RNA, amplification of VP-2 protein encoding gene by RT-PCR, separation of RT-PCR product by agarose gel electrophoresis, DNA sequencing and data analysis.

Results: Amplification products of the VP-2 encoding gene of AEV by RT-PCR methods of various types of poultry from field specimens showed a positive results on sample code 499/4/12 which generated DNA fragment in the size of 619 bp. Sensitivity test of RT-PCR amplification showed that the minimum concentration of RNA template is 127.75 ng/μl. The multiple alignments of DNA sequencing product indicated that positive sample with code 499/4/12 has 92% nucleotide homology compared with AEV with accession number AV1775/07 and 85% nucleotide homology with accession number ZCHP2/0912695 from Genbank database. Analysis of VP-2 gene sequence showed that it found 46 nucleotides difference between isolate 499/4/12 compared with accession number AV1775/07 and 93 nucleotides different with accession number ZCHP2/0912695.

Conclusions: Analyses of the VP-2 encoding gene of AEV with RT-PCR method from 13 samples from field specimen generated the DNA fragment in the size of 619 bp from one sample with sample code 499/4/12. The sensitivity rate of RT-PCR is to amplify the VP-2 gene of AEV until 127.75 ng/μl of RNA template. Compared to Genbank databases, isolate 499/4/12 has 85% and 92% nucleotide homology.

Keywords: avian encephalomyelitis, reverse transcription polymerase chain reaction, viral protein 2 gene.

Introduction

Avian encephalomyelitis (AE) is a viral disease which can infect chickens, especially young chickens, birds, quails and turkeys [1-3]. The incidence of AE in Indonesia has been reported since 2009, namely in Lampung Province, Banten Province, Central Java Province, Yogyakarta Province and East Kalimantan Province on Indonesia. In general, the clinical symptoms in infected chickens are ataxia, incoordination, paralysis, and rapid tremor of the head and neck. Transmission of AE virus (AEV) infection generally occurs through infected eggs (egg transmission) and

fecal-oral route [2]. AE incidence is always accompanied by a drastic decrease of egg production in laying hens and an increase in morbidity and mortality up to 80%. AEV infection may also increase the susceptibility of poultry to other infection agents, therefore, it is extremely harmful, especially in the commercial layer and broiler industry.

AEV causes disease in poultry worldwide, and flocks must be vaccinated for protection. Based on its protein composition, AEV is most closely related to those of hepatitis A virus (HAV) [4]. AEV is a member of the family Picornaviridae, which is classified into six genus, *Enterovirus, Rhinovirus, Cardiovirus, Aphthovirus, Hepatovirus,* and *Parechovirus* [5]. Member of the family Picornaviridae consists of small positive sense single-stranded RNA genome of more than 9.243 nucleotides excluding poly(A) tail, the kind of viruses which are capable of infecting various vertebrate species, including birds [6,7]. Chicken are an important reservoir for diverse picornaviruses that may cross avian species barriers through mutation and recombination [8]. AEV could be detected as a novel picornavirus in domesticated common quail (*Coturnix coturnix*) [9] while the novel turkey picornaviruses have been reported to be metagenomically detected, and the complete genome is characterized in fecal samples from healthy and affected turkeys in Hungary and USA [10,11].

Viral particles AEV has a diameter of 24-32 nm, non-enveloped with a sedimentation co-efficient of 148 Svenberg. AEV consists of 7.032 nucleotides, single sequence and open reading frame (ORF) that encodes a large polyprotein. It has four structural proteins in the region of P1 (VP-4, VP-2, VP-3, VP-1) and seven nonstructural proteins in P2 and P3 regions. Gene that encodes viral protein 2 (VP-2) in AEV is a more conserve and it does not have any similarity with VP-2 gene of other viruses [12]. Therefore, the use of a specific primer with VP-2 gene target is a more appropriate for diagnosis of AE disease than other genes. VP-1 protein is a major host-protective immunogenic against AEV challenge and demonstrates further that the antibody raised against VP-1 protein could neutralize AEV infection the more effective than antibody against the VP-3 or VP-0 protein in a virus neutralization (NV) test. Based on its sensitivity and specificity, it is indicated that VP-1 protein has a highly promising and reliable diagnostic potential and a suitable antigen for enzyme-linked immunosorbent assay (ELISA) detection of AEV antibodies in chickens [13].

In the field, the diagnosis of AE is still quite difficult, because a lot of poultry disease have very similar clinical symptoms, such as Newcastle Disease (ND), Marek's Disease, Ricketsia, deficiency of B1 and B2 vitamins, *Aspergillosis, Salmonellosis, Coccidiosis, Omphalitis,* and *Mycoplasmosis.* Diagnosis of the disease is still confusing, and the serological tests do not show any difference between various kinds of AEV isolates [2]. A variety of diagnostic methods has been developed to diagnose AEV, which include AEV isolation using intracerebral inoculation into day old chicken, inoculation and propagation into embryonated fowl eggs (yolk sac). The serological diagnosis has also been developed such as hemagglutination (HA) test, complement fixation (CF), indirect fluorescence antibody, ELISA, VN, and agar gel precipitation (AGP) [14]. Serological test by ELISA for detection of antibodies against AEV in the chicken serum is prone to errors due to blood samples mishandling, such as heat treatment, repetitive freezing and thawing and hemolysis severity so it can affect ELISA results [15]. In commonly occurring and economically influential poultry disease, such as infectious bronchitis (IB), chicken anemia (CA) and AE, the commercially available ELISAs are routinely used as diagnostic tools to determine whether an individual bird or a flock has been previously exposed to IBV, CAV, or AEV [16]. Besides that, a rapid non-radioactive digoxigenin DNA probe is used to detect AEV.

This probe hybridized specially with a DNA fragment of VP-1 gene with the sensitivity rate as little as 10 pg of targeted DNA fragment [17]. However, these diagnostic methods still have weakness and deficiencies, namely requiring a long time and skilled laboratory personnel, cross-reaction, false positive or false negative, less sensitive and expensive.

The routine AEV diagnosis which is performed in the laboratory is serological tests, by using HA test, HI test, and CF test (CFT) to detect the presence of antibodies against the hemagglutinin protein. Another laboratory test is AGP test. Serological methods are less effective in poultry because poultry is often infected by other viruses which have the same protein. Some viruses are often found to have some serotypes and genotypes so that the sensitivity and specificity of these tests are low [18]. Another diagnostic method is routinely performed by viral isolation from embryonated chicken eggs.

Although serological test and virus isolation from embryonated chicken egg have a high specificity and sensitivity, they have some disadvantages, such as taking long time, requiring modern laboratory facilities, requiring skilled human resources, and high cost. Molecular-based diagnostic method has some advantages in terms of rapidly, sensitivity and specificity to diagnose viral diseases [19].

The objective of this research was to analyze VP-2 encoding gene of AEV from various species of birds in field specimen by reverse transcription polymerase chain reaction (RT-PCR) amplification using specific nucleotides primer for confirmation of AE diagnosis. By this molecular method, it was expected to detect AEV rapidly, accurately and sensitively. It could be confirmed the differential diagnosis of AE in the field specimen and commercially poultry industry, it could be used as a basic study for viral disease surveillance and molecular epidemiology study in poultry diseases.

Materials and Methods

Ethical approval

AEV isolates were propagated and approved by the ethical committee in Animal Disease Investigation Center (ADIC) in Wates, Yogyakarta. All laboratory protocols and research procedures were supervised and approved by the ethical committee in Laboratorium Penelitian dan Pengujian Terpadu (LPPT), Universitas Gadjah Mada, Yogyakarta, Indonesia.

Virus samples

The virus samples were collected from field specimens by ADIC in Wates, Yogyakarta, Indonesia during the period 2011-2012. AEV were isolated from brain organ of chickens showing neurologic symptoms such as tremor and ataxia. They were inoculated and propagated into the yolk sac of 9-11 days old specific antibody negative embryonated chicken eggs. After 3-5 days post-inoculation, the embryos were removed from eggs. The embryo brains were harvested and collected into phosphate buffered saline (PBS) pH. 7.2, then they were homogenized by a sterile homogenizer. The homogenized brain tissues were then centrifuged at 14.000 rpm for 1 h. The supernatant was collected as a viral suspension for viral RNA extracting. The list of AEV isolates are presented in Table-1.

Research materials and primer for RT-PCR

The main research materials of this study consists of High Pure Viral Nucleic Acid Kit (cat. no: 11-858-874-001) from Roche, SuperScript™ III One-Step RT-PCR with Platinum Taq (cat. no: 12574-026) from Invitrogen, UltraPure™ agarose gel from (cat. no:16500-100) from Invitrogen, 1x Buffer Tris base-Boric acid-EDTA, PBS, RedSafe nucleic acid dye from Intron, aquabidest, distilled water, Blue Loading dye (cat. no: 10816-015), 1 kb DNA Ladder (cat. no: 29,278,801) from Promega, and the specific oligonucleotide primers (Table-2).

Viral RNA extraction

Extraction of AEV RNA was performed by High Pure Viral Nucleic Acid Kit based on standard procedures from Roche. A total of 200 µl viral suspension was extracted in 50 µl end volume of viral RNA.

Amplification of VP-2 gene of AEV by RT-PCR

Amplification of VP-2 gene of AEV was performed by SuperScript™ III One-Step RT-PCR with Platinum Taq-based on the standard procedure from Invitrogen. RT-PCR amplification which begins by a single cycle of RT at 50°C for 30 min, followed by a pre-denaturation step at 94°C for 2 min. PCR amplification stages consist of three stages: Denaturation at 94°C for 15 s, annealing at 57°C for 30 s, and extension at 68°C for 45 s. Stages of PCR amplification is done repeatedly in 40 cycles. Amplification process was ended by a final extension at 68°C for 5 min. AE

commercial live vaccine is used as a positive control in this amplification, whereas the negative control derived from sterile dH$_2$O contains no virus.

Electrophoresis of RT-PCR products

RT-PCR products were electrophoresed in 1.5% agarose gel (Invitrogen) with RedSafe dye (Intron) staining. Fragments DNA were visualized in the dark room by UV-Transilluminator. The positive result of RT-PCR product from VP-2 gene was indicated as a DNA fragment in the size of 619 bp.

Sensitivity test of RT-PCR

RNA of sample code 499/4/12 was used as template for RT-PCR amplification. Initial RNA concentration of 1022 ng/µl then was adjusted by serial dilution as many as 7 times with the concentration of 1022 ng/µl, 511 ng/µl, 255.5 ng/µl, 127.75 ng/µl, 63.88 ng/µl, 31.94 ng/µl, and 15,97 ng/µl. Then, to determine the sensitivity of RT-PCR, each serial dilution of RNA was used as template for RT-PCR amplification with amplification condition similar to amplification condition for the VP-2 gene of AEV.

DNA sequencing

DNA sequencing to determine the nucleotide sequence of VP-2 gene was carried out in Genetika Science Indonesia Co., by chain termination method (Sanger Method). Then, the DNA sequencing products were analyzed in multiple alignments and compared by the sequence of VP-2 gene of AEV database from Genbank by MEGA 5.05 software program.

Results

In this work, the analysis of VP-2 gene from AEV was conducted using RT-PCR. The amplification product was a fragment DNA in size of 619 bp. Electrophoresis of DNA fragments from RT-PCR products was presented in Figure-1.

Table-1: The AEV isolates from field specimens which were collected from several district in Indonesia.

Sample number	Sample code	Type of bird	Area in Indonesia
1	1341/8/11	Layer	Ambarawa, Semarang
2	1340/8/11	Layer	Tengaran, Semarang
3	17/I/12 (P. 03/I/12)	Layer	Mlati, Sleman
4	1785/X/11	Layer	Karanganyar, Karanganyar
5	499/4/12	Layer	Danurejan, Yogyakarta
6	1443/09/2012	Duck	Sanden, Bantul
7	1428/09/2012	Duck	Gatak, Sukoharjo
8	1132/07/2012	Broiler	Ngaglik, Sleman
9	1019/06/2012	Layer	Karanglewas, Banyumas
10	1018/06/2012	Layer	Laweyan, Surakarta
11	958/06/2012	Layer	Jatinegara, Tegal
12	922/06/2012	Layer	Purwokerto Timur, Banyumas
13	921/06/2012	Layer	Jurang, Temanggung

AEV=Avian encephalomyelitis virus

Table-2: Primer used for amplification of VP-2 gene of AEV [20].

Gene target	Primer sequence	RT-PCR product	Temperature
VP-2 gene	AE-1: 5'-CTTATGCTGGCCCTGATCGT-3'	619 bp	57°C
	AE-2: 5'-TCCCAAATCCACAAACCTAGCC-3'		61°C

VP-2=Viral protein 2, RT-PCR=Reverse transcription polymerase chain reaction, AEV=Avian encephalomyelitis virus

The RT-PCR technique provides a faster and sensitive detection of AEV that might require some days and consecutive passages in cell culture for virus isolation. The application of RT-PCR method in molecular virology research for diagnosis of viral disease is expected to be more widespread. Then, the all 13 virus samples were also analyzed by serological test for detection of avian influenza (AI), ND viruses and molecular tested. The recapitulation of the serological and molecular test was presented in Table-3.

Sensitivity test to the RT-PCR methods was conducted by serial dilution of sample no. 5 with the sample code 499/4/12 by the initial RNA concentration of 1022 ng/μl. The serial dilution was performed 7 times with the concentration of 1022 ng/μl, 511 ng/μl, 255.5 ng/μl, 127.75 ng/μl, 63.88 ng/μl, 31.94 ng/μl, 15.97 ng/μl. The RNA of serial dilution with this certain concentration then was used as a template for RT-PCR amplification. Amplification results using RNA template from serial dilution to determine the sensitivity test of sample code 499/4/12 was shown in Figure-2.

Forward primer consists of 22 nucleotides and reverse primer consists of 20 nucleotides. The length of RT-PCR products was 619 bp, it is in accordance with the findings of the previous Xie et al. [20]. Location of forward primer annealing is into the VP-4 protein encoding gene region, while the location of reverse primer annealing is into the VP-3 protein encoding gene. Scheme of primers annealing and amplified region is presented in Figure-3.

Discussion

Genome of AEV consists of around 7.5 kb with a single ORF encoding of 2.143 amino acids. As the other picornavirus, the ORF of AEV is divided into three regions, namely P1, P2 and P3 region. P1 region, especially encodes VP, VP-1, VP-2, VP-3 and VP-4 [21,22]. VP-1, VP-2, VP-3 and VP-4 proteins of AEV have a molecular weight in size of 43 kDa, 35 kDa, 33 kDa and 14 kDa respectively [1]. In this study, we analyze of VP-2 encoding gene of AEV by

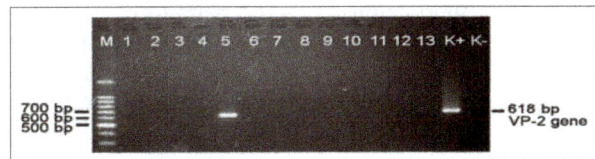

Figure-1: Electrophoresis of avian encephalomyelitis products of viral protein-2 gene from avian encephalomyelitis virus in agarose gel 1.5%. Fragments DNA of amplification products has the size of 619 bp. M is DNA ladder 100 bp, lane 1-13 are samples, K+ is positive control and K− is negative control. Sample No. 5 (sample code 499/4/12) is positive sample.

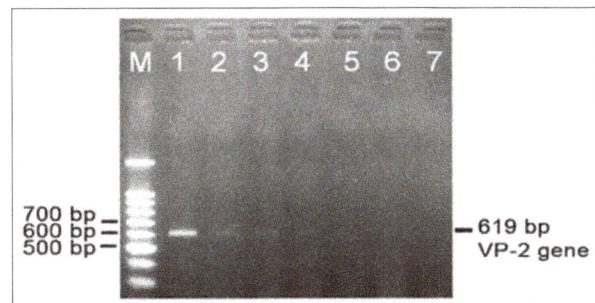

Figure-2: The sensitivity of RT-PCR method for detecting VP-2 gene of avian encephalomyelitis virus using RNA template from serial dilution of sample code 499/4/12 in agarose gel 1.5%. Lane M is marker DNA Ladder, lane 1-7 are number of serial dilution of RNA template with the concentration 1=1022 ng/μl, 2=511 ng/μl, 3=255.5 ng/μl, 4=127.75 ng/μl, 5=63.5 ng/μl, 6=31.94 ng/μl, and 7=15.97 ng/μl respectively.

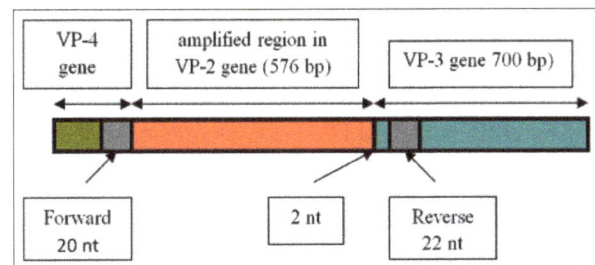

Figure-3: Schema of primers annealing and amplified region in VP-2 encoding gene of AEV.

Table-3: Serological and molecular tests of 13 AEV isolates from field specimens.

Number	Sample code	Serological test	Molecular test (RT-PCR)
1	1341/8/11	AI (+), ND (−)	NT
2	1340/8/11	AI (+), ND (−)	NT
3	17/I/12, (P. 03/I/12)	AI, ND (−)	NT
4	1785/X/11	AI, ND (−)	NT
5	499/4/12	AI, ND (−), AE Suspect	AE (+)
6	1443/09/2012	AI (+), ND (−)	AE, ND (−), H5 (+)
7	1428/09/2012	AI (+), ND (−)	AE (−), ND, H5 (+)
8	1132/07/2012	AI, ND (−)	AE, AI (−)
9	1019/06/2012	AI, ND (−)	AE, AI (−)
10	1018/06/2012	AI, ND (−)	AE (−)
11	958/06/2012	AI, ND (−)	AE (−)
12	922/06/2012	AI (+), ND (−)	AE (−)
13	921/06/2012	AI, ND (−)	AE (−)

NT=Not tested, +=Positive result, -=Negative result, AI=Avian influenza, RT-PCR=Reverse transcription polymerase chain reaction, AEV=Avian encephalomyelitis virus

RT-PCR method using a specific pairs of oligonucleotide primer which were designed previously by Xie et al., [20]. From 13 virus isolate samples of field specimens, a sample in lane 5 (sample code 499/4/12) is positive sample with clear DNA fragment of RT-PCR product in size of 619 bp, whereas 12 others samples from field specimens have no DNA fragment of RT-PCR product. Perhaps, these samples are not infected by AEV but infected by other avian pathogens or infectious agents, which have similar clinical symptom with AE. In lane K+ (positive control) also indicated DNA fragment in size 619 bp, this positive control originates from live vaccine AEV (CEVA). In lane K− (negative control) it is shown that there is no amplification product of VP-2 gene. Amplification products of the VP-2 encoding gene of AEV by RT-PCR methods of various type of poultry from field specimens showed a positive results on sample code 499/4/12 which generated DNA fragment in the size of 619 bp. This amplification results was in accordance with Xie et al. [20] who stated that RT-PCR method can detect AEV in more simple, sensitive and specific ways compared to AEV isolation and various immunologic methods. The use of fecal specimen has also been performed by Farkas et al. [23], who collected swabs and litter extracts from chickens, domestic ducks, turkeys and Canadian geese to detect novel picornaviruses by RT-PCR amplification, Liao et al. [24] detected and completely sequenced a novel picornavirus from Peking ducks (Anas platyrhynchos domesitica). Liu et al. [25] developed the rapid detection and quantification for AEV by using an SYBR Green real-time RT-PCR method for amplify VP-1 gene. Compared to conventional RT-PCR this method was 100 times more sensitive. It could detect levels as low as 10 standard DNA copies of the AEV from SX strain, so it was effective for AEV diagnosis and surveillance.

In Table-3, a total of 13 field specimen samples were serologically and molecularly tested for possible infection by ND and AI viruses (AIVs). The recapitulation showed that some of the field specimens were negatively infected by ND virus but positively infected by AIV. Molecular test for AEV using ELISA showed that only sample code 499/4/12 is positively infected by AEV, whereas others 12 samples are negative and not infected by AEV.

Then using positive sample (sample code 499/4/12), we further tested the sensitivity of RT-PCR method using serial dilution RNA template for RT-PCR amplification. This sensitivity test using RT-PCR methods was performed by serial dilution of RNA template using sample code 499/4/12. The initial RNA concentration for serial dilution using sample code no 499/4/12 was 1022 ng/μl. The serial dilution was performed 7 times with the concentration of 1022 ng/μl, 511 ng/μl, 255.5 ng/μl, 127.75 ng/μl, 63.88 ng/μl, 31.94 ng/μl, 15.97 ng/μl respectively. The RNA of serial dilution with this certain concentration then was used as template for RT-PCR amplification. Amplification results using RNA template from serial dilution to determine the sensitivity test of sample code 499/4/12 was shown in Figure-2. In this study, the sensitivity of RT-PCR method is 127.75 ng/μl, while according to Haryanto et al. [26] was 10 pg/μl. This result difference may due to differences in the conditions of field sample purity, method difference of viral RNA extraction and different conditions for RT-PCR amplification.

Manoharan et al. [27] have conducted PCR sensitivity tests to assess of VP-1 gene of CA virus (CAV) using three different primer sets. This study proved that PCR method is a useful technique for CAV DNA detection in field specimen, this study also demonstrates that the field CAV detection limit could be extended further to the level of detecting subclinical infection due to the use of the most sensitive primer. RT-PCR method was also performed to directly amplify from field specimens of fusion (F) protein encoding genes of NDV [26], the matrix (M) and hemaglutinin (H5) protein encoding genes of AIV H5N1 subtype [28], and viral protein-2 (VP-2) encoding gene of infectoius bursal disease virus (IBDV) [29].

Based on the RT-PCR product for sensitivity test by serial dilution of RNA template of sample code 499/4/12 (Figure-3). The sensitivity of RT-PCR amplification could be obtained until 4 times serial dilution which produced as little as 127.75 ng/μl of RNA template. It showed that the sensitivity of RT-PCR for amplification of VP-2 gene of AEV by serial dilution of RNA sample as template was high. That means a small amount of RNA template which was extracted directly from field specimens could be well amplified and visualized as a clear DNA fragment in agarose gel.

In this study, we did not have field samples from young birds of less than 4 weeks, because in this collecting period, all collected field samples derived from adults birds with neurological symptoms. There is a marked age resistance to clinical signs in birds exposed after they are 2-3 weeks of age. The clinical signs in exposed young chicks to have a minimum incubation period of 10-11 days, at the same time, that VN antibodies can be detected in adult birds [2]. Infection of AEV in mature birds may experience a temporary drop in egg production (5-10%) but it did not develop to the neurological symptoms [30].

Specificity of nucleotide primers used in this work was shown by DNA sequencing products of positive sample which was then analyzed using NCBI BLAST program. This analysis showed that nucleotides primers for amplification of VP-2 gene of this work has 92% homology to the AEV isolate (accession number AV1775/0/), and 85% identical to the AEV strain (accession number ZCHP2/0912695). It is indicated that RT-PCR method is specific to identify AEV from field specimen. Welchman de et al. [31] reported that AEV infecting pheasants were distinct from AEV infecting chickens. RT-PCR amplification for detecting of AEV in a non-standard host species should be supported by the appearance of the minimal lesion in central nervous system. Apart from that, immunohistochemistry would have been a useful diagnostic aid to demonstrate AEV in pigeons [32].

Based on the multiple alignments of VP-2 gene of AEV (isolate 499/4/12) in comparing with Genbank database, it found 46 nucleotides difference between 499/4/12 isolate with AV 1775/07 isolate from Genbank, whereas with ZCHP2/0912695 isolate found 93 nucleotides difference. Using MEGA version 5.05 software program, it was shown that positive isolate (499/4/12) is really positive amplification of VP-2 protein encoding gene from AEV. It strengthened the highly homologous nucleotides composition of tested positive sample with Genbank databases.

The common problem for AEV diagnosis is less rapid and time-consuming. The diagnosis of AE in field cases was just based on anamnesis of infected chickens in a flock, histopathological changes, and specific clinical symptoms from the infected chickens. RT-PCR method has advantages compared to other diagnostic methods, in AE cases, amplification of VP-2 gene can detect and identify the presence of AEVes more rapidly and specificcally, especially for field specimen samples. The high specificity and sensitivity of RT-PCR method indicated that this method can be used to detect VP-2 gene of AEV from field specimens. Reagents which are used for RT-PCR amplification can be prepared easily and take less amount. Inoculation and propagation of AEV into embryonated chicken eggs takes a long time, whereas molecular technique such as RT-PCR can provide the result within a day. For diagnosis of AEV, the RT-PCR method is more effective, efficient and specific compared to others diagnostic tests. RT-PCR method targeting VP-2 gene of AEV has some advantages and it is a quantitative diagnostic method, so it can not be used to determine the quantity of infectious agents.

Proper diagnosis of AE disease should be done early and rapidly to prevent the spreading of AEV to poultry that has not been infected yet. Rapid, sensitive and specific method for laboratory diagnosis of AE disease in poultry is needed. Laboratory diagnosis for AEV was conducted by virus isolation into embryonated chicken eggs and various immunological methods which required a lot of money, complicated laboratory apparatus and consumed a lot of time. This study indicated that the RT-PCR method targeting VP-2 gene of AEV can be used to detect and identify AEV from field specimen rapidly, effectively and efficiently so it has provided a significant contribution in AEV detection and AE disease spread control.

Currently, laboratory diagnosis of AE disease is performed by AEV isolation and detection with various immunologic methods that are laborious, highly costly and time-consuming. A rapid, sensitive, and specific method to diagnose of AE disease is still required for diagnosis confirmation. Xie *et al*. [20]

have developed an RT-PCR method for AEV detection which is simple to employ as well as sensitive and specific.

Conclusion

Analyses of the VP-2 encoding gene of AEV with RT-PCR method from 13 samples from field specimen generated the DNA fragment in the size of 619 bp from one sample with sample code 499/4/12. The sensitivity rate of RT-PCR is to amplify the VP-2 gene of AEV until 127.75 ng/µl of RNA template. Compared to Genbank databases, isolate 499/4/12 has 85% and 92% nucleotide homology.

Authors' Contributions

AH was responsible for the overall stage of research (research preparation, execution, completing), RE did the RT-PCR amplification and phylogenetic analysis, VW did the serological and molecular test, SHI did the virus isolation and MDT quantification, NW drafted and revised the manuscript. All authors contributed to support the research datas, they read and approved the final manuscript.

Acknowledgments

The authors would like to thank Head of the Department of Biochemistry, Faculty of Veterinary Medicine, Universitas Gadjah Mada, Yogyakarta and Head of the Animal Disease Investigation Center (ADIC) in Wates, Daerah Istimewa Yogyakarta Province, Indonesia for the opportunity, virus samples and laboratory facilities to finish this research. This research was supported by research schema of Institutional Collaboration Research Grant (Hibah Penelitian Kerjasama Institusi), LPPM Universitas Gadjah Mada, Yogyakarta 2012, awarded to Aris Haryanto.

Competing Interests

The authors declare that they have no competing interests

References

1. Tannock, G.A. and Shafren, D.R. (1994) Avian encephalomyelitis: A review. *Avian Pathol.*, 23: 603-620.
2. Calnek, B.W., Barnes, J.H., Beard, C.W., Reid, W.M. and Yoder, H.W. (2005) Disease of Poultry. Iowa State University Press, Ames Iowa, USA.
3. Ingram, D.R., Miller, D.L., Baldwin, C.A., Turco, J. and Lockhart, J.M. (2015) Serologic survey of wild turkeys (*Meleagris gallopavo*) and evidence of exposure to avian encephalomyelitis virus in Georgia and Florida, USA. *J. Wildlife Dis.*, 51(2): 374-379.
4. Bakhshesh, M., Groppelli, E., Willcocks, M.M., Royall, E., Belsham, G.J. and Roberts, L.O. (2008) The picornavirus avian encephalomyelitis virus possesses a Hepatitis C virus-like internal ribosome entry site element. *J. Virol.*, 82(4): 1993-2003.
5. Boros, A., Pankovics, P. and Reuters, G. (2014) Avian picornavirus: Molecular evolution, genome diversity and unusual genome features of a rapidly expanding group of virus in birds. *Infect. Genet. Evol.*, 28: 151-166.
6. Boros, A., Pankovics, P., Knowles, N.J., Nemes, C.,

Delwart, E. and Reuter, G. (2014) Comparative complete genome analysis of chicken and turkey Megriviruses (family Picornaviridae): Long 3' untranslated regions with a potential second open reading frame and evidence for possible recombination. *J. Virol.*, 88(11): 6434-6443.

7.   Bullman, S.I., Kearney, K., O'Mahony, M., Kelly, L., Whyte, P., Fanning, S. and Morgan, J.G. (2014) Identification and genetic characterization of a novel picornavirus from chickens. *J. Gen. Virol.*, 95(5): 1094-1103.

8.   Lau, S.K., Woo, P.C., Yip, C.G., Li, K.S., Fan, R.Y., Bai, R., Huang, Y., Chan, K.H. and Yuen, K.Y. (2014) Chickens host diverse picornaviruses originated from potential interspesies transmission with recombination. *J. Gen. Virol.*, 95: 1924-1944.

9.   Pankovics, P., Boros, A. and Reuter, G. (2012) Novel picornavirus in domesticated common quail (*Coturnix coturnix*) in Hungary. *Arch. Virol.*, 157(3): 525-530.

10. Boros, A., Nemes, C., Pankovics, P., Kapusinszky, B., Delwart, E. and Reuter, G. (2012) Identification and complete genome characterization of a novel picornavirus in turkey (*Meleagris gallopavo*). *J. Gen. Virol.*, 93(10): 2171-2182.

11. Boros, A., Nemes, C., Pankovics, P., Kapusinszky, B., Delwart, E. and Reuter, G. (2013) Genetic characterization of a novel picornaviruses in turkey (*Meleagris gallopavo*) distinct from turkey galliviruses and megriviruses and distantly related to the members of the genus avihepatovirus. *J. Gen. Virol.*, 94(7): 1496-1509.

12. Buenz, E.J. and Howe, C.L. (2006) Picornaviruses and cell death. *Trends Microbiol.*, 14: 28-36.

13. Wei, L., Chee, L.L., Wei, T., Kwang, J., Zhou, J., Wang, J., Shi, L. and Liu, J. (2008) The VP1 protein of avian encephalomyelitis virus is a major host-protective immunogenic that serves as diagnostic potential. *J. Virol. Methods*, 149(1): 56-62.

14. Xie, Z., Fadl, A.A., Girshick, T. and Khan, M.I. (1999) Detection of avian adenovirus by polymerase chain reaction. *Avian Dis.*, 43: 98-105.

15. Kurian, A., Neumann, E.J., Hall, W.F. and Marks, D. (2012) Effects of blood sample mishandling on ELISA results for infectious bronchitis virus, avian encephalomyelitis and chicken anemia virus. *Vet. J.*, 192(3): 378-381.

16. Pattison, M., Mc Mullin, P.F., Bradbury, J.M. and Alexander, D.J. (2008) Poultry Diseases. Saunders Elsevier, Philadelphia, USA.

17. Wie, L., Zhou, J., Wang, J., Shi, L. and Liu, J. (2008) Development of a non-radioactive digoxigenin cDNA probe for the detection of avian encephalomyelitis virus. *Avian Pathol.*, 37(2): 187-191.

18. Fenner, F.J., Gibbs, E.J., Frederick, A.M., Rott, R., Michael, J.S., White, D.O. (1993) Veterinary Virology. 2nd ed., Vol. 29. Academic Press, Inc., San Diego. p511-515.

19. Gavin, P.J. and Thomson, R.B. (2003) Review of rapid diagnostic tests for influenza. *Clin. Appl. Immunol. Rev.*, 4: 151-172.

20. Xie, Z., Khan, M.I., Girshick, T. and Xie, Z. (2005) Reverse transcriptase-polymerase chain reaction to detect avian encephalomyelitis virus. *Avian Dis.*, 49: 227-230.

21. Marvil, P., Knowles, N.J., Mockett, A.P.A., Britton, P., Brown, T.D.K. and Cavanagh, D. (1999) Avian encephalomyelitis virus is a picornavirus and is most closely related to hepatitis A virus. *J. Gen. Virol.*, 80: 653-662.

22. Wei, L., Liu, J., Yao, W.G., Zhang, F.L. and Zhou, J. (2004) Determination of the whole genome of avian encephalomyelitis virus isolate in China. *Chin. J. Virol.*, 20: 230-236.

23. Farkas, T., Fey, B., Hargitt, E., Parcells, M., Ladman, B., Murgia, M. and Saif, Y. (2012) Molecular detection of novel picornaviruses in chickens and turkeys. *Virus Genes*, 44(2): 262-272.

24. Liao, Q., Zheng, L., Yuan, Y., Shi, J. and Zhang, D. (2014) Molecular characterization of a novel picornavirus in Pekin ducks. *Vet. Microbiol.*, 172(1-2): 78-91.

25. Liu, Q., Yang, Z., Hao, H., Cheng, S., Fan, W., Du, E., Xiao, S., Wang, X. and Zhang, S.J. (2014) Development of a SYBR Green real-time RT-PCR assay for the detection of avian encephalomyelitis virus. *J. Virol. Methods*, 206: 46-50.

26. Haryanto, A., Kristiawan, D., Irianingsih, S.H. and Yudianingtyas, D.W. (2013) Amplification of fusion protein encoding gene of Newcastle Disease Virus from field specimens by onestep RT-PCR method. *J. Vet.*, 14(3): 387-393.

27. Manoharan, A.S., Ramadas, P. and Kumanan, K. (2012) Assessment of polymerase chain reaction sensitivity for the detection of chicken anaemia virus using different primers for three genes. *Vet. Arch.*, 82(1): 89-102.

28. Haryanto, A., Krisanti, B., Irianingsih, S.H. and Yudianingtyas, D.W. (2012) Molecular diagnosis of avian influenza virus A subtipe H5N1 based on amplification of M and H5 genes by onestep simplex RT-PCR method. *J. Vet.*, 13(2): 92-101.

29. Haryanto, A., Irianingsih, S.H., Yudianingtyas, D.W., Wijayanti, N. and Budipitojo, T. (2013) Single step multiplex RT-PCR for detection and differential diagnosis of avian influenza virus, newcastle disease and infectious bursal disease viruses in chicken. *Int. Res. J. Biotechnol.* 4(2): 34-39.

30. Calnek, B.W. (2008) Avian encephalomyelitis. In: Saif, Y.M., Fadly, A.M., Glisson, J.R., Mc Douglas, L.R., Nolan, L.K., Swayne, D.E., editors. Diseases of Poultry. 12th ed. Wiley-Blackwell, Ames, IA, USA. p430-441.

31. Welchman de, B.D., Cox, W.J., Gough, R.E., Wood, A.M., Smyth, V.J., Todd, D. and Spackman, D. (2009) Avian encephalomyelitis virus in reared pheasants: A case study. *Avian Pathol.*, 38(3): 251-256.

32. Toplu, N. and Alcigir, G. (2004) Avian encephalomyelitis in naturally infected pigeons in turkey. *Avian Pathol.*, 33: 381-386.

19

Histomorphological studies of broiler chicken fed diets supplemented with either raw or enzyme treated dandelion leaves and fenugreek seeds

Saim Qureshi[1], Mohammed Tufail Banday[1], Irfan Shakeel[1], Sheikh Adil[1], Masood Saleem Mir[2], Yasir Afzal Beigh[3] and Umar Amin[2]

1. Division of Livestock Production and Management, Faculty of Veterinary Sciences and Animal Husbandry, Sher-e-Kashmir University of Agricultural Sciences & Technology of Kashmir, Shuhama - 190 006, Srinagar, Jammu and Kashmir, India; 2. Division of Veterinary Pathology, Faculty of Veterinary Sciences and Animal Husbandry, Sher-e-Kashmir University of Agricultural Sciences & Technology of Kashmir, Shuhama - 190 006, Srinagar, Jammu and Kashmir, India; 3. Division of Animal Nutrition, Faculty of Veterinary Sciences and Animal Husbandry, Sher-e-Kashmir University of Agricultural Sciences & Technology of Kashmir, Shuhama -190 006, Srinagar, Jammu and Kashmir, India.
Corresponding author: Sheikh Adil, email: aadilsheikh5@gmail.com,
SQ: s.qureshi619@gmail.com, MTB: mtbanday5@gmail.com, IS: erfaanshakeel3@gmail.com,
MSM: masoodmir11@gmail.com, YAB: vetyasir10@gmail.com, UA: umaramin146@gmail.com

Abstract

Aim: Herbal plants and their derived products are extensively used particularly in many Asian, African, and other countries of the world as they are considered as ideal feed additives because of their non-residual effect and ability to influence the ecosystem of gastrointestinal microbiota in a positive way. Further, the enzymatic treatment of these herbs helps in their efficient utilization by the host. Dandelion leaves and fenugreek seeds have been reported to have positive effect in terms of improving the performance of broiler chicken, but not much literature is available regarding their effect on gut histomorphology; therefore, the present study was conducted to explore the effect of these herbs either alone or in combination with or without enzyme treatment on histomorphology of liver and small intestine of broiler chicken.

Materials and Methods: To achieve the envisaged objective, 273-day-old commercial broiler chicks were procured from a reputed source and reared together until 7 days of age. On the 7th day, the chicks were individually weighed, distributed randomly into 7 groups of 3 replicates with 13 chicks each. Birds in the control group were fed diets without additives (T_1). The other six treatment groups were fed the basal diet supplemented with 0.5% dandelion leaves (T_2), 1% fenugreek seeds (T_3), combination of 0.5% dandelion leaves and 1% fenugreek seeds (T_4), enzyme treated dandelion leaves 0.5% (T_5), enzyme treated fenugreek seeds 1% (T_6), and combination of enzyme treated dandelion leaves (0.5%) and (1%) fenugreek seeds (T_7). The histomorphological study of liver and small intestines was conducted among different treatment groups.

Results: The results revealed the hepato-protective nature of both dandelion leaves and fenugreek seeds either alone or in combination with or without enzyme treatment when compared with the control group. Moreover, the histomorphological findings of jejunum revealed the beneficial effect of dandelion leaves, fenugreek seeds and enzymes on the intestinal mucosa in terms of cellular infiltration, architecture of villi, villus height/crypt depth ratio, thereby improving the intestinal health.

Conclusion: The dandelion leaves and fenugreek seeds have hepato-protective nature and beneficial effect on the intestinal morphology particularly when included along with enzymes in the diet of broiler chicken.

Keywords: broiler chicken, dandelion, fenugreek, histomorphology.

Introduction

Phytogenics are a group of natural growth promoters or non-antibiotic growth promoters derived from herbs, spices, or other plants. Compared with synthetic antibiotics or inorganic chemicals, these plant-derived products have proven to be safe, less toxic, residue free and are thought to be ideal feed additives in food animal production. Phytogenic feed additives have gained increasing interest, especially for their application in poultry diets [1]. They beneficially affect the ecosystem of gastrointestinal microbiota through controlling potential pathogens and improving digestive capacity in the small intestine and stabilizing the microbial eubiosis in the gut [2]. The herbal plant extracts help in the alteration of intestinal microbiota, increase of enzyme secretion, improvement of the immune response, and histomorphological maintenance of the gastrointestinal tract [3].

Kashmir, often referred to as paradise on earth, is located at the northwestern tip of Himalayan biodiversity hotspot [4]. The region supports a rich and spectacular plant biodiversity of great scientific curiosity and promising economic benefits. Among the herbal flora available in the region, two herbal plants, i.e., dandelion leaves (*Taraxacum officinale*) and seeds of fenugreek (*Trigonella foenum-graecum*) were utilized for the study of the diets of the broiler chicken. Dandelion is a well-known medicinal plant that grows in nature in Asia, Europe, and North America [5]. The roots of the herb are primarily considered for supporting digestion and liver function, while as its leaves are used as diuretic and digestive stimulant [6]. Fenugreek is grown mainly in India, Pakistan, and China. Its seeds have many therapeutical effects such as hypoglycemic, anti-helminthic, anti-inflammatory, and anti-microbial properties [7]. It also contains lecithin and choline that help to dissolve cholesterol and fatty substances. It also contains neurin, biotin, and trimethylamine which tends to stimulate the appetite by their action on the nervous system [8]. The dietary supplementation of dandelion leaves and fenugreek seeds have been reported to increase the performance of broiler chicken [9-11]. Enzyme supplementation in poultry diets has been reported to improve the performance [12] by degrading non-starchy polysaccharides, improving the digestion and absorption of nutrients [13], and improving their intestinal morphology [14].

Since, dandelion leaves and fenugreek seeds were reported to have positive effect in terms of improving the performance of broiler chicken, but not much literature is available regarding their effect on gut histomorphology; therefore, the present study was conducted to explore the effect of these herbs either alone or in combination with or without enzyme treatment on histomorphology of liver and small intestine of broiler chicken.

Materials and Methods

Ethical approval

The study was conducted after approval of research committee and institutional ethical committee.

Methodology

273-day-old commercial broiler chicks procured from a reputed source were utilized for the study which lasted 42 days. Chicks were reared in battery cages until 7 days of age. During this period, all the birds were provided with a pre-starter mash (23% crude protein and 2800 Kcal/kg metabolizable energy). Birds had free access to feed and water throughout and were maintained on a constant 24 h light schedule. On the 8th day, the chicks were individually weighed, distributed into seven treatment groups of three replicates with 13 chicks in each in a completely randomized design so that the treatment means differ as little as possible. Birds in the control group were fed diets without additives (T_1). The other six treatment groups were fed the basal diet supplemented with 0.5% dandelion leaves (T_2), 1% fenugreek seeds (T_3), combination of 0.5% dandelion leaves and 1% fenugreek seeds (T_4), enzyme treated dandelion leaves 0.5% (T_5), enzyme treated fenugreek seeds 1% (T_6), and combination of enzyme treated dandelion leaves (0.5%) and (1%) fenugreek seeds (T_7). The diets were formulated to meet the recommendations of the Bureau of Indian standards [15]. Dandelion leaves (*T. officinale*) and fenugreek seeds (*T. foenum-graecum*) were procured, dried and in powder form mixed thoroughly in aforesaid quantities to a small amount of feed (1 kg) in a premixer. The resultant mixture was then mixed with the rest of the feed in a mechanical blender until a thorough and consistent mixture was obtained. All chicks were vaccinated against Ranikhet disease on the 5th day with F1 strain vaccine and infectious bronchitis virus-95 vaccine against infectious bursal disease on the 16th day. Chicks were checked twice daily for mortality if any. Birds were kept under the same managerial, hygienic, and environmental conditions.

Parameters recorded

For the histopathological analysis, the tissue samples from liver (main organ of biotransformation) jejunum (main site for absorption) were collected from the slaughtered birds (6 birds per treatment) at the end of experimental period (42 days) and fixed in 10% buffered formalin saline. Tissues were dehydrated by immersing through a series of alcohols of increasing concentrations (from 70% to absolute), infiltrated with xylene, and embedded in paraffin. The casting of blocks was carried out in L-molds (two L-shaped pieces) which facilitated the manipulation of size as per the requirement. The rotary type microtome was used for cutting the paraffin sections. The blocks were properly trimmed, and the sections of 5 mm thickness were cut. Continuous ribbons (6-7 inches long) of the material were cut and laid on the surface of constant temperature water bath (around 55°C). The sections were separated with a heated scalpel after they spread completely. The cut sections were mounted on the clean glass slides using Mayer's egg albumin as the section adhesive. The mounted slides were dried in paraffin oven at 60°C for 1 h. The tissue sections were stained by the Harris hematoxylin and eosin staining method. The paraffin sections were deparaffinized with the xylene before hydration through graded alcohol to distilled water. This was followed by the dehydration in ascending grades of alcohol. The clearing was performed in the xylene, and a drop of distrene plasticizer xylene mountant was placed on a coverslip and the section on the slide pressed on it. The slide was inverted, and the cover slip was pressed with a rod to remove the air bubbles if any trapped. The values were measured with an oculometer at a magnification of ×10 under a light microscope fitted with the stage micrometer.

Results

Liver

The histomorphological examination of liver from the control group (T_1) showed a mild degree of hepatocellular degeneration with occasional distortion of hepatic cords associated with Kupffer cell hyperplasia. Frequently marked mononuclear cell infiltration was observed in perivascular area and occasional heterophil forming aggregates of various sizes were noted in the liver parenchyma (Figures-1 and 2). Compared to control, T_2 group had occasional and only mild perivascular mononuclear cell infiltration (Figure-3). The T_3 group showed less hepatocellular degeneration, Kupffer cell hyperplasia and perivascular mononuclear cell infiltration and occasional heterophil aggravate in the parenchyma, but the changes were less severe than the control group (Figure-4). Liver from T_4 showed hepatocyte regeneration (Figure-5), T_5 (Figure-6), and T_6 (Figure-7) had less hepatocellular degenerative changes and diffuse inflammatory cell infiltration. The Group T_7 showed normal architecture and beneficial effect on liver (Figure-8).

Small intestine

The histological examination of jejunum showed an improvement in the jejunal villus height (p<0.05) and villus height/crypt depth ratio in all the groups fed dandelion leaves and fenugreek seeds with or without enzyme treatment compared to control (Table-1). The control group (T_1) showed mucous degeneration of glandular epithelium at certain places, diffuse infiltration of inflammatory cells, predominantly heterophils in mucosa in addition to clubbing of villi (Figures-9 and 10). The T_2 group had normal villus architecture with mild cellular infiltration in mucosa and sub-mucosa; occasional clubbing of villi with less severe infiltration of inflammatory cells than control group was noted (Figure-11). The Group T3 revealed an increase in thickness and height of villi as compared to control

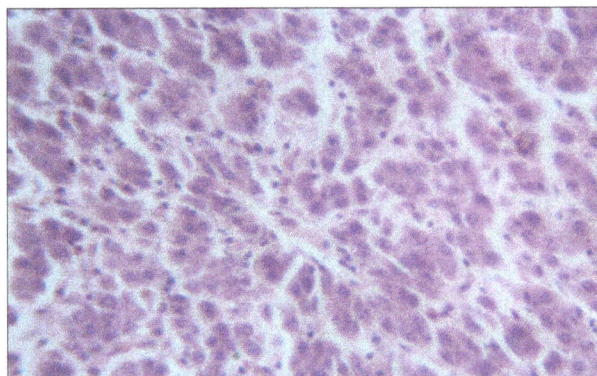

Figure-1: Liver from control group (T_1) showing mild degree of inflammation with occasional Kupffer cell hyperplasia and distortion of hepatic cords (H and E, ×4).

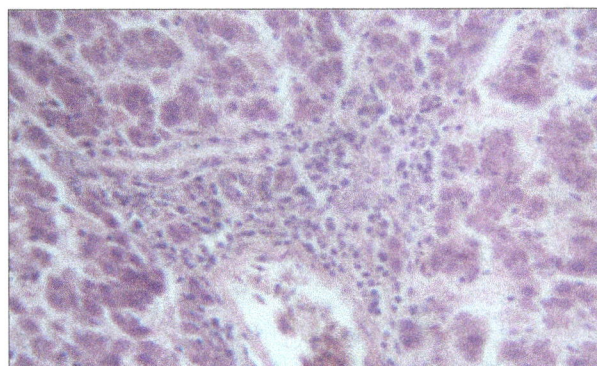

Figure-2: Liver from control group (T_1) showing heterophil aggregates (H and E, ×4).

Table-1: Effect of dandelion leaves and fenugreek seeds on jejunal histomorphology of broiler chicken.

Parameter	Treatments						
	T_1	T_2	T_3	T_4	T_5	T_6	T_7
Villus height (μm)	995.7±14.55[a]	1019.4±10.24[ab]	1032.3±11.54[abc]	1064.2±12.53[cd]	1042.3±8.48[bc]	1038.0±14.87[bc]	1088.3±5.93[d]
Crypt depth (μm)	158.3±3.27	156.4.1±1.54	157.7±5.32	152.4±5.68	155.6±4.97	152.4.±5.91	151.1±3.05
Villus height/crypt depth ratio	6.29±0.07	6.51±0.10	6.55±0.15	7.01±0.35	6.71±0.24	6.83±0.32	7.20±0.13

Means within the same row with different superscripts are significantly different (p<0.05)

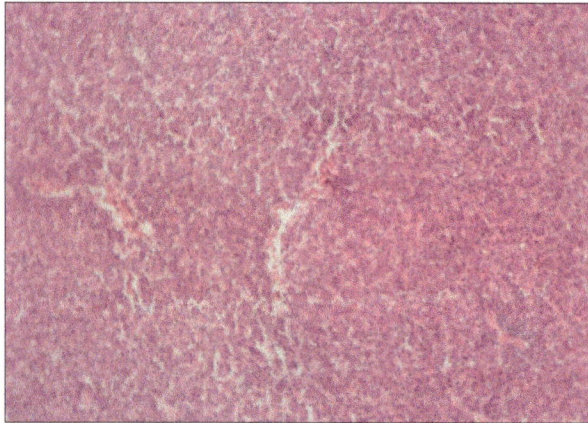

Figure-3: Liver from T_2 showing occasional and only mild perivascular mononuclear cell infiltration (H and E, ×4).

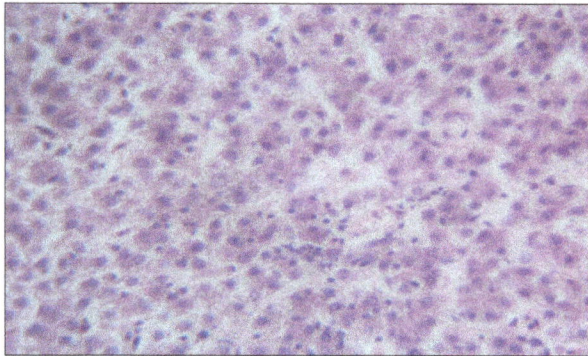

Figure-4: Liver from T_3 showing less Kupffer cell hyperplasia and perivascular mononuclear cell infiltration (H and E, ×4).

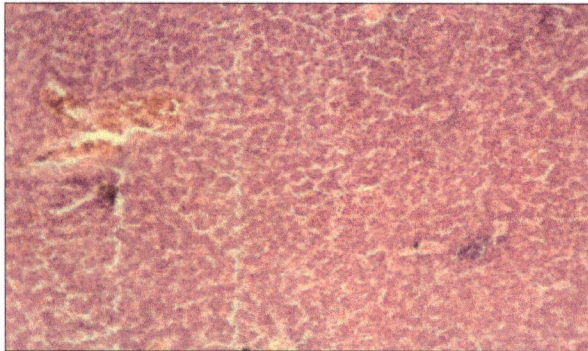

Figure-5: Liver from T_4 showing hepatocyte regeneration and less heterophil infiltration (H and E, ×4).

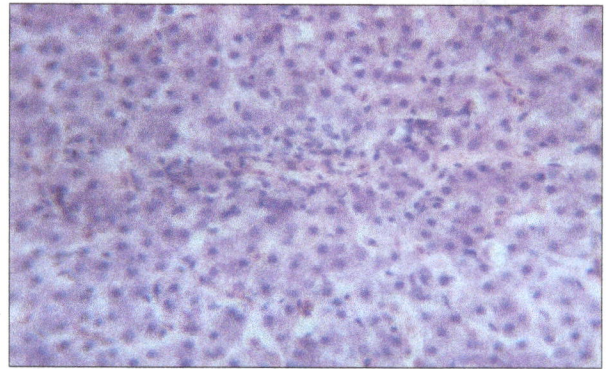

Figure-6: Liver from T_5 showing less hepatocellular degenerative changes and diffuse inflammatory cell infiltration (H and E, ×4).

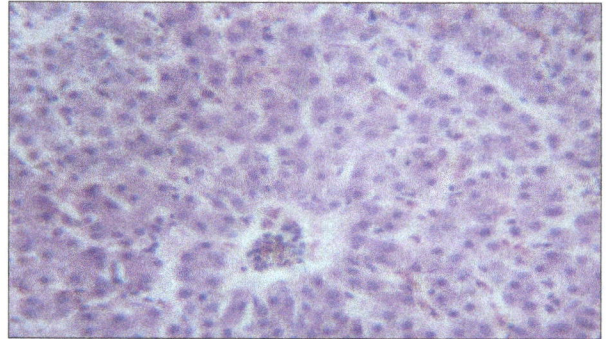

Figure-7: Liver from T_6 showing less hepatocellular degenerative changes and diffuse inflammatory cell infiltration (H and E, ×4).

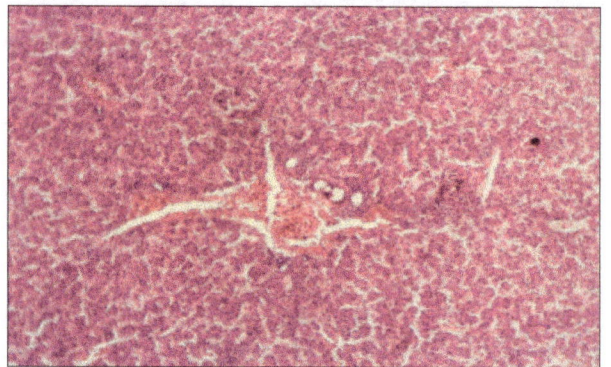

Figure-8: Liver from T_7 showing normal architecture and beneficial effect on liver (H and E, ×4).

and mild cellular infiltration with occasional distortion of villi was also observed (Figure-12). Compared to control, T_4 showed normal villus architecture and increase in height of villi (Figure-13). Jejunum from T_5, T_6, and T_7 had normal villus architecture, increase in height of villus and occasional areas of cellular infiltration than T_1 (Figures-14-16).

Discussion

Liver

The histological examination of liver in different treatment groups revealed the hepato-protective role of both dandelion leaves and fenugreek seeds. There

was increased hepato-regeneration in the treatment groups where dandelion leaves and fenugreek seeds were supplemented in the diet when compared to the control group. Further, there was a decrease in Kupffer cell hyperplasia and perivascular mononuclear cell infiltration. Best results were observed where both dandelion leaves and fenugreek seeds were used along with enzymes (T_7). The results of the present study coincide with the results of Park *et al*. [16], Tabassum *et al*. [17], Al-Malki *et al*. [18], and Gulfraz *et al*. [19] who reported the hepato-protective role of dandelion leaves. Likewise, fenugreek seeds have also been reported to have a hepato-protective impact [20,21]. The hepato-protective role of dandelion leaves might

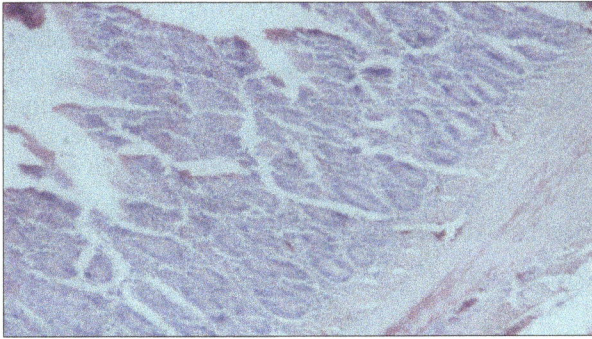

Figure-9: Jejunum from control group (T$_1$) showing mucous degeneration of glandular epithelium at certain places (H and E, ×2.5).

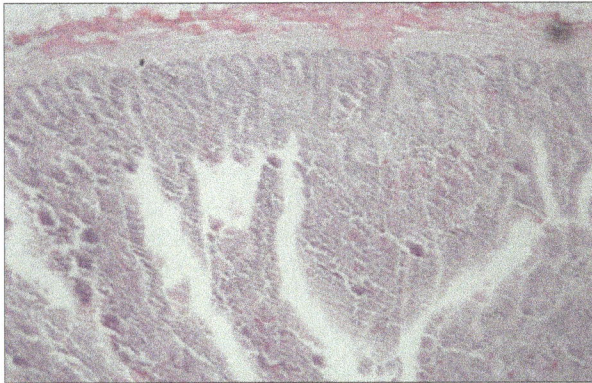

Figure-12: Jejunum from T$_3$ showing normal villus architecture with increase in thickness of villus, less and occasional areas of distortion (H and E, ×2.5).

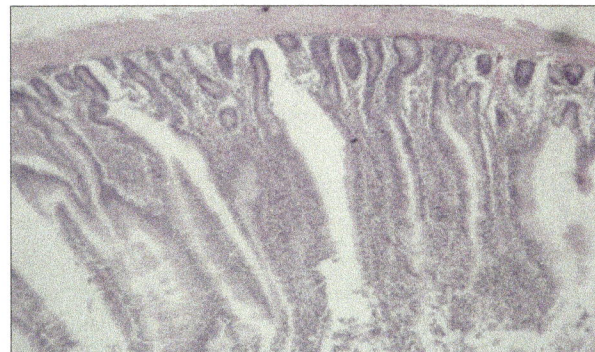

Figure-10: Jejunum from control group (T$_1$) showing diffuse infiltration of inflammatory cells, predominantly heterophils and clubbing of villi (H and E, ×2.5).

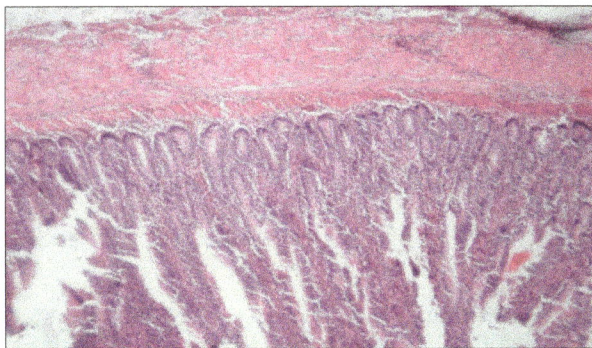

Figure-13: Jejunum from T$_4$ showing normal villus architecture, increase in height of villi (H and E, ×2.5).

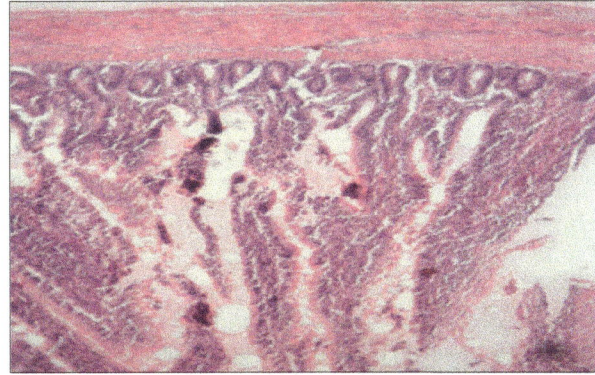

Figure-11: Jejunum from T$_2$ showing normal villus architecture with mild cellular infiltration in mucosa and sub-mucosa (H and E, ×2.5).

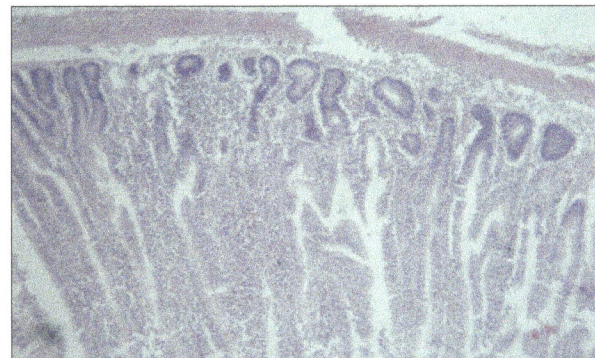

Figure-14: Jejunum from T$_5$ showing normal villus architecture, increase in height of villus, occasional areas of cellular infiltration (H and E, ×2.5).

be attributed to the bioactive components present in it such as Vitamins (A, C, thiamine, and riboflavin), sesquiterpene lactones, triterpenes, carotenoids (lutein), fatty acids (myristic), and flavonoids (apigenin and luteolin) present in it [17,22,23]. Bitter compounds present in dandelion leaves have been reported to increase the production of bile from gall bladder thereby improving the liver function [24]. Further, the hepato-protective role of fenugreek seeds might be attributed to the bioactive ingredients present in it, which enhance hepatic function and due to its antioxidant activity as reported by Bukhari *et al.*, [25] who

reported the antioxidant capacity of the fenugreek extracts.

Small intestine

The histological examination of jejunum revealed an improvement in villus height, villus height/crypt depth ratio, and less mononuclear cellular infiltration in all the groups fed either dandelion leaves or fenugreek seeds alone or in combination with or without enzyme treatment when compared with the control group. Best results were obtained in the treatment group where the combination of enzyme treated dandelion leaves and fenugreek seeds were used. Increased villus height helps to enhance the absorptive surface area for better

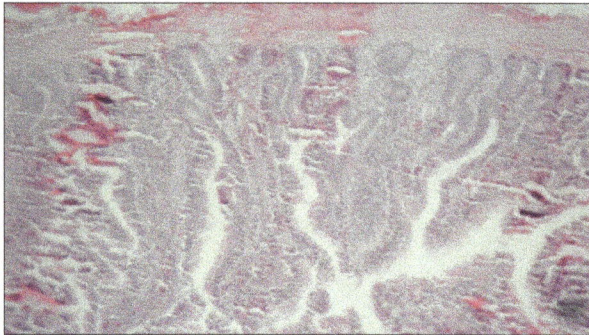

Figure-15: Jejunum from T$_6$ showing thickening of villi and increase in height of villi (H and E, ×2.5).

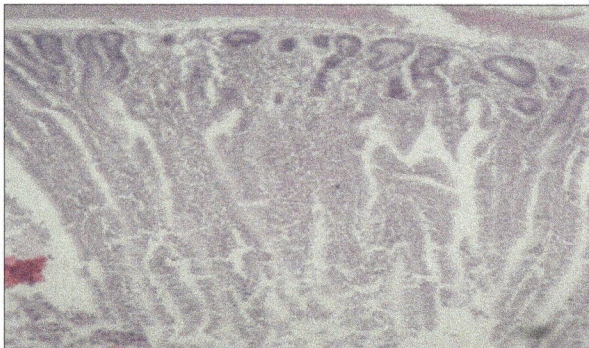

Figure-16: Jejunum from T$_7$ showing normal villus architecture with increase in thickness and height of villus, occasional areas of cellular infiltration compared to control group (H and E, ×2.5).

utilization of nutrients as reported by Adil *et al.* [26] with the use of feed additives in broiler chicken. Similarly, Abdel-Rahman *et al.* [27] and Debnath *et al.* [28] reported that the supplementation of herbal products in the diet of broiler chicken enhance intestinal villus height and surface area, resulting in better intestinal health. The short or damaged villi impair the absorption of the intestine, which might lead to poor performance of birds [29]. In addition, enzyme supplementation has been reported to improve villus height and villus height/crypt depth ratio in poultry [14,30]. Moreover, in the present study, the jejunal crypt depth decreased non-significantly in the treatment groups compared to control. The crypts are responsible for production of enterocytes required for renewal of villi and the more the crypt is demanded in terms of cell renewal, the greater its depth [31], thus indicating that the villi were not compromised in any way in all the treatment groups fed dandelion leaves and fenugreek seeds either alone or in combination with or without enzyme addition. Furthermore, there was an improvement in the villus height/crypt depth ratio in all the treatment groups which has been regarded as a good indicator of better intestinal health [31]. The beneficial effect on jejunal histomorphology by dandelion leaves and fenugreek seeds might be attributed to their anti-microbial action which in turn has been reported to decreases the inflammatory reactions at the mucosa, thereby increasing the villus height [32,33]. Additional improvement in the intestinal morphology by the addition of enzymes may be because dietary inclusion of the enzymes helps to degrade the non-starch polysaccharides and diminish their negative impact on the gut morphology as they have been reported to suppress the gut morphological development at higher levels [14].

Conclusion

The dandelion leaves and fenugreek seeds have hepato-protective nature and beneficial effect on the intestinal morphology, particularly when included along with enzymes in the diet of broiler chicken.

Authors' Contributions

This study is the part of M.V.Sc. Thesis of the first author SQ, who carried out the research under the guidance of MTB. IS, UA helped during the trial and MSM in the processing of samples. SA provided necessary guidelines during the work and helped in the technical writing of the article. YAB helped in thorough revision of the manuscript. All authors have read and approved the final version of the manuscript.

Acknowledgments

The authors are thankful to the Directorate of Research, Sher-e-Kashmir University of Agricultural Sciences and Technology of Kashmir for providing necessary funding for the work.

Competing Interests

The authors declare that they have no competing interests.

References

1. Windisch, W., Schedle, K., Plitzner, C. and Kroismayr, A. (2008) Use of phytogenic products as feed additives for swine and poultry. *J. Anim. Sci.,* 86: 140-148.

2. Hashemi, S.R. and Davoodi, H. (2010) Phytogenics as new class of feed additive in poultry industry. *J. Anim. Vet. Adv.,* 9(17): 2295-2304.

3. Brugalli, I. (2003) Alternative power: The use of herbal and nutraceutical as modulators of immunity and animal performance. In: Symposium on Management and Nutrition Poultry and Pigs, Campinas. Proceedings: Brazilian Animal Nutrition College. p167-182.

4. Husain, M. (2001) Geography of Jammu and Kashmir. Rajesh Publication, New Delhi, India. p28.

5. Malik, H.A., Khuroo, A.A. and Dar, G.H. (2011) Ethnomedicinal uses of some plants in the Kashmir Himalayas. *Indian J. Tradit. Knowl.,* 10(2): 362-366.

6. Mir, M.A., Sawhney, S.S. and Jassal, M.M.S. (2013) Qualitative and quantitative analysis of phytochemicals of *Taraxacum officinale. Wudpeck. J. Pharm. Pharmacol.,* 2(1): 1-5.

7. Bash, E., Ulbricht, C., Kuo, G. and Smith, M. (2003) Therapeutic applications of fenugreek. *Altern. Med. Rev.,* 8: 20-27.

8. Michael, D. and Kumawat, D. (2003) Legend and Archeology of Fenugreek, Constitutions and Modern Applications of Fenugreek Seeds. International Symposium, USA. p41-42.

9. Galib, A.M., Al-Kassi, A. and Noor, M.W. (2010) A

Comparative study on diet supplementation with a mixture of herbal plants and dandelion as a source of prebiotics on the performance of broilers. *Pak. J. Nutr.,* 9(1): 67-71.

10. Rabia, J.A. (2010) Effect of using fenugreek, parsley and sweet basil seeds as feed additives on the performance of broiler chickens. *Int. J. Poult. Sci.,* 9(3): 278-282.

11. Raziq, F., Khan, S., Naila, C. and Asad, S. (2012) Effect of water based infusion of *Lycium, Aloe barbedensis, Pimpinella anisum, Berberis Trigonella foenum-graecum* and *Allium sativum* on the performance of broiler chicks. *Pak. Vet. J.,* 32(4): 593-596.

12. Yousuf, S., Banday, M.T., Adil, S., Salahuddin, M. and Rehman, M. (2012) Efficacy of enzyme and yeast supplements on performance of broiler chicken fed high fiber diets. *Indian J. Anim. Sci.,* 82(4): 410-414.

13. Tufarelli, V., Dario, M. and Laudadio, V. (2007) Effect of xylanase supplementation and particle-size on performance of guinea fowl broilers fed wheat-based diets. *Int. J. Poult. Sci.,* 6: 302-307.

14. Ayoola, A.A., Malheiros, R.D., Grimes, J.L. and Ferket, P.R. (2015) Effect of dietary exogenous enzyme supplementation on enteric mucosal morphological development and adherent mucin thickness in Turkeys. *Front. Vet. Sci.,* 2(45): 1-8.

15. BIS (1992). Poultry Feeds Specification. 4th Revision. Bureau of Indian Standards. New Delhi, pp. 4.

16. Park, C., Yusi, Z. and Youngsun, S. (2007) Hepatoprotective effect of Dandelion *(Taraxacum officinale)* against acute liver injury induced by carbon tetrachloride in Sprague-Dawley rats. *Fed. Am. Soc. Exp. Biol.,* 21(1): 862.

17. Tabassum, N., Shah, M.Y. and Qazi, M.A. (2010) Prophylactic activity of extract of *Taraxacum officinale* against hepatocellular injury induced in mice. *Pharmacol. Online.,* 2: 344-352.

18. Al-Malki, A., Kamel, A.A., Gamal, A. and Hassan, A. (2013) Hepatoprotective effect of dandelion *(Taraxacum officinale)* against induced chronic liver cirrhosis. *J. Med. Plants Res.,* 7(20): 26-35.

19. Gulfraz, M., Dawood, A. and Sheeraz, A. (2014) Effect of leaf extracts of *Taraxacum officinale* on CCl₄ induced hepatotoxicity in rats, *in vivo* study. *Pak. J. Pharm.,* 27(4): 825-829.

20. Onera, A., Cihat, U., Mercan, H., Onturkb, H. and Cengizc, R. (2008) Anti-inflammatory and hepatoprotective activities of *Trigonella foenum-graecum. Pharmacol. Online.,* 2(1): 126-132.

21. Eman, A. (2011) Pathological and biochemical studies on the effect of *Trigonella foenum-graecum* and *Lupinus termis* in alloxan induced diabetic rats. *World Appl. Sci. J.,* 12(10): 1839-1850.

22. Schmidt, M. (1979) The delightful Dandelion. *J. Organ. Gard.,* 26: 112-117.

23. Jackson, B.S. (1982) The lowly dandelion deserves more respect. *Can. Geogr. Mag.,* 102: 54-59.

24. Jassim, M.N., Safanah, A.F. and Omar, M.N. (2012) Identification of dandelion *Taraxacum officinale* leaves components and study its extracts effect on different microorganisms. *J. Al-Nahrain Univ.,* 15(3): 7-14.

25. Bukhari, S.A., Bhanger, M.I. and Shahabuddin, M. (2008) Antioxidative activity of extracts from fenugreek seeds *(Trigonella foenum-graecum). Pak. J. Anal. Environ. Chem.,* 9(2): 78-83.

26. Adil, S., Banday, M.T., Bhat, G.A., Mir, M.S. and Rehman, M. (2010) Effect of dietary supplementation of organic acids on performance, intestinal, histomorphology and serum biochemistry of broiler chicken. *Vet. Med. Int.,* 2010: 479485, 1-7.

27. Abdel-Rahman, H.A., Fathallah, S.I. and Helal, A.A. (2014) Effect of turmeric (*Curcuma longa*), fenugreek *(Trigonella foenum-graecum* L.) and/or bioflavonoid supplementation to the broiler chicks diet and drinking water on the growth performance and intestinal morphometeric parameters. *Glob. Vet.,* 12(5): 627-635.

28. Debnath, B.C., Choudhary, K.B.D., Ravikanth, K., Thakur, A. and Maini, S. (2014) Comparative efficacy of natural growth promoter with antibiotic growth promoter on growth performance and intestinal morphometry in broiler birds. *Int. J. Pharmacol. Sci. Health Care,* 4: 155-168.

29. Samanya, M. and Yamauchi, K. (2002) Histological alteration of intestinal villi in chickens fed dried *Bacillus subtilis var natto. Comp. Biochem. Physiol.,* 133(4): 95-104.

30. Luo, D., Yanga, F., Yang, X., Yao, J., Shi, B. and Zhou, Z. (2009) Effects of xylanase on performance, blood parameters, intestinal morphology, microflora and digestive enzyme activities of broilers fed wheat-based diets. *Asian-Aust. J. Anim. Sci.,* 22(9): 1288-1295.

31. Petrolli, T.G., Albino, L.F.T., Rostagno, H.S., Gomes, P.C., Tavernari, F. and Balbino, E.M. (2012) Herbal extracts in diets for broilers. *R. Bras. Zootech.,* 41(7): 1683-1690.

32. Loddi, M.M., Moraes, V.M.B., Nakaghi, L.S.O., Tucci, F.M., Hannas, M.I. and Ariki, J.A. (2004) Mannan oligosaccharide and organic acids on performance and intestinal morphometric characteristics of broiler chickens. In: Proceedings of the 20th Annual Symposium. p45.

33. Mahmood, S., Rehman, A., Yousaf, M., Akhtar, P., Abbas, G., Hayat, K., Mahmood, A. and Shahzad, M.K. (2015) Comparative efficacy of different herbal plant's leaf extract on haematology, intestinal histomorphology and nutrient digestibility in broilers. *Adv. Zool. Bot.,* 3(2): 11-16.

20

Test day variability in yield and composition of Surti and Mehsani buffaloes milk at day 15 and 60 postpartum

K. K. Tyagi[1], B. P. Brahmkshtri[2], U. V. Ramani[3], V. B. Kharadi[1], G. M. Pandaya[2], M. Janmeda[2], K. J. Ankuya[4], M. D. Patel[1] and L. M. Sorathiya[1]

1. Livestock Research Station, Navsari Agricultural University, Navsari, Gujarat, India; 2. Department of Animal Genetics and Breeding, College of Veterinary Sciences, Navsari Agricultural University, Navsari, Gujarat, India; 3. Department of Animal Biotechnology, College of Veterinary Sciences, Navsari Agricultural University, Navsari, Gujarat, India; 4. Livestock Research Station, Sardarkrushinagar Dantiwada Agricultural University, Sardarkrushinagar, Gujarat, India.
Corresponding author: K. K. Tyagi, e-mail: naulrs@gmail.com,
BPB: bpbkhatri@gmail.com, UVR: umedramani@yahoo.co.in, VBK: vishnukharadi2@gmail.com,
GMP: gmp2004@gmail.com, MJ: mamtajanmeda@yahoo.co.in, KJA: ankuya@rediffmail.com,
MDP: drmanish911@yahoo.com, LMS: lmsorthiya@yahoo.co.in

Abstract

Aim: To estimate individual test day variability in yield and composition of Surti and Mehsani buffaloes milk at day 15 and 60 postpartum (pp).

Materials and Methods: A total of 13 normally calved Surti and Mehsani buffaloes each maintained at Livestock Research Stations of Navsari and Sardarkrushinagar Dantiwada Agricultural Universities, respectively, were selected for the study. Milk sample was collected from each selected buffalo at day 15 and 60 pp to study milk yield and composition variability between these two breeds. Buffaloes were categorized for the ease of data analysis and comparisons into four groups, viz., S15 (Surti buffaloes 15th day pp), S60 (Surti buffaloes 60th day pp), M15 (Mehsani buffaloes 15th day pp), and M60 (Mehsani buffaloes 60th day pp).

Results: There were 37.20% and 25.03% significant ($p \leq 0.05$) increase in mean test day milk yield (TDMY) of S60 and M60 as compared to S15 and M15 groups, respectively. The mean TDMY of Mehsani buffalo was 99.19% and 81.53% significantly ($p \leq 0.05$) higher than Surti buffaloes at day 15 and 60 pp, respectively. The mean fat and protein corrected test day milk yield (FPCTDMY) of all the groups was found to be significantly different ($p \leq 0.05$) from each other. There was significant ($p \leq 0.05$) increase of 1.94 and 3.45 kg in mean FPCTDMY with the progression of lactation between day 15 and 60 pp in Surti and Mehsani buffaloes, respectively. Similarly, the mean FPCTDMY of Mehsani buffaloes were approximately double with 103.27% and 96.36% higher yield as compared to Surti buffaloes at day 15 and 60 pp, respectively. Among milk composition, significant differences were observed for solid not fat (SNF) and protein%, whereas fat and lactose% were steady among four groups. The only significant ($p \leq 0.05$) difference was observed for SNF in M60 group, which was 8.29%, 6.85%, and 10.70% higher as compared to S15, S60, and M15 groups, respectively. The mean protein% in milk of Mehsani buffaloes was 21.01% and 33.05% significantly ($p \leq 0.05$) higher than Surti buffaloes milk at day 15 and 60 pp, respectively. However, there was a significant difference in protein% observed with the advancement of lactation in Mehsani buffaloes, but it was not so in the case of Surti buffaloes.

Conclusion: Major consistent finding of the present study reveals that milk yield and protein% of Mehsani buffalo was significantly higher than Surti buffalo at day 15 and 60 pp.

Keywords: buffalo, Mehsani, milk composition, milk yield, Surti.

Introduction

Buffaloes are imperative sources of edible milk for human consumption in several parts of the world including India. The current buffalo population in India as per latest 19th livestock census is 108.7 million which accounts for 21.23% of the total livestock population [1]. Gujarat had around 9.55% contemporary buffalo population of the country and bestowed with high milk producing breeds. Milk production in India grew at an annual growth rate of 5.0% and reached a volume of 127.9 million tons milk in the year 2011-2012 [2]. Buffalo was the prime contributor with 58.34% share to the total milk pool in Gujarat state [3]. Genetic improvement for milk production remained precedence of animal breeders for which they primarily utilize milk yield records.

One of the important milk yield records is test day milk yield (TDMY). Individual test date effect is one of the key advantages of using TDMY records. It becomes much more vital when gene expression studies interrelated to milk yield is sought by investigators on a particular day. Similarly, it is indispensable to know bioactive constituents of milk for maximum value addition. The composition of buffalo milk is mainly determined by fat, protein, solid not fat, (SNF) and lactose. Buffalo milk is characterized by higher solids contents for being a richer source of lipids, protein, lactose, and minerals.

Genetic variability remained the prime focus of breeders to explore reasons for differential production potential among different breeds. Keeping this in view, Surti and Mehsani buffalo breeds maintained at organized farms of state agricultural universities in their breeding tract were selected for the present study. The experiment was designed to understand TDMY and composition dynamics during early lactation in Surti and Mehsani buffaloes at organized farms situated in their home tracts.

Materials and Methods

Ethical approval

The prior approval from the Institutional Animal Ethics Committee was obtained for the use of Surti and Mehsani buffalo breeds maintained at Livestock Research Stations of Navsari and Sardarkrushinagar Dantiwada Agricultural Universities, respectively.

Selection of experimental animals

About 13 normally calved Surti and Mehsani buffaloes each maintained at Livestock Research Stations of Navsari and Sardarkrushinagar Dantiwada Agricultural Universities, respectively, were selected for the study. Milk samples were collected repeatedly from the same buffaloes at 15th and 60th day postpartum (pp). Buffaloes were categorized for the ease of data analysis and interpretations into four groups, viz., S15 (Surti buffaloes 15th day pp), S60 (Surti buffaloes 60th day pp), M15 (Mehsani buffaloes 15th day pp), and M60 (Mehsani buffaloes 60th day pp).

Sample collection

Whole milk sample from each selected animal was collected during milking into a sterile bucket, and milk yield was determined using electronic balance. 50 ml aliquot was taken in polypropylene tube and was subjected to milk composition analysis immediately after collection.

Estimation of parameters

TDMY in kg was calculated by combining morning and evening milk yield of collection day. Cumulative milk yield in first 15 (CMY15) and 60 days pp (CMY60) was calculated by summing up TDMY of first 15 and 60 days pp, respectively. Milk composition of samples such as milk protein, fat, and SNF and lactose% was analyzed using Lactoscan milk analyzer as per manufacturer instructions. Fat and protein corrected TDMY (FPCTDMY) was calculated by correcting TDMY to 4.0% fat and 3.3% protein using the formula:

$$FPCTDMY (kg)=TDMY (kg)\times[0.337+(0.116 \times fat\%)+(0.06\times protein\%)] [4]$$

Statistical analysis

The data on milk yield and milk composition was subjected to statistical analysis using Statistical Package for Social Sciences (SPSS, Version 20.0) software. Descriptive statistics specifying mean ± standard error of mean, highest and lowest value were calculated for each group. One-way ANOVA procedure was undertaken to compare means. *Post-hoc* multiple comparisons were made using Duncan multiple new range test. Independent sample t-test was used for two-group comparisons. Bivariate correlations were calculated using Pearson correlation coefficient. The size of correlation (very high, high, moderate, low, and negligible) was interpreted as per the standard classification [5].

Results and Discussion

TDMY

The TDMY recorded in present study ranged from 2.00 to 5.50 kg, 4.10 to 7.40 kg, 5.16 to 10.59 kg, and 6.49 to 12.52 kg among S15, S60, M15, and M60 groups, respectively. There were 37.20% and 25.03% significant (p≤0.05) increase in mean TDMY of S60 and M60 as compared to S15 and M15 groups, respectively. The mean TDMY of Mehsani buffalo was 99.19% and 81.53% significantly (p≤0.05) higher than Surti buffaloes at day 15 and 60 pp, respectively. This may be attributed to the superiority of genes accountable for milk production in Mehsani buffaloes compared to Surti buffaloes. In this context, the subsistence of the Mehsana breed in North Gujarat, India had been reported way back to 1940s. These buffaloes were obtained through selection of cross-bred buffaloes having characteristics intermediate between Surti and Murrah [6,7]. The genetic preeminence of Murrah buffalo breed for milk yield in comparison to other buffalo breeds had been advocated by several authors [8-10]. Thus, higher milk yield in Mehsani buffaloes in comparison to Surti buffaloes may partially be credited to introgression of higher milk-producing genes from Murrah buffaloes into this breed and their ensuing fixation in gene pool. Steady significant increase in milk yield was observed from 15th day (2nd week) to 60th day (9th week) in Surti and Mehsani buffaloes with the progression of lactation. The similar steady increasing trend of TDMY with 5.52±0.06 kg in 2nd week to 7.90±0.06 kg in 9th week of lactation had been reported in Murrah buffaloes [9]. Milk production was also found to augment between days 16 and 60 (11.35 kg/head) in Mediterranean buffaloes [11]. Similarly, a raise of 6.63 kg in weekly milk yield from 2nd week (29.64 kg) to 9th week (36.27 kg) had also been reported in Nagpuri buffaloes [12].

Fat and protein corrected test day milk yield (FPCTDMY)

The mean FPCTDMY of all the groups was found to be significantly different (p≤0.05) from each other. The range of FPCTDMY observed among S15, S60, M15, and M60 groups was 2.84-7.60, 5.66-9.64, 7.41-15.21, and 10.06-18.47 kg, respectively. There was significant (p≤0.05) increase of 1.94 and 3.45 kg in mean FPCTDMY with the advancement of lactation between day 15 and 60 pp in Surti and Mehsani buffaloes, respectively. Correspondingly, the mean FPCTDMY of Mehsani buffaloes were almost double with 103.27% and 96.36% higher yield as compared to Surti buffaloes at day 15 and 60 pp, respectively. The mean FPCTDMY reflected genuine milk yield irrespective of protein and fat contents of the milk because these two major factors were corrected using a formula [4]. The mean FPCTDMY was 40.16%, 40.28%, 43.03%, and 51.73% higher as compared to mean TDMY of S15, S60, M15, and M60 groups, respectively. This can be due to higher protein and fat% in Surti and Mehsani buffaloes milk compared to normalized values used in correction formula. The percent increase for mean FPCTDMY compared to mean TDMY was higher in Mehsani buffaloes because of their plausibly higher protein and fat% increase with progression of lactation (Table-1).

Cumulative milk yield of first 15 and 60 days

The CMY15 had ranged from 28.26-87.14 to 73.25-134.15 kg among Surti and Mehsani buffaloes, respectively. The lowest to highest CMY60 observed among Surti and Mehsani buffaloes were 172.06-384.44 kg and 364.58-641.45 kg, respectively. The mean CMY15 and CMY60 of Mehsani buffalo were just about 87% significantly (p≤0.05) higher than Surti buffalo. Higher, mean CMY60 (313.89 kg) had been reported in Surti buffaloes maintained at Livestock Research Station, Vallabhnagar, Rajasthan [13]. This may be ascribed to variation in various non-genetic factors such as location, period of study, size of data sets, and parity. In the present study, the CMY15 and CMY60 were also significantly higher in Mehsani as compared to Surti buffaloes. These findings were in agreement with the higher standard lactation yield of 1984.17±81.78 kg reported for Mehsani buffaloes [14] as compared to 1450.07±43.99 kg of Surti buffaloes [15]. Lactation yield of 1610 kg (1308-1838) was also reported for Mehsani buffaloes under Indian conditions [16]. Average milk production of around 2000 kg per lactation with lactation length of 315 days in Mehsani buffaloes had also been cited [17]. The higher cumulative milk yield in Mehsani buffaloes compared to Surti buffaloes may be endorsed to

various genetic and non-genetic factors as discussed previously for similar differences observed in TDMY and FPCTDMY in these two breeds.

Milk composition

The milk composition in Surti and Mehsani buffaloes at different stages of lactation was analyzed. While reviewing, it was observed that data pertaining to milk yield at different lactation stages were available; however, very few studies had described composition traits around day 15 and 60 pp. Accordingly, data obtained in the present study have been discussed about the overall and stage wise composition data available in different lactation studies.

Fat%

The fat% was found to be steady without any notable significant differences among the four groups. The fat% ranged from 6.23% to 7.92%, 6.52% to 8.82%, 6.46% to 7.99%, and 6.92% to 8.80% in milk of S15, S60, M15, and M60 groups, respectively. In the present study, the mean fat% among S15, S60, M15, and M60 groups was in the range of 7.2-7.79%. The mean fat% among the groups did not differ significantly. The mean fat% data observed under this study was higher than earlier published reports of 6.17% and 6.46% for Surti and Mehsani buffaloes [18]. However, fat% reported in the present study was lower than 8.59%, 8.10%, and 8.40% fat reported for water buffaloes in Italy [19], Turkey [20], and Europe [21], respectively. Some of the reports of lower fat (6.59%) as compared to present study were also reported in Mediterranean breed [22]. Complementary to our results, significantly higher fat content (8.64%) at the end of the peak production period in Mediterranean buffaloes was also been reported [11]. Compared to four groups of present study, the higher fat contents of 8.71% [23] and 9.01% [24] were also reported in Mediterranean buffaloes. Nevertheless, comparable fat (7.0-7.7%) was reported in other several studies [25-29].

SNF%

The lowest SNF% observed was 9.30%, 9.25%, 6.46%, and 8.83% among milk of S15, S60, M15, and M60 groups, respectively. The highest SNF% observed was 10.45%, 10.38%, 10.15%, and 11.27%

Table-1: Mean milk yield and composition traits of Surti and Mehsani buffaloes at day 15 and 60 postpartum.

Traits/Groups	S15	S60	M15	M60	F/t values
N	13	13	13	13	
TDMY (kg)	3.71[a]±0.26	5.09[b]±0.26	7.39[c]±0.45	9.24[d]±0.48	42.43**
FPCTDMY (kg)	5.20[a]±0.37	7.14[b]±0.35	10.57[c]±0.62	14.02[d]±0.71	52.69**
CMY15 (kg)	52.04[a]±4.00	-	97.27[b]±5.33	-	6.79**
CMY60 (kg)	-	255.55[a]±14.60	-	477.52[b]±24.46	7.79**
Fat%	7.34±0.11	7.39±0.20	7.2±0.14	7.79±0.16	2.63
SNF%	9.65[a]±0.09	9.78[a]±0.10	9.44[a]±0.14	10.45[b]±0.17	11.48**
Protein%	3.57[a]±0.04	3.51[a]±0.04	4.32[b]±0.05	4.67[c]±0.07	124.14**
Lactose%	5.12±0.07	5.24±0.09	5.07±0.06	5.32±0.08	2.20

**significant at p≤0.01, N=Number of observations. Means bearing different superscripts between groups differed significantly. TDMY=Test day milk yield, FPCTDMY=Fat and protein corrected test day milk yield, CMY15=Cumulative milk yield in first 15 days pp, CMY60=Cumulative milk yield in first 60 days pp, SNF=Solid not fat

among milk of S15, S60, M15, and M60 groups, respectively. The only significant (p≤0.05) difference was observed in the M60 group which was 8.29, 6.85, and 10.70% higher as compared to S15, S60, and M15 groups, respectively. Mean SNF content obtained in milk of S15, S60, and M15 groups in our experiment was nearly similar to mean SNF of 9.57±0.03% during the first month reported in Murrah buffaloes [30]. However, in contrast to the present study, they reported a decrease in mean SNF to 9.38±0.03% in successive second month. The mean SNF of 9.4-9.5% roughly similar to that of M15 group had been reported in Murrah buffaloes of Punjab [31] and Swamp buffaloes of Bangladesh [32]. Although, mean SNF of 9.9% that comes in between the mean SNF% reported in the present study for S60 and M60 was also reported in Bulgarian buffaloes [33]. The higher mean SNF of 10.45% had been observed for the M60 group in the present study. Earlier a range of 9.8-10.1% SNF had been reported for Egyptian buffaloes [34], which was nearly comparable to the SNF% reported in the present study among S60 and M60 group. Mean SNF of 8.3% compared to all four groups of present study had also been reported in non-descript buffaloes reared at high altitudes in the Kumaon hills of the central Himalayas [35]. Similarly, mean SNF of 9.2% had also been reported in water buffaloes of Bangladesh [32]. The only reference of high SNF% comparable to that of M60 group was cited in Brazilian buffaloes producing milk with 10.4% SNF [22].

Protein%

The mean protein% in milk of Mehsani buffaloes was 21.01% and 33.05% significantly (p≤0.05) higher than Surti buffaloes milk at day 15 and 60 pp, respectively. However, there was a significant difference in protein% observed with the advancement of lactation in Mehsani buffaloes, but it was not so in the case of Surti buffaloes. There was 8.10% significant (p≤0.05) increase in mean protein% observed from day 15 to 60 pp in Mehsani buffalo. The protein% ranged from 3.30% to 3.92%, 3.36% to 3.71%, 4.05% to 4.62%, and 4.33% to 5.06% among milk of S15, S60, M15, and M60 groups, respectively. The lowest mean protein content in the present study was observed in the S60 group and that of highest was observed in M60 group. The protein% observed in the present study was higher than 2.70% protein reported in non-descript buffaloes reared at high altitudes in the Kumaon hills of the central Himalayas [35]. Slightly higher protein (3.6-3.85%) as compared to S15 and S60 were reported in Egyptian buffaloes [34,36]. Protein content within the range of 3.73-3.97% which was in between the observed protein% in milk of Surti and Mehsani buffaloes had been reported in Murrah buffaloes of India [30,31] and Argentina [37,38] as well as water buffaloes of Bangladesh [32]. Slightly lower protein of 4.11% and 4.13% as compared to the M15 group was reported in buffaloes of Pakistan [39]

and Brazil [22], respectively. The protein content of 4.24-4.45% in Azerbiajan [40], while 4.35% in buffaloes of Pakistan [41] and France [27], comparable to M15 had also been reported. The protein content of 4.40% and 4.49% in between the range of M15 and M60 group was reported in buffaloes of Turkey [42] and Bulgaria [33], respectively. The protein content of 4.74% and 4.65% comparable to that of M60 group was reported in buffaloes of China [43] and Italy [44]. Higher protein% as compared to the present study to the tune of 4.90% and 5.20% had also been reported in buffaloes of Germany [45] and Jaffarabadi buffaloes reared in Argentina [38], respectively.

Lactose%

The lowest to highest lactose% observed was 4.69-5.54%, 4.85-5.80%, 4.84-5.51%, and 5.02-5.86% among milk of S15, S60, M15, and M60 groups, respectively. There was no significant difference observed for mean lactose% within and between breeds. Lactose% in the range of 4.99-5.24 was reported in buffaloes of Egypt [34,36] that are in agreement with the findings of the present experiment. Lactose% in between 4.5% and 5.0% had been reported in buffaloes of India [30,31], Italy [44], Pakistan [39], Bangladesh [32], Azerbiajan [40], Murrah breed in Argentina [37,38], Jaffarabadi breed in Argentina [38], and Bulgaria [33]. However, lactose% higher than 5.0% in concurrence to present study was also reported in buffaloes of Pakistan [41] and France [27].

Correlation coefficients among milk yield and composition traits

The correlation coefficients among milk yield and composition traits of Surti and Mehsani buffaloes are presented in Tables-2 and 3. The moderate positive significant (p≤0.05) correlation was observed between protein and fat% in Surti buffaloes at day 60 pp. However, at day 60 pp moderate positive non-significant correlation was observed between protein and SNF% in Mehsani buffaloes. The only moderate positive non-significant correlation at day 15 was observed in Surti buffaloes between TDMY and lactose%. All remaining correlations were of low to the negligible magnitude between different traits among the four groups.

Similar to S60 group, a significant correlation between fat and protein% had also been reported with moderate positive significant correlation (0.60) in mixed buffalo milk [46]. Most of the correlations in the present study were low to the negligible magnitude and were non-significant to draw out any valid and repeatable inference. Comparable non-significant correlations of low to negligible magnitude among milk yield and composition traits had also been reported by several authors [46-48].

Conclusion

In the present study, it was found that Mehsani buffaloes were significantly higher milk producer in terms of TDMY and FPCTDMY as compared to Surti

Table-2: Correlation coefficients between milk yield and composition traits at day 15 (above diagonal) and day 60 postpartum (below diagonal) in Surti buffaloes.

Traits	TDMY (kg)	%			
		Fat	SNF	Protein	Lactose
TDMY (kg)	-	0.02	−0.16	0.25	0.52
Fat%	−0.27	-	0.26	−0.22	0.19
SNF%	−0.15	0.26	-	−0.09	0.17
Protein%	0.33	0.63*	0.22	-	−0.30
Lactose%	0.01	−0.22	0.24	0.14	-

*Significant at p≤0.05. TDMY=Test day milk yield, SNF=Solid not fat

Table-3: Correlation coefficients between milk yield and composition traits at day 15 (above diagonal) and day 60 postpartum (below diagonal) in Mehsani buffaloes.

Traits	TDMY (kg)	%			
		Fat	SNF	Protein	Lactose
TDMY (kg)	-	−0.33	−0.35	0.36	0.15
Fat%	−0.36	-	0.33	0.05	0.08
SNF%	−0.22	0.46	-	−0.11	−0.18
Protein%	0.28	0.36	0.53	-	−0.09
Lactose%	0.01	−0.06	0.13	0.21	-

TDMY=Test day milk yield, SNF=Solid not fat

buffaloes at day 15 and 60 pp. The major consistent finding of the present study reveals that milk yield and protein% of Mehsani buffalo was significantly higher than Surti buffalo at day 15 and 60 pp.

Authors' Contributions

KKT, BPB, UVR, and VBK designed the study. The experiment was done by KKT, GMP, MJ, KJA, MDP, and LMS, whereas laboratory work was done by KKT, GMP, and MJ. All the authors participated in data analysis, draft, and revision of the manuscript. All authors read and approved the final manuscript.

Acknowledgments

We acknowledge the Dean, College of Veterinary Sciences and Animal Husbandry, NAU, Navsari, for providing necessary financial support and laboratory facilities to carry out the research work. In addition, we thank Research Scientist, Livestock Research Station, SDAU, for providing necessary help in samples and data collection.

Competing Interests

The authors declare that they have no competing interests.

References

1. GOI. (2012) 19 Livestock Census-2012. Government of India, Ministry of Agriculture, Department of Animal Husbandry, Dairying and Fisheries. Krishi Bhawan, New Delhi, India.
2. Anonymous. (2013) Annual Report - 2012-13. New Delhi, India: Deparment of Dairying Fisheries and Animal Husbandary, Ministry of Agriculture. Government of India, New Delhi.
3. Anonymous. (2012) 29th Survey Report on Estimates of Major Livestock Products for the Year 2011-2012. Sector 10-A Gandhinagar - 382 010. Gujarat State, India.
4. Anonymous. (2008) Feeding Standards, Feeding Advice and Nutrition Value of Feeding Ingredients. Product Board Animal Feed, CVB Series No. 43.
5. Hinkle, D.E., Wiersma, W. and Jurs, S.G. (2003) Applied Statistics for the Behavioral Sciences. V. Houghton, Mifflin, Boston.
6. Trivedi, K.R. (2000) Buffalo recording systems in India. In: Proceeding Workshop on Animal. Recording and Management Strategies for Buffaloes. ICAR Technical Series. p5-12.
7. Sethi, R.K. (2003) Buffalo Breeds of India. Proceeding Fourth Asian Buffalo Congress. 25-28 February.
8. Sastry, N.S.R. and Thomas, C.K. (2005) Livestock Production and Management. IV Revised. Kalyani Publishers, New Delhi, India.
9. Sahoo, S.K., Singh, A., Gupta, A.K., Chakravarty, A.K., Singh, M. and Ambhore, G.S. (2014) Estimation of genetic parameters of weekly test-day milk yields and first lactation 305-day milk yield in Murrah buffaloes. *Vet. World*, 7: 1094-1098.
10. Thiruvenkadan, A.K., Panneerselvam, S., Murali, N., Selvam, S. and Saravanakumar, V.R. (2014) Milk production and reproduction performance of Murrah buffaloes of Tamil Nadu, India. *Buffalo Bull.*, 33: 291-300.
11. Salari, F., Altomonte, I. and Martini, M. (2013) Buffalo milk: A case study of some parameters related to milk production. *Large Anim. Rev.*, 19: 17-20.
12. Sahare, M.G., Sawaimul, A.D., Ali, S.Z., Sirothia, A.R. and Bhojane, G.R. (2009) Weekly milk producation trends in early lactation period of Nagpuri buffalo. *Vet. World*, 2: 278-279.
13. Singh, B. and Tailor, S.P. (2014) Genetic evaluation of Surti sires for part and complete lactation milk yield. *Indian J. Anim. Sci.*, 84: 789-791.
14. Anonymous. (2015) Annual Progress Report of AGRESCO Sub-Committee on Animal Production and Fisheries Sciences, Sardarkrushinagar Dantiwada Agricultural University, Sardarkrushinagar, Gujarat.
15. Anonymous. (2015) Annual Progress Report of AGRESCO Sub-Committee on Animal Production and Fisheries Sciences. Navsari Agricultural University, Navsari, Gujarat.
16. Rao, M.K. and Nagarcenkar, R. (1997) Potentialities of the buffalo. *World Rev. Anim. Prod.*, 13: 53-62.
17. Jakhesara, S.J., Rank, D.N., Kansara, J.D., Parikh, R.C., Vataliya, P.H. and Solanki, J.V (2010) Microsatellite DNA typing for assessment of genetic variability in Mehsana buffalo breed of. *Buffalo Bull.*, 29: 262-269.
18. Misra, S.S., Sharma, A., Bhattacharya, T.K., Kumar, P. and Saha, R.S. (2008) Association of breed and polymorphism of α-s1 and α-s2 casein genes with milk quality and daily milk and constituent yield traits of buffaloes (*Bubalus bubalis*). *Buffalo Bull.*, 27: 294-301.
19. Rosati, A. and Van Vleck, L.D. (2002) Estimation of genetic parameters for milk, fat, protein and mozzarella cheese production for the Italian river buffalo *Bubalus bubalis* population. *Livest. Prod. Sci.*, 74: 185-190.
20. Yilmaz, O., Ertugrul, M. and Wilson, R.T. (2012) Domestic livestock resources of Turkey: Water buffalo. *Trop. Anim. Health Prod.*, 44: 707-714.
21. Borghese, A. (2013) Buffalo livestock and products in Europe. *Buffalo Bull.*, 32: 50-74.
22. Macedo, M.P., Wechesler, F.S., Ramos, A.A., Macado, M.P., Wechesler, F.S., Ramos, A.A., do Amaral, J.B., de Souza, J.C., de Resende, F.D. and De Oliveria, J.V. (2001) Chemical composition and production of milk from Mediterranean buffalo cows raised in western São Paulo State, Brazil (In Portuguese). *Rev. Bras. Zootec.*, 30: 1084-1088.
23. Bartocci, S., Tripaldi, C. and Terramoccia, S. (2002) Characteristics of foodstuffs and diets, and the quanti-qualitative milk parameters of Mediterranean buffaloes

bred in Italy using the intensive system. *Livest. Prod. Sci.*, 77: 45-58.

24. Tonhati, H., Lima, A.L., Lanna, D.P., de Camargo, G.M., Baldi, F., de Albuquerque, L.G. and Montrezor, J.M. (2011) Milk fatty acid characterization and genetic parameter estimates for milk conjugated linoleic acid in buffaloes. *J. Dairy Res.*, 78(2): 1-6.

25. Altman, P.L. and Dittmer, D.K. (1961) Blood and Other Body Fluids. Federation of American Societies for Experimental Biology, Washington, DC.

26. Sindhu, J.S. and Singhal, O.P. (1988) Qualitative aspects of buffalo milk constituents for products technology. Buffalo Production and Health – A Compendium of Latest Research Information Based on Indian Studies.

27. Ahmad, S., Gaucher, I., Rousseau, F., Beaucher, E., Piot, M., Grongnet, J.F. and Gaucheron, F. (2008) Effects of acidification on physico-chemical characteristics of buffalo milk: A comparison with cow's milk. *Food Chem.*, 106: 11-17.

28. Ménard, O., Ahmad, S., Rousseau, F., Briard-Bion, V., Gaucheron, F. and Lopez, C. (2010) Buffalo vs. Cow milk fat globules: Size distribution, zeta-potential, compositions in total fatty acids and in polar lipids from the milk fat globule membrane. *Food Chem.*, 120: 544-551.

29. Han, X., Lee, F.L., Zhang, L. and Guo, M.R. (2012) Chemical composition of water buffalo milk and its low-fat symbiotic yogurt development. *Funct. Foods Health. Dis.*, 2: 86-106.

30. Dubey, P.C., Suman, C.L., Sanyal, M.K., Pandey, H.S., Saxena, M.M. and Yadav, P.L. (1997) Factors affecting composition of milk of buffaloes. *Indian J. Anim. Sci.*, 67: 802-804.

31. Sodi, S.S., Mehra, M.L., Jain, A.K. and Trehan, P.K. (2008) Effect of non-genetic factors on the composition of milk of Murrah buffaloes. *Indian Vet. J.*, 85: 950-952.

32. Khan, M.A.S., Islam, M.N. and Siddiki, M.S.R. (2007) Physical and chemical composition of swamp and water buffalo milk: A comparative study. *Ital. J. Anim. Sci.*, 6: 1067-1070.

33. Peeva, T. (2001) Composition of buffalo milk: Sources of specific effects on the separate components. *Bulg. J. Agric. Sci.*, 7: 329-335.

34. Abd El-Salam, M.H. and El-Shibiny, S. (1966) The chemical composition of buffalo milk I General composition. *Indian J. Dairy Sci.*, 19: 151-154.

35. Meena, H.R., Ram, H. and Rasool, T.J. (2007) Milk constituents in non-descript buffaloes reared at high altitudes in the Kumaon hills of the centeral Himalayas. *Buffalo Bull.*, 26: 72-76.

36. Kholif, A.M. (1997) Effect of number and stage of lactation on the yield, composition and properties of buffalo's milk. *Egypt. J. Dairy Sci.*, 25: 25-39.

37. Patino, E.M., Medez, F.I., Faisal, E.L., Cedres, J.F., Gomez, L.G. and Stafani, M.C.G. (2003) Buffalo milk composition of murrah and half-breed murrah x mediterraneo in corrientes, Argentina. *Buffalo Newsl.*, 18: 8-10.

38. Patino, E.M. and Stefani, Y.M.C. (2005) Milk composition of breed Jafarabadi in corrientes, Argentina (In Spanish). *Rev. Electrón. Vet. REDVET*, 6: 1-4.

39. Imran, M., Khan, H., Hassan, S.S. and Khan, R. (2008) Physicochemical characteristics of various milk samples available in Pakistan. *J. Zhejiang Univ. Sci. B.*, 9: 546-551.

40. Akhundov, D.M. and Farzalieva, R.R. (1979) Composition and properties of milk of heifer buffaloes. *Agamaliogly Zootekhnil.*, 1: 6-8.

41. Arian, H.H., Khaskhali, M., Arian, M.A., Soomro, A.H. and Nizamani, A.H. (2008) Heat stability and quality characteristics of postpartum buffalo milk. *Pak. J Nutr.*, 7: 303-307.

42. Sekerden, Ö., Erdem, H., Kankurda, B. and Özlü, B. (1999) Factors affecting milk composition and changes in milk composition with lactation stage in anatolian buffaloes (In Turkish). *Turk. J. Vet. Anim. Sci.*, 23: 505-509.

43. Han, B.Z., Meng, Y., Li, M., Yang, Y.X., Ren, F.Z., Zeng, Q.K. and Robert Nout, M.J. (2007) A survey on the microbiological and chemical composition of buffalo milk in China. *Food Control.*, 18: 742-746.

44. Tufarelli, V., Dario, M. and Laudadio, V. (2008) Diet composition and milk characteristics of Mediterranean water buffaloes reared in South Eastern Italy during spring season. *Livest. Res. Rural Dev.*, 20: 1-7.

45. Braun, P.G. and Preuss, S.E. (2008) Nutritional composition and chemico-physical parameters of water buffalo milk and milk products in Germany. *Milchwissenschaft*, 63: 70-72.

46. Gâjâilă, I., Gâjâilă, G., Dobrea, M. and Cotor, G. (2014) Determination of relationships between milk composition and cheese yield using principal component analysis and logit model. *Bull. UASVM Vet. Med.*, 71: 62-65.

47. Khalid, J., Abdullah, M., Khalid, M.S., Ahmad, N., Bhatti, J.A. and Younas, U. (2013) Inter-relationship of milk constituents with body and udder measurements in Nili-Ravi buffaloes raised at commercial farms of Pakistan. *Buffalo Bull.*, 32: 1170-1173.

48. Hamad, M.N.E., El-Moghazy, M.M. and Abdel-Aziz, M.E. (2014) Phenotypic correlations among Egyptian buffalo milk production and its major chemical constituents. *J. Agric. Sci. Mansoura Univ.*, 10: 1-8.

21

Congenital and inherited neurologic diseases in dogs and cats: Legislation and its effect on purchase in Italy

Annamaria Passantino and Marisa Masucci

Department of Veterinary Sciences, University of Messina, Polo Universitario Annunziata, 98168 Messina, Italy.
Corresponding author: Annamaria Passantino, e-mail: passanna@unime.it,
MM: masucci@unime.it

Abstract

Many of the congenital neurologic diseases can result in incapacity or death of the animal. Some of them, such as idiopathic epilepsy and hydrocephalus, exhibit breed or familial predisposition and a genetic basis was proved or suggested. Some diseases can be presumptively diagnosed after a detailed signalment (breed predisposition), history (e.g. family history because many of these defects have familial tendencies), and through physical exam; other diagnostic methods (radiography, computed tomography, magnetic resonance, electrophysiologic tests, etc.) can provide supportive evidence for the congenital defect and help to confirm the diagnosis. Some cases can lead to civil law-suits when the lesions are congenital, but not easily recognizable, or when the lesions are hereditary but tend to became manifest only after some time (more than 12 months after the date of purchase, e.g., after the vice-free guarantee period has expired). Moreover, quite frequently an early diagnosis is not made because there are delays in consulting the veterinarian or the general practitioner veterinarian does not perceive subtle signs. This study was designed to focus on the medico-legal aspects concerning the buying and selling in Italy of dogs and cats affected by congenital and hereditary neurologic diseases that could constitute vice in these animals. While adequate provisions to regulate in detail the various aspects of pet sale have still to be drawn up by legislators, it may be helpful to involve breeders, by obliging them by contract to extend guarantees in the case of hereditary lesions, including neurologic diseases.

Keywords: buy/sell, cat, dog, hereditary disease, nervous system.

Introduction

To most European citizens, companion animals become more than just animals in the home. Cats, dogs, and other companion animals often occupy the status of the beloved family member. Despite this status which most of these animals gain in the home, they are legally considered mere goods [1] or commodities during the sales process (purchase). Indeed, companion animals have no independent status or personhood in the legal world. In the eyes of the law, animals are property: They are goods to be bought and sold, acquired, and maintained.

The term "goods" is meant to afford buyers and sellers certain rights and responsibilities in the transaction. The terms "possession" and "property" are often used synonymously. Nevertheless, there is an important difference. The term "property" (*dominium, proprietas*) refers to the right to dispose of a thing, while the term "possession" (*possessio*) designates the actual power over a thing.

The Italian Civil Code (article 812) at present considers animals as *res,* i.e., a thing (as property) as opposed to a person, who has rights [2,3].

The purchase (*emptio venditio*) is a contract that obliges one party (*venditor*) to provide a thing (a commodity) and the other party (*emptor)* to provide payment. It is a bilateral contract since both parties are creditors and debtors at the same time - the *venditor* owes the commodity and the *emptor* owes the money.

The seller is always liable for defects of the commodities (including animals). For redhibitory defects (vice), however, he/she is only liable if he kept them secret on purpose or if he guaranteed a faultless product.

In veterinary legal medicine, the illness must be considered a vice [4] in those cases where it renders an animal unsuitable for its specified use or significantly reduces its value.

An animal, which is unsuitable for its specified use, must be affected with a behavioral character defect or illness. The illness causes a disturbance in normal organic functioning, which may be localized or generalized, following an anatomic alteration which will inevitably cause an appreciable permanent or temporary impairment.

To qualify as vice, however, illness must be [4,5]:
1. Pre-existing or have a pre-existing cause. It is clear that congenital and hereditary neurologic diseases can come under this heading since most of them are typically primary; for this reason, it is difficult to demonstrate that environmental factors have contributed to their phenotypization;
2. Hidden. This means that it cannot be discovered

by an ordinary inspection or examination; or rather, it is not easily recognized at the moment of purchase, and it cannot be detected using the normal due diligence.

3. Serious or chronic so as to affect the use of the animal or such that, if the buyer knew of the disease, he/she would not enter into the contract. In fact, defect renders the thing sold unfit for the use for which it is intended or diminishes its fitness for the intended use to such an extent that the vendee would not have bought or would have given a lower price if he had been aware of the defect.

In dogs and cats, there are many neurologic conditions of proven or suspected hereditary origin, both congenital and non-congenital, which may constitute vice in the buying and selling of these animals.

These cases would be lead to civil law-suits when the lesions are congenital, but not easily recognizable, or when the lesions are hereditary but tend to became manifest only after some time (more than 12 months after the date of purchase, i.e., after the vice-free guarantee period has expired). Moreover, an early diagnosis quite frequently is not made because there are delays in consulting a veterinarian or the general practitioner veterinarian does not perceive subtle signs.

This study will present an overview of general contract law related to sales of dogs and cats as well as the rights and remedies of buyers under Italian law. Finally, the study will highlight some concerns facing buyers, especially when purchasing companion animals (dogs and cats) affected by congenital and hereditary neurologic diseases.

Current Italian Law

In Italy, the purchase of animals is regulated by the Civil Code (article 1470 and subsequent) and dated back to 1942. These articles regulate the purchase of real property, and they are also adopted in the field of the purchase of animals.

In fact, the only article concerning animal purchase in Italy is article 1496 of the Italian Civil Code. It states that the guarantee against vices in the sale of animals is regulated by special laws or by local usage or, if these are lacking, by article 1490 of the Civil Code and subsequent. The latter reads as follows: "The seller is obliged to guarantee that the object sold is immune from vices which make it unsuitable for the usage to which it is destined or that decrease the value of it in an appreciable way."

In Italy, only when the animal is affected by a serious or chronic vice that is pre-existing and not easily recognizable, will the buyer be able, with respect to the terms of expiry and to rules contained in article 1495 of the Italian Civil Code, to exercise one of the two legal actions foreseen by the Code, namely, redhibitory action or estimatory action (remedies of the vendee). "Redhibitory action" (*actio redhibitoria*) means rescission of sale, and "estimatory action" (*actio estimatoria* or *quanti minoris*) means reduction of the price (article 1492 Civil Code).

The time limits for rescission or exaction of proportionate reduction of the purchase price against the vendor under article 1495 are 8 days from the day of delivery and 1 year from the date of purchase.

Congenital and Inherited Neurological Diseases

Physiologic nervous system development may be affected by inherited or congenital factors, e.g., *in utero* exposure to viral (parvovirus-induced cerebellar hypoplasia) or teratogenic substances (cranium bifidum, spina bifida, abnormal atlanto-occipital articulation, exencephaly, and hydrocephalus associated with griseofulvin therapy) [6,7].

Many kinds of anomaly result from pathologic nervous system development:

i. Macroscopic malformations (hydrocephalus, cerebellar hypoplasia, lissencephaly, hydromyelia, syringomyelia, spinal dysraphism) [8-15];

ii. Microscopic lesions (involving the inner ear in congenital deafness and vestibular syndrome and the gray or white matter in degenerative diseases) [9,16,17];

iii. Alterations involving molecular structures only (decreased number of acetylcholine receptors in congenital myasthenia gravis, enzymatic deficiency in storage diseases, abnormalities of neurotransmitters or their receptors in narcolepsy) [9,18-24].

In some cases, the involvement of the nervous system results from malformations of the skull or the spine (meningocele and myelomeningocele in association with spina bifida, spinal cord compressions caused by hemivertebrae, butterfly vertebrae, transitional vertebrae, and malformation of the dens of the axis) [9,10,12,25-30].

In many cases, the clinical signs are apparent at birth and there is no progression of the disease, but sometimes, e.g., in degenerative diseases, the onset of symptoms occurs in the first few months or years of life, and they are slowly progressive and lead to the animal's death (Table-1). Clinical signs related to idiopathic epilepsy and spinal cord compression due to congenital vertebral anomalies can develop in adult animals (Table-1) [25,31]. Mild neurologic signs, although present at birth, can be mistaken for the normal awkwardness of the puppies by their owner.

Some congenital diseases may be diagnosed by physical examination because there are typical signs (e.g., hydrocephalus, myelomeningocele, and meningoencephalocele). Appropriate diagnostic tests are required for many congenital neurologic diseases (Table-1). In some cases, the diagnosis can be made

Table-1: Breeds affected by inherited neurologic diseases [9,10,34-38].

Disease	Dog	Cat
Abiotrophies Incidence: Rare Prognosis: Guarded to poor (there are different degrees of the disease, which is slowly progressive) Age of onset of clinical signs: 6 weeks to 5 years Clinical signs: Cerebellar ataxia, paresis/paralysis Diagnosis ante mortem: Genetic (American Staffordshire Terrier); in other breeds only post mortem	American Staffordshire Terrier, Australian Kelpie, Beagle, Bernese Mountain Dog, Blue Terrier, Bobtail, Border Collie, Breton Spaniel, Cairn Terrier, Chow Chow, Cocker Spaniel, Doberman Pinscher, Fox Terrier, German Shepherd Dog, Golden Retriever, Gordon Setter, Kerry Samoyed, Labrador Retriever, Lapland, Pointer, Poodle, Rhodesian Ridgeback, Saluki, Wire-haired Great Dane	Domestic, Siamese
Ceroid lipofuscinosis Incidence: Rare Prognosis: Guarded to poor Age of onset of clinical signs: 4 months to 9 years (most animal<2 years) Clinical signs: Personality change, visual impairment, ataxia, seizures Diagnosis ante mortem: Yes (genetic, histopathology of skin biopsies)	Australian Cattle Dog, Blue Heelers, Blue Heelers, Border Collie, Chihuahua, Cocker Spaniels, Dachshund, English Setter, Salukis, Tibetan Terrier, Yugoslavian Sheep Dog	Domestic, Siamese
Congenital myasthenia gravis Incidence: Rare Prognosis: Guarded Age of onset of clinical signs: 6-8 weeks Clinical signs: Weakness worsening after exercise Diagnosis ante mortem: Yes (electrodiagnostic tests, pharmacological tests, muscle biopsy)	Fox Terrier, Jack Russel Terrier, Samoyed, Springer Spaniel	Siamese
Demyelinating diseases of peripheral nerves Incidence: Rare Prognosis: Poor Age of onset of clinical signs: 3 weeks to 3 months Clinical signs: LMN paresis/paralysis Diagnosis ante mortem: Yes (peripheral nerve biopsy)	Alaskan Malamute, Golden Retriever, Tibetan Mastiff	Siamese
Fucosidosis Incidence: Rare Prognosis: Poor Age of onset of clinical signs: 6 months to 2 years Clinical signs: Various, predominantly behavioral and motor Diagnosis ante mortem: Yes (enzyme analysis, genetic tests)	Springer Spaniel	
Gangliosidosis Incidence: Rare Prognosis: Poor Age of onset of clinical signs: 2 months to 1.5 years Clinical signs: Vision deficits, lethargy, gait disturbances Diagnosis ante mortem: Yes (blood cytology, genetic tests)	Alaskan Husky (controlla denominazione), Beagle, German Shorthaired Pointer, Japanese Spaniel, Portuguese Water Dog, Shiba, Springer Spaniel	Domestic, Korat, Siamese
Globoid cell leukodystrophy Incidence: Rare Prognosis: Poor Age of onset of clinical signs: 5 weeks to 2 years Clinical signs: Cerebellar ataxia, paraparesis/plegia amaurosis, behavior disturbance Diagnosis ante mortem: Yes (genetic tests)	Basset Hound, Beagle, Blue Tick Coonhound, Cairn Terrier, Pomeranian, Poodle, West Highland White Terrier	Domestic
Glucocerebrosidosis Incidence: Rare Prognosis: Poor Age of onset of clinical signs: 6-8 months Clinical signs: Ataxia Diagnosis ante mortem: Yes (enzyme assay)	Silky Terrier	Abyssinian
Glycogenosis Incidence: Rare Prognosis: Poor Age of onset of clinical signs: 5 months to 1.5 years Clinical signs: Two forms: Early neonatal death or progressive neuromuscular weakness Diagnosis ante mortem: Yes (genetic test in IV type in the cat)	German Shepherd Dog, Lapland Dog, Springer Spaniel	Domestic, Norwegian Forest Cat

(Contd...)

Table-1: (*Continued*)

Disease	Dog	Cat
Hemivertebrae, Butterfly vertebrae Incidence: Common Prognosis: Good to poor Age of onset of clinical signs: Variable Clinical signs: Asymptomatic or ataxia, paresis/paralysis due to acute or chronic spinal cord compression Diagnosis ante mortem: Yes (RX, CT)	"Screw-tailed" brachycephalic breeds: Boston Terrier, French and English Bulldog, Pug	
Hydrocephalus Incidence: Common Prognosis: Guarded Age of onset of clinical signs: Shortly after birth Clinical signs: Enlargement of the skull, open sutures, and fontanelles, behavioral changes, depression, seizures, amaurosis, ataxia Diagnosis ante mortem: Yes (ultrasonography, TC, MR, EEG)	Toy breeds: Chihuahua, Maltese, Pomeranian, Yorkshire Terrier, Toy Poodle Brachycephalic breeds: Boston terrier, English Bulldog, Lhasa Apso, Pekingese, Pug Bernese Mountain Dog, Chow Chow, Dalmatian, Samoyed, Springer Spaniel, Weimaraner	Siamese
Hypomyelinating diseases Incidence: Rare Prognosis: Guarded (not progressive and improvement can occur) Age of onset of clinical signs: Shortly after birth Clinical signs: Tremors Diagnosis ante mortem: No (post mortem histopathology)		
Idiopathic epilepsy Incidence: Very common in dogs, rare in cats Prognosis: Guarded Age of onset of clinical signs: 6 months to 5 years Clinical signs: Seizures Diagnosis ante mortem: Yes (by excluding other causes of seizures. No positive diagnostic signs can substantiate the diagnosis)	Beagle, Bernese Mountain Dog, Boxer, Cocker Spaniel, Collie, Dachshund, German Shepherd Dog, Golden Retriever, Irish Setter, Keeshond, Labrador Retriever, Poodle, Saint Bernard, Siberian Husky, Tervuren, Wire Fox Terrier	
Inherited deafness Incidence: Common Prognosis: Good *quoad vitam* Age of onset of clinical signs: Shortly after birth Clinical signs: Deafness Diagnosis ante mortem: Yes (electrodiagnostic tests)	Argentine Dogo, Australian Shepherd, Bobtail, Dalmatian, Doberman Pinscher, English Bulldog, English Setter, Foxhound, Great Dane, Great Pyrenees, Maltese, Pointer	*White blue-eyed cats*
Leukodystrophies Incidence: Rare Prognosis: Poor Age of onset of clinical signs: Few weeks to few years Clinical signs: Ataxia, paresis/paralysis, seizures Diagnosis ante mortem: No (post mortem histopathology)	Afghan Hound, Dalmatian, Kookier, Labrador Retriever, Poodle, Rottweiler, Scottish Terrier	
Lissencephaly Incidence: Rare Prognosis: Guarded Age of onset of clinical signs: Shortly after birth-12 months Clinical signs: Behavioral changes, seizures, amaurosis, visual deficit Diagnosis ante mortem: Yes (CT, MR)	Fox Terrier, Irish Setter, Lhasa Apso	Domestic
Malformations of the dens of the axis Incidence: Common Prognosis: Guarded Age of onset of clinical signs: <1 year Clinical signs: Cervical pain, tetraparesis/paralysis Diagnosis ante mortem: Yes (RX, CT)	Toy breeds	Domestic
Mannosidosis Incidence: Rare Prognosis: Poor Age of onset of clinical signs: 2-7 months Clinical signs: Facial dysmorphism, ataxia, tremors, altered behavior, seizures Diagnosis ante mortem: Yes (genetic tests)		Domestic, Persian
Mucopolysaccharidosis Incidence: Rare Prognosis: Poor Age of onset of clinical signs: 3-10 months Clinical signs: Progressive paresis Diagnosis ante mortem: Yes (urinary biochemical tests, genetic tests (in mucopolysaccharidosis VI of the cat)	Dachshund, Labrador Retriever, Doberman Pinscher, Plott Hound	Domestic, Siamese

(*Contd...*)

Table-1: (*Continued*)

Disease	Dog	Cat
Narcolepsy Incidence: Rare Prognosis: Good quoad vitam (the severe forms can be invalidating) Age of onset of clinical signs: <6 months Clinical signs: Recurring sudden attacks of sleep and/or loss of muscle tone Diagnosis ante mortem: Yes (clinical diagnosis, electrodiagnostic tests, genetic tests)	Doberman Pinscher, Labrador Retriever	
Peripheral axonopathies Incidence: Rare Prognosis: Guarded to poor Clinical signs: Tetraparesis/paralysis Diagnosis ante mortem: Yes (peripheral nerve histopathology)	Boxer, German Shepherd Dog, Rottweiler	
Sfingomyelinosis Incidence: Rare Prognosis: Poor Age of onset of clinical signs: 2-4 months Clinical signs: Ataxia, tremors, paresis/paralysis Diagnosis ante mortem: Yes (enzyme assay)	Boxer, Poodle	Balinese, Domestic Siamese
Spina bifida/meningomyelocele Incidence: No common Prognosis: Good (spina bifida only) guarded to poor (spina bifida with meningomyelocele) Age of onset of clinical signs: Shortly after birth Clinical signs: Spina bifida can be asymptomatic, meningomyelocele: Incontinence, paraparesis/paralysis Diagnosis ante mortem: Yes (clinical signs, RX, CT)	English Bulldog	Manx Cat
Spongiform degeneration of gray or white matter Incidence: Rare Prognosis: Poor Age of onset of clinical signs: 1-6 months Clinical signs: Tremors, ataxia, behavioral changes, mental status alterations, visual deficit Diagnosis ante mortem: No (histopathology post mortem)	Bull Mastiff, Cocker Spaniel, Labrador Retriever, Rottweiler, Saluki, Samoyed, Silky Terrier	Birman, Egyptian Mau

LMN=Lower motor neuron, CT=Computed tomography, EEG=Electroencephalogram, MR=Magnetic resonance

only by excluding other causes (e.g., idiopathic epilepsy) or only after the death of the animal because it requires anatomic and histopathologic evaluations (e.g. degenerative diseases) (Table-1) [9,10].

Inherited neurologic diseases usually affect specific breeds (Table-1).

An Approach to the Problem: Proposals

The authors propose to make eradication plans for hereditary and/or congenital neurologic disease official and, indeed, obligatory for legal and ethical reasons. Genetic selection giving preference to certain characteristics can result in hereditary neurologic defects, which may cause problems of varying entity and this shows a lack of respect animals as sentient beings [32]. In this context, there are emotional and psychological implications for the owner who is made aware of the fact that his animal suffers from hereditary and genetic neurologic defects.

To reduce the incidence of congenital and/or hereditary neurologic disease in pets, it would also be useful that:

a. Practicing veterinarians discourage reproduction in animals with neurologic alterations for which inherited etiology is recognized or suspected.

b. Breeders and geneticists work together on eradication of hereditary anomalies. Genetic tests, in particular, make possible a rapid, accurate, and early confirmation of diagnosis in sick animals even before the clinical signs are evident; the carriers can thus be removed from breeding programs [33]. When genetic tests are not available, detailed information on pedigrees will make identification of carriers possible so as to carry out selective and rational breeding.

Another useful development could be to enhance breeders' responsibility by enforcing the inclusion of a lengthening of guarantee time in the case of hereditary defects, including neurologic defects, which may only become evident after the age of 12 months (Table-1), that is, beyond the validity of the guarantee.

Conclusions

Cooperation among dog breeders, researchers, prospective purchasers, and purebreed dog organizations at all levels is essential if genetically healthy dogs are to become a reality.

Breeders should understand the implications of genetic diseases recognized as affecting their breeds and take steps to breed only those dogs/cats that will minimize the propagation of unwanted characteristics.

Prospective buyers should be made aware of the genetic diseases related to the breed they are considering. They should also ask a physical exam and test results or genetic histories for the animals they are planning to purchase.

Veterinarians should inform owners, breeders, and prospective breeders about congenital/hereditary neurologic diseases.

Authors' Contributions

AP and MM generated the concept, collected materials, draft, and revised the manuscript. Both authors read and approved the final manuscript.

Acknowledgments

The authors are grateful to prof. Caroline Keir for the assistance in review of English language.

Competing Interests

The authors declare that they have no competing interests.

References

1. Favre, D. (2010) Living property: A new status for animals within the legal system. *Marq. L. Rev.*, 93: 1021-1071.
2. Passantino, A. and De Vico, G. (2006) Our mate animals. *Biol. Forum.*, 99(2): 200-204.
3. Passantino, A. (2007) The legal protection of human feeling for animals. Aracne publisher, Roma, Italy, p 1-108.
4. Passantino, A. (2006) Medico-legal considerations of canine leishmaniasis in Italy: An overview of an emerging disease with reference to the purchase. *Rev. Sci. Tech.*, 25(3): 1111-1123.
5. Quartarone, V., Quartuccio, M., Cristarella, S. and Passantino, A. (2012) Technical consultation in purchase of animals: Case report. *Veterinaria*, 26(5): 45-53.
6. Scott, F.W., de Lahunta, A., Schultz, R.D., Bistner, S.I. and Riis, R.C. (1975) Teratogenesis in cats associated with griseofulvin therapy. *Teratology*, 11(1): 79-86.
7. Stuetzer, B. and Hartmann, K. (2014) Feline parvovirus infection and associated diseases. *Vet. J.*, 201(82): 150-155.
8. Green, C.E., Vandevelde, M. and Braund, K. (1976) Lissencephaly in two Lhasa Apso dogs. *JAVMA*, 169(4): 405-410.
9. Bernardini, M. (2010) Neurology of the dog and cat. 2nd edition. Poletto publisher, Milan, Italy.
10. Lorenz, M.D., Coates, J.R. and Kent, M. (2011) Handbook of Veterinary Neurology. 5th ed. Saunders, Elsevier, St. Louis.
11. Thomas, W.B. (2010) Hydrocephalus in dogs and cats. *Vet. Clin. N. Am. Small.*, 40(1): 143-159.
12. Berlanda, M., Zotti, A., Brandazza, G., Poser, H., Calò, P. and Bernardini, M. (2011) Magnetic resonance and computed tomographic features of 4 cases of canine congenital thoracic vertebral anomalies. *Can. Vet. J.*, 52: 1334-1338.
13. Lee, K.I., Lim, C.Y., Kang, B.T. and Park, H.M. (2011) Clinical and MRI findings of lissencephaly in a mixed breed dog. *J. Vet. Med. Sci.*, 73(10): 1385-1388.
14. MacKillop, E. (2011) Magnetic resonance imaging of intracranial malformations in dogs and cats. *Vet. Radiol. Ultrasound*, 52(1): S42-S51.
15. Kromhout, K., van Bree, H., Broeckx, B.J.C., Bhatti, S., De Decker, S., Polis, I. and Gielen, I. (2015) Low-field magnetic resonance imaging and multislice computed tomography for the detection of cervical syringomyelia in dogs. *J. Vet. Intern. Med.*, 29: 1354-1359.
16. Lee, M. (1993) Congenital vestibular disease in a German shepherd dog. *Vet. Rec.*, 113(24): 571.
17. Branis, M. and Burda, H. (1985) Inner ear structure in deaf and normally hearing Dalmatian dogs. *J. Comp. Pathol.*, 95(2): 295-299.
18. Oda, K., Lambert, E.H., Lennon, V.A. and Palmer, A.C. (1984) Congenital canine myasthenia gravis: I. Deficient junctional acetylcholine receptors. *Muscle Nerve*, 7(9): 705-716.
19. Lin, L., Faraco, J., Li, R., Kadotani, H., Rogers, W., Lin, X., Qiu, X., de Jong, P.J., Nishino, S. and Mignon, E. (1999) The sleep disorder canine narcolepsy is caused by a mutation in the hypocretin (orexin) receptor 2 gene. *Cell*, 98(3): 365-376.
20. Masucci, M. (2008) Narcolepsy in dogs: Etiology, pahtogenesis and clinical managment. *Summa animali da compagnia*, 3: 11-20.
21. Hemsley, K.M. and Hopwood, J.J. (2010) Lesson learnt from animal models: Pathophysiology of neuropathic lysosomal storage disorders. *J. Inherit. Metab. Dis.*, 33(4): 363-371.
22. Shelton, G.D. (2010) Routine and specialized laboratory testing for the diagnosis of neuromuscular diseases in dogs and cats. *Vet. Clin. Path.*, 39(3): 278-295.
23. Mignot, E.J.M. (2014) History of narcolepsy at Stanford University. *Immunol. Res.*, 58: 315-339.
24. Rinz, C.J., Levine, J.L., Minor, K.M., Humphires, H.D., Lara, R., Starr-Moss, A.N., Guo, L.T., Williams, D.C., Shelton, G.D. and Clark, L.A. (2014) A *COLQ* missense mutation in labrador retrievers having congenital myasthenic syndrome. *PLoS One*, 9(8): e106425.
25. Masucci, M., Giudice, E., Di Pietro, S. and Pugliese, A. (2002) Emivertebra in dogs. Description on three cases. *Summa*, 4: 53-58.
26. Dewey, C.W., Marino, D.J. and Loughin, C.A. (2013) Craniocervical junction abnormalities in dogs. *N. Z. Vet. J.*, 61(84): 202-211.
27. Charalambous, M., Jeffery, N.D., Smith, P.M., Goncalves, R., Barker, A., Hayes, G., Ives, E. and Vanhaesebrouck, A.E. (2014) Surgical treatment of dorsal hemivertebrae associated with kyphosis by spinal segmental stabilization, with o without decompression. *Vet. J.*, 202(2): 267-273.
28. Guitierrez-Quintana, R., Guevar, J., Stalin, C., Faller, K., Yeamans, C. and Penderis, J. (2014) A proposed radiographic classification scheme for congenital thoracic vertebral malformations in brachycephalic "screw-tailed" dog breeds. *Vet. Radiol. Ultrasound*, 55(6): 585-591.
29. Song, R.B., Glass, E.N., Kent, M., Sánchez, M.D., Smith, D.M. and de Lahunta, A. (2014) Surgical correction of a sacral meningomyelocele in a dog. *J. Am. Anim. Hosp. Assoc.*, 50(6): 436-443.
30. Voorbij, A.M.W., Meij, B.P., van Bruggen, L.W.L., Grinwis, G.C.M., Stassen, Q.E.M. and Kooistra, H.S. (2015) Atlanto-axial malformation and instability in dogs with pituitary dwarfism due to an *LHX3* mutation. *J. Vet. Intern. Med.*, 29: 207-213.
31. De Risio, L., Bhatti, S., Muñana, K., Penderis, J., Stein, V., Tipold, A., Berendt, M., Farqhuar, R., Fisher, A., Long, S., Mandigers, P.J.J., Matiasek, K., Packer, R.M.A., Pakozdy, A., Patterson, N., Platt, S., Modell, M., Potschka, H., Pumarola Batlle, M., Rusbridge, C. and Volk, H.A. (2015) International veterinary epilepsy task force consensus proposal: Diagnostic approach to epilepsy in dogs. *BMC Vet. Res.*, 11: 148.
32. European Community. (2007) Treaty of lisbon amending the treaty on European Union and the treaty establishing the European community, signed at Lisbon, 13 December 2007. *Off. J. EU.*, C306: 1-271.
33. Sargan, D.R. (2007) Inherited metabolic disease in companion animals: Prospects for their diagnosis and elimination in the next decade. *Vet. J.*, 174(2): 223-224.
34. Abitbol, M. (2009) Cerebellar ataxia of American staffordshire terrier. *Summa animali da compagnia*, 3: 6-8.
35. Braund, K.G. (2003) Storage disorders. In: Vite, C.H., editor. Braund's Clinical Neurology in Small Animals: Localization, Diagnosis and Treatment. International

Veterinary Information Service, Ithaca NY. pA3219.0203. Available from: http//:www.ivis.org, Accessed on 20-01-2016.

36.   deLahunta, A. and Glass, E. (2009) Veterinary Neuroanatomy and Clinical Neurology. Saunders Elsevier, St. Louis.

37.   LeCouter, R.A. (2007) Genetic markers in the diagnosis and prevention of neurological diseases. Proceedings of the 32nd WSAVA Congress, Sydney, Australia, 19-23 August; 2007.

38.   Penderis, J. (2008) Genetic advances in neurological disease. Proceedings of the 33rd WSAVA Congress, Dublin, Ireland, 20-24 August; 2008. p489-491.

22

Diversity of *Meq* gene from clinical Marek's disease virus infection in Saudi Arabia

Mahmoud H. A. Mohamed[1,2], Ibrahim M. El-Sabagh[3,4], Malik A. Al-Habeeb[5] and Yousef M. Al-Hammady[6]

1. Department of Clinical Studies, College of Veterinary Medicine, King Faisal University, Al-Hufof, 31982, Saudi Arabia;
2. Department of Avian and Rabbit Medicine, Faculty of Veterinary Medicine, Zagazig University, 44519, Zagazig, Egypt;
3. Central Biotechnology Laboratory, College of Veterinary Medicine, King Faisal University, Al-Hufof, 31982, Saudi Arabia; 4. Department of Virology, Faculty of Veterinary Medicine, Cairo University, 12211, Giza, Egypt; 5. Excutive Department of Risk Assessment, Saudi Food and Drug Authority, Saudi Arabia; 6. Central Veterinary Laboratory, Riyadh, Saudi Arabia.
Corresponding author: Ibrahim M. El-Sabagh, e-mail: ibrahimelsabagh@yahoo.com,
MHAM: mahmoudhassanain@yahoo.com, MAA: mxm0063@hotmail.com, YMA: ymh_82_01@hotmail.com

Abstract

Aim: The aim of this study was to demonstrate the genomic features of *Meq* gene of Marek's disease virus (MDV) recently circulating in Saudi Arabia (SA).

Materials and Methods: Two poultry flocks suffering from mortalities and visceral tumors were presented to the Veterinary Teaching Hospital, King Faisal University, SA. Subjected to different diagnostic procedures: Case history, clinical signs, and necropsy as well as polymerase chain reaction followed by *Meq* gene sequence analysis.

Results: Case history, clinical signs, and necropsy were suggestive of MDV infection. The *Meq* gene was successfully detected in liver and spleen of infected chickens. A 1062 bp band including the native *Meq* ORF in addition to a 939 bp of *S-Meq* (short isoform of *Meq*) were amplified from Saudi 01-13 and Saudi 02-13, respectively. The nucleotide and deduced amino acids sequences of the amplified *Meq* genes of both Saudi isolates showed distinct polymorphism when compared with the standard USA virulent isolates Md5 and GA. The sequence analysis of the *S-Meq* gene showed a 123 bp deletion representing 41 amino acids between two proline-rich areas without any frameshift. The *Meq* gene encoded four repeats of proline-rich repeats (PRRs sequences), whereas the *S-Meq* contains only two PRRs. Interestingly, the phylogenetic analysis revealed that both of SA MDV isolates are closely related to the MDV strains from Poland.

Conclusion: The two MDV isolates contain several nucleotide polymorphisms resulting in distinct amino acid substitutions. It is suggested that migratory and wild birds, as well as world trading of poultry and its by-products, have a great contribution in the transmission of MDVs overseas.

Keywords: deletion, Marek's disease virus, *Meq* gene sequence, phylogenic analysis, Saudi Arabia.

Introduction

Marek's disease (MD) is lymphoproliferative disease of chickens caused by the highly infectious cell-associated alphaherpesvirus MD virus serotype 1 (MDV1) or Gallid herpesvirus 2 and induces malignant lymphomas in chickens [1]. Currently, MD has been effectively controlled using the vaccines along with good management practice, and major losses to the poultry industry as a result of the disease have largely been averted [2-4].

The MDV genome of Md5 strain is about 177,874 bp linear dsDNA; it is predicted to encode 103 proteins [5]. The genetic basis and molecular mechanisms underlying viral virulence and oncogenicity remain poorly understood. The search for viral factors related to oncogenicity identified the viral genes encoding proteins involved in T-cell transformation (*Meq*) and others with potential involvement in tumorigenicity, viral virulence, and host range (pp24, pp38, viral interleukin 8) [6,7].

The *Meq* gene encodes a 339-amino acid protein with an N-terminal basic region leucine zipper (bZIP) domain and a C-terminal transactivation domain [8]. The bZIP domain, similar to that of the Jun/Fos family of oncoprotein, consists of two stretches of basic residues basic regions 1 and 2 (BR1 and BR2) and a leucine zipper [8]. The transactivation domain is characterized by 2.5 proline-rich repeats (PRRs), which contain several SH3-binding motifs [8]. Several studies showed that the attenuated MDV shows some deletions in the BamHI-D and H fragments and has an inserted repeat sequence in the unique long region (UL) of the genome compared to the parent [9]. On the other hand, attenuated strains of MDV1 are not oncogenic although no structural or transcriptional changes have been reported concerning *Meq* gene [10]. Several reports suggested that the number of PRRs and point mutations in PPPP stretches might provide an indication of the isolate pathogenicity [4,11]. As a requirement for the disease control in Saudi Arabia (SA), vaccination with a cell associated modified live CVI988 and herpesvirus of turkey (HVT) strain FC 126 are frequently used in broiler and layers chickens at 1-day old. The vaccination failure and inability of the vaccine to protect chickens against overt clinical signs following field infection may be due to increasing in the virulence of the virus or early exposure [12].

In this study, we aimed to characterize MDVs circulated in the eastern region of SA using polymerase chain reaction (PCR) and genomic sequencing and detect the diversity of the *Meq* gene structure between two oncogenic MDVs from field cases.

Materials and Methods

Ethical approval

This study was carried out after the necessary permission of Institutional Animal Ethics committee, King Faisal University, Saudi Arabia.

Case history and clinical specimens

12-15 weeks old layer chickens from two farms in the eastern region, SA, vaccinated with commercial MDV vaccines (contains cell associated modified live Marek's Rispens CVI988 strain virus and HVT strain FC 126), were represented to the Avian Clinic, Veterinary Teaching Hospital, King Faisal University, Al-Hassa, SA. Birds showing high mortality (10%) with signs of depression and general weakness. Birds subjected to routine postmortem examination. Samples of liver, spleen, kidneys, and proventriculus were collected aseptically and subjected to molecular detection and characterization of MDV in the Central Biotechnology Laboratory.

DNA extraction

Total DNA was extracted from up to 25 mg spleen samples as well as commercial live attenuated MDV as a positive control using DNeasy Blood and Tissue Kit (QIAGEN, USA). After complete lysis of the specimens by ATL buffer and proteinase K, absolute ethanol was added then the mixture was transferred to a spin column according to manufacturer's protocol. Purified DNAs were recovered in 150 μl AE buffer and stored at −20°C for further testing.

Detection of the *Meq* oncoprotein gene

The extracted DNAs were screened for presence of MDV using HotStartTaq® Plus Master Mix Kit (QIAGEN, USA). 2 μl sample of each purified genomic DNAs was amplified in 20 μl of the final volume of a 2X HotStartTaq Plus Master Mix containing 1.5 mM MgCl₂, 200 μM of each dNTP, 1 unit HotStartTaq Plus DNA polymerase, and 10 μM of each forward (F:GCACTCTAGAGTGTA AAGAGATGTC TCAG) and reverse (R:TAACTCG AGGAGAAGAAACATGG GGCATAG) primers [13]. Thermo-cycling conditions were enzyme activation and initial denaturation at 95°C for 5 min followed by

35 cycles of 94°C for 30 s, 55°C for 30 s, and 72°C for 30 s and a final extension step at 72°C for 10 min. The amplified PCR products were electrophoresed in 1.5% agarose gel stained with ethidium bromide and documented using ultraviolet gel documentation system (BIORAD).

Sequencing and construction of phylogenetic tree

Meq gene specific bands were excised from the agarose gel, purified using Montàge DNA gel extraction kit (Millipore, USA) and sequenced in an automated ABI 3730 DNA sequencer (Applied Biosystems, USA). The obtained sequence was aligned by the Clustal W method. The obtained nucleotide sequences were compared with MDV sequences available in Genbank by BLAST web tool of the Genbank (Table-1). A phylogenetic tree was constructed using MEGA version 5.20 software.

Genbank accession number

The obtained *Meq* gene sequences of the detected MDV were submitted to the GenBank database with the accession number (Saudi 01-13; KJ949617 and Saudi 02-13; KJ949618).

Results

Clinical examination

Birds necropsy and morphological observations of the visceral organs revealed enlarged liver with

Table-1: MDV reference strains used in construction the phylogenetic tree.

Accession No.	Country	Name	Reference
HM991861	China	MDV/BY/China	[30]
HQ638151	China	MDV/TQ20/CH	[31]
EF546430	China	MDV/GXY2/CH	Unpublished
HQ658624	China	MDV/HLJ/07/II	[7]
HQ658619	China	MDV/LN/08/V	[7]
HQ658627	China	MDV/HLJ/06/I	[7]
AY362712	USA	MDV/617A	[21]
KJ464784	Poland	MDV/12_08 LORF7	Unpublished
KJ464771	Poland	MDV/5_06 LORF7	Unpublished
HQ204815	Poland	MDV/73_08_PL	Unpublished
AY362725	USA	MDV/648A	[21]
AF243438	USA	MDV/Md5	[5]
HM749326	India	MDV/tn-n3	Unpublished
AB638844	Japan	MDV/Tokachi-s1	[28]
KC243264	Iraq	MDV/10A	[11]
KC243266	Iraq	MDV/51C	[11]
KC243266	Iraq	MDV/95E	[11]
EF523775	Australia	MDV/Woodsland1	Unpublished
EF523775	Australia	MDV/FT158	Unpublished
AF493558	China	MDV/648A	Unpublished
AF493555	Netherland	MDV/CVI988	Unpublished
HF546085	China	MDV/HNGS201	[12]
KC161221	Egypt	MDV/Egypt_5	[32]
EF523390	USA	MDV/RB-1B	Unpublished
AF147806	USA	MDV/GA	[22]
EF523774	Australia	MDV/MPF75	Unpublished
JX467678	Egypt	MDV/Egypt_1	[32]
JN808272	India	MDV/ABT/HSR/5253	Unpublished
JN808280	India	MDV/ABT/HSR/7158	Unpublished
KJ464769	Poland	Wroclaw_06 LORF7	Unpublished

MDV=Marek's disease virus

rounded edges multiple grayish tumors and the spleen were enlarged with grayish nodules.

Molecular detection of *Meq* gene

PCR analysis of *Meq* gene ORF specific for MDV serotypes 1 was done to detect MVD in DNA of tested samples. A 1062 bp fragment was detected in sample 1, whereas in sample 2, a smaller fragment was observed (939 bp).

Sequence and phylogenetic analysis of different *Meq* gene fragments

Nucleotide gene sequence of the *Meq* gene ORF detected in Saudi 01-13 was 1062 bp encoding for a polypeptide of 339 amino acids, whereas the *S-Meq* ORF of Saudi 02-13 (939 bp) showed deletion of about 123 bp between the nucleotides 538 and 660 of the ORF. The deleted area encoding for a polypeptide 41 amino acids without frameshift (Figures-1 and 2). The deletion site was identified between two PRR regions in C-terminal proline-rich domain. Nucleotide and deduced amino acid sequences of the MDV isolates from SA were highly conserved when compared to MDV strains worldwide (CVI988/NLT, GA/USA, Md5/USA, 12_08LO-RF7/PL, and RB-1B/USA). Three amino acid substitutions: Asp.80Tyr., Cys.110Ser., and Pro.218Ser. were identified in the *Meq* of MDVs isolated from SA and MDV strain from Poland (12_08LO-RF7/POL), in addition, eight amino acids substitutions were identified among the Saudi strains and MDVs from Iraq (Table-2).

Phylogenetic analysis

The obtained nucleotide sequences of *Meq* gene (Saudi 01-13 and Saudi 02-13) were compared with those of 30 references MDVs summarized in Table-1 for homology analysis using MEGA version 5.2. These 30 reference MDVs representing different regions all over the world. The Saudi 01-13 and Saudi 02-13 had the highest nucleotide homology (99.8% and 99.6%) with 12 08LORF7/PL, respectively (Figure-3). Comparing the antigenic peaks (index) of both Saudi MDVs, Iraq 95 and 12_08/LORF7/POL, the data showed that they are quite similar although the Saudi 02-13 and Iraq 95 showing a deletion of 123 nucleotide representing 41 amino acid which support the hypothesis that the deletion did not cause frame shift (Figure-4).

Discussion

In the last 40 years, the incidence and interest to MDV has been increasing because of the intensive use of vaccination to control the disease [14]. The virus isolation, genomic sequencing as well as monitoring the oncogenic genes changes are played an important role in the prevention and control of MDV infection in chickens [15]. The polymorphism of *Meq* gene amino

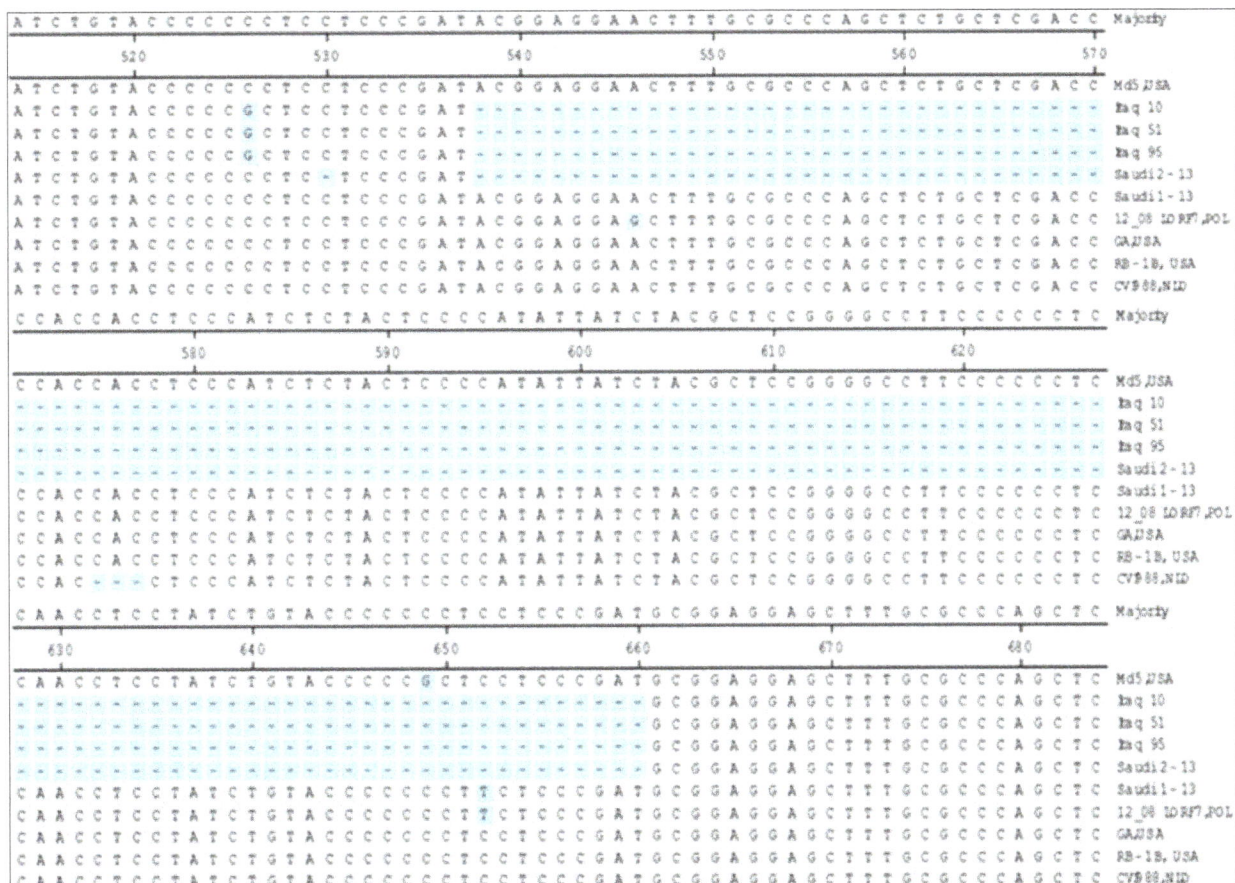

Figure-1: Alignment of *Meq* gene sequences. The nucleotides alignment of *Meq* genes from the strains listed at the right. Unmatched sequences represented by dashes (−). Deletion of nucleotides (538-660) in Saudi 02-13 without frameshifting.

Table-2: Amino acid substitution of Meq gene protein.

Strain/country	Basic region			Leu Zip	Transactivation domain								
	71	77	80	110	141	168	194	200	217	218	283	320	328
CVI988/NLD	S	E	D	C	H	S	-	I	P	P	A	I	S
GA/USA	A	K	D	C	H	S	P	I	P	P	A	I	S
Md5/USA	A	K	D	C	H	S	P	I	A	P	V	T	S
Saudi 01-13	A	E	Y	S	P	S	P	I	P	S	A	I	S
Saudi 02-13*	A	E	Y	S	P	S	-	-	-	S	A	I	S
12_08/LORF7/POL	A	E	Y	S	P	S	P	I	P	S	A	I	L
RB-1B/USA	A	K	D	C	H	S	P	I	P	P	A	I	S
Iraq 10*	S	E	D	C	H	P	-	-	A	P	A	I	S
Iraq 51*	S	E	D	C	H	S	-	-	A	P	A	I	S
Iraq 95*	S	E	D	C	H	S	-	-	A	P	A	I	S

*MDVs isolates with S-Meq. MDV=Marek's disease virus

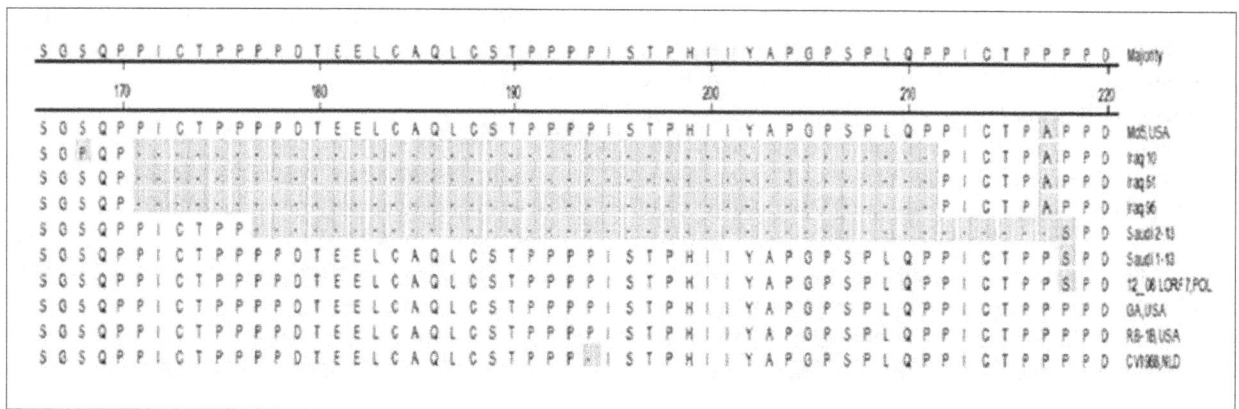

Figure-2: Alignment of *Meq* gene amino acids sequences. The amino acid alignment of *Meq* genes from the strains listed at the right. Unmatched sequences represented by dashes (−). Deletion of amino acids (177-217) in Saudi 02-13 without frameshifting.

acids sequences, as well as point mutations, was found to be correlated to MDV1 virulence [16-18]. The *Meq* gene product is a transcription factor with N-terminal bZIP proteins homologs to Jun/Fos oncoproteins [6].

Meq can interact with itself and cellular proteins such as p53 and C-terminal binding protein and can contribute to cellular oncogenesis [19]. Analysis of MDV genome showed several changes including the expansion of the 132 bp direct repeats located in the internal repeat regions flanking the long unique region [20,21]. On the other hand, differences in the *Meq* gene between oncogenic and non-oncogenic MDV1 have been reported as a result of 177 or 180 bp insertion in the *Meq* gene that may postulate as a cause of biological changes results in attenuation of the MDV1 oncogenic strains [16,18,22].

In this study, the main complaint of the owners of two layer flocks aged 12 and 15 weeks old chickens were uneven growth and about 10% mortalities. Following necropsy, there have been found enlargement of the liver and spleen with grayish, yellowish nodules. No lesions were seen on the skin as well as nervous tissues. In addition, gross lesions associated with emaciation were recorded as previously reported [23-26]. Lesions were suggestive for MD [27]. For further diagnosis, samples were tested

using conventional PCR [13]. PCR was positive for *Meq* gene of MDVs. Unlikely, predicted the size of the PCR products from Saudi 01-13 and Saudi 02-13 were different. The reason why the two bands are different may be due to genetic diversity (deletion or insertion) of the amplified *Meq* gene as reported by Chang et al. [18] and Lee et al. [22].

The *Meq* gene of both MDV isolates was compared with five standard MDVs, deletion of 123 bp in the *Meq* ORF (538-660) between two PRRs in the C-terminal proline-rich domain was detected in Saudi 02-13. The deletion did not cause any frameshift in the *Meq* gene ORF. Wajid et al. [11] reported a 123 bp deletion in *Meq* gene from Iraq. Surprisingly, the deletion in the *Meq* gene of Iraq strains starts from the same nucleotide positions as Saudi isolates (Figure-1). Whereas, on the corresponding amino acid sequence, the deletion occurred between 2 proline residues $^{170}P{\downarrow}P^{171}$ while in Saudi isolates the deletion was in PRR $^{175}PP{\downarrow}PP^{178}$ this may be due to the missed nucleotide at position 530 in the Saudi 02-13 (Figure-2). Previous studies showed that the *Meq* gene is considered the most important molecule in MDV oncogenicity and among the notable finding related to the virulence was distinct diversity and point mutation in the *Meq* proteins [4,18,21-28]. Structural changes in

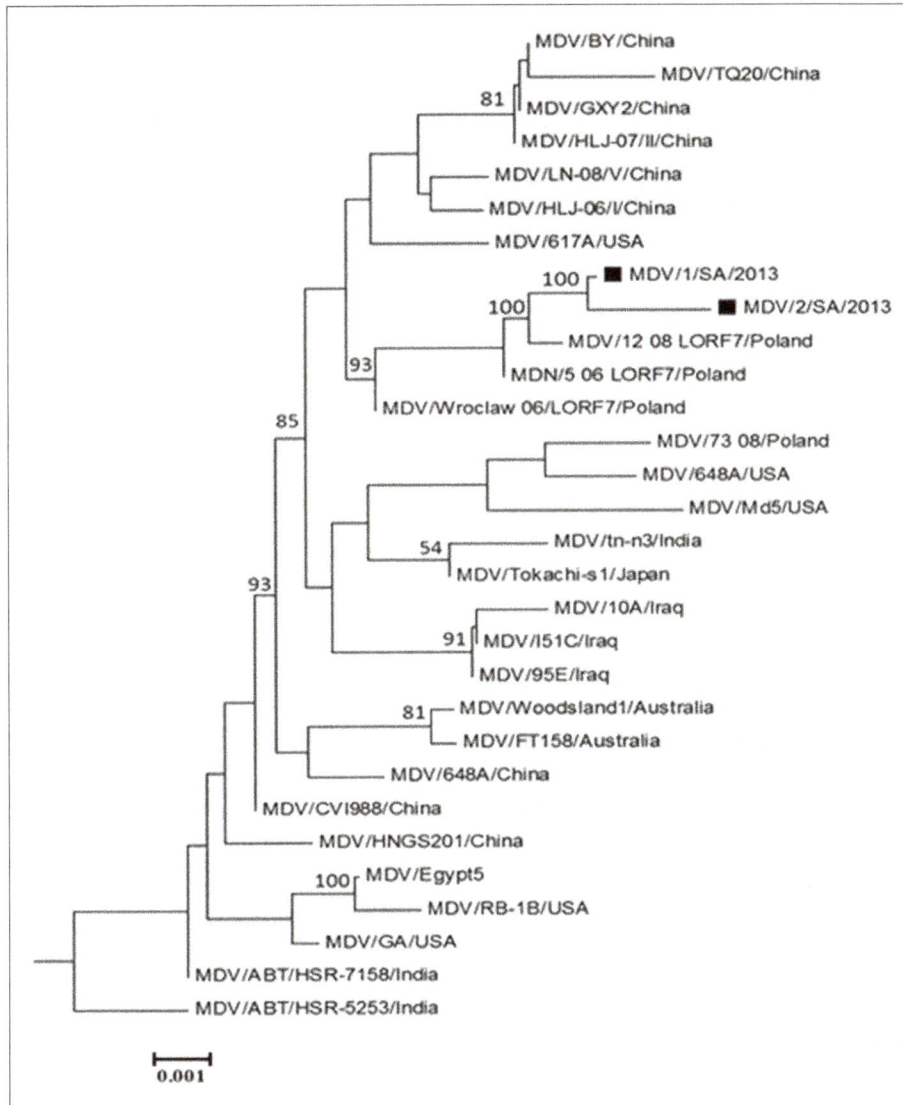

Figure-3: Phylogenetic analysis on *Meq* gene sequences of 2 Saudi Arabian isolates and other 30 references Marek's disease virus. The phylogenetic tree was constructed using the MEGA version 5.0 by the neighbor-joining method with 1000 bootstrap replicates. Black squares indicate the two isolates from Saudi Arabia.

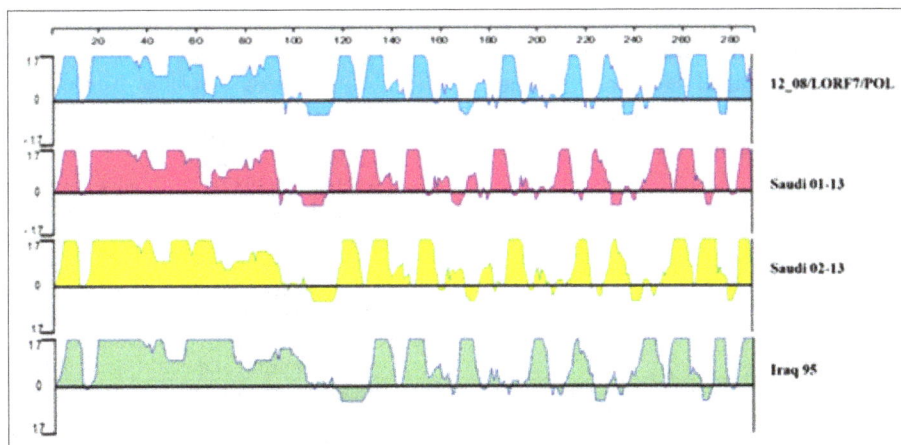

Figure-4: Antigenic index according to Jameson-Wolf for both Saudi Marek's disease virus, Iraq 95 and 12_08/LORF7/POL. Using Protean analysis DNASTAR Software Package.

the MDV genome were previously reported including 200-bp deletion in *Bam*HI/L of MDV strain MD11 and 400 bp deletion in the *Bam*HI-A region of MDV strain CVI988 [29]. On the hand, insertion of 177 or 180 bp in the *Meq* gene of CVI988 was reported and does not cause any frameshift in *Meq* gene ORF that may result in attenuation [21,22]. The number of PPPP motif in the PRRs was 4 in the Saudi 01-13 and 2 in the Saudi 02-13; this previously reported as a virulence dependent factor the low number of PRRs is correlated to the high in virulence [4,11]. Both Saudi isolates had point mutations that interrupted extensions of four proline at position 3 ^{216}PPPP^{219} to ^{216}PPSP^{219} which are a unique substitution in Saudi isolates and 12_08LORF7/POL. Comparison of *Meq* gene sequence of the studied strains with 30 reference MDV1 strains revealed that the SA MDV strains clustered with the MDV strains from Europe (12_08LORF7/POL) that may be contributed to the importation of poultry and/or poultry by-products from European countries or due to movement of birds during migration.

Conclusion

For our knowledge, this is the first comprehensive study describe the incidence of MDV in SA. Both of the detected MDV strains causing lymphomas in layer chickens. Based on the clinical picture and the genomic sequencing both of the MDV isolates found to have characteristics of virulent MDVs although the Saudi 02-13 showed deletion of 123 bp without causing any frameshift. The antigenic index of Saudi MDVs and certain regional and international isolates were quite similar. In Saudi 02-13, the amino acid deletion started at position 177 is due to the short isoform of *Meq*. More concern should be given to the imported poultry and poultry by-products, migratory birds as well as vaccination process to control the MDV infection.

Authors' Contributions

MHM and IME: Study design, PCR, Genomic analysis and prepared the manuscript. MA and YA: Collected samples. All authors read and approved the final manuscript.

Acknowledgments

The authors are highly thankful to Collage of Veterinary Medicine, King Faisal University, Saudi Arabia, for providing necessary support to carry out the work by the Scientific Research Deanship [Project # 150047].

Competing Interests

The authors declare that they have no competing interests.

References

1. Calnek, B.W. and Witter, R.L. (1991) Marek's disease. In: Calnek, B.W., editor. Diseases of Poultry. 10th ed. Iowa State University Press, Ames, Iowa, p369-413.

2. Chang, S., Dunn, J.R., Heidari, M., Lee, L.F., Ernst, C.W., Song, J. and Zhang, J. (2012) Vaccine by chicken line interaction alters the protective efficacy against challenge with a very virulent plus strain of Marek's disease virus in White Leghorn chickens. *World J. Vac.*, 2: 1-11.

3. Gimeno, I.M., Witter, R.L., Cortes, A.L., Reddy, S.M. and Pandiri, A.R. (2012) Standardization of a model to study

revaccination against Marek's disease under laboratory conditions. *Avian Pathol.*, 41: 59-68.

4. Renz, K., Cooke, J., Cheetham, B., Hussain, Z., Islam, A., Tannock, G. and Brown, S. (2012) Pathotyping of Australian isolates of Mareks disease virus and association of pathogenicity with MEQ gene polymorphism. *Avian Pathol.*, 41: 161-176.

5. Tulman, E.R., Afonso, C.L., Lu, Z., Zsak, L.D., Rock, L. and Kutish, G.F. (2000) The genome of a very virulent Marek's disease virus. *J. Virol.*, 74(17): 7980-7988.

6. Jones, D., Lee, L., Liu, J.L., Kung, H.J. and Tillotson, J.K. (1992) Marek's disease virus encodes a basic-leucine zipper gene resembling the fos/jun oncogenes that is highly expressed in lymphoblastoid tumors. *Proc. Natl. Acad. Sci. U.S.A.*, 89: 4042-4046.

7. Zhang, Y.P., Liu, C.J., Zhang, F., Shi, W. and Li, J. (2011) Sequence analysis of the MEQ gene in the predominant Marek's disease virus strains isolated in China during 2006-2008. *Virus Genes.*, 43: 353-357.

8. Liu, J.L. and Kung, H.J. (2000) Marek's disease herpesvirus transforming protein MEQ: A C-Jun analogue with an alternative life style. *Virus Genes.* 21: 51-64.

9. Peng, Q., Zeng, M., Bhuiyan, Z.A., Ubukata, E., Tanaka, A., Nonoyama, M. and Shirazi, Y. (1995) Isolation and characterization of Marek's disease virus (MDV) cDNAs mapping to the BamHI-I2, BamHI-Q2, and BamHI-L fragments of the MDV genome from lymphoblastoid cells transformed and persistently infected with MDV. *Virology*, 213: 590-599.

10. Sung, H.W. (2002) Recent increase of Marek's disease in Korea related to the virulence increase of the virus. *Avian Dis.*, 46: 517-524.

11. Wajid, S.J., Katz, M.E., Renz, K.G. and Walkden-Brown, S.W. (2013) Prevalence of Marek's disease virus in different chicken populations in Iraq and indicative virulence based on sequence variation in the EcoRI-Q (MEQ) gene. *Avian Dis.*, 57: 562-568.

12. Yu, Z.H., Teng, M., Luo, J., Wang, X.W., Ding, K., Yu, L.L., Su, J.W., Chi, J.Q., Zhao, P., Hu, B., Zhang, G.P. and Liu, J.X. (2013) Molecular characteristics and evolutionary analysis of field Marek's disease virus prevalent in vaccinated chicken flocks in recent years in China. *Virus Genes.*, 47(2): 282-291.

13. Król, K., Samorek-Salmonowicz, E., Kozdruń, W. and Woźniakowski, G. (2007) Duplex PCR assay for detection and differentiation of pathogenic and vaccine strains serotype 1. *Bull. Vet. Inst. Pulawy.*, 51: 331-335.

14. Witter, R.L., Calnek, B.W., Buscagli, C., Gimeno, I.M. and Schat, K.A. (2005) Classification of Marek's disease viruses according to pathotype: Philosophy and methodology. *Avian Pathol.*, 34: 75-90.

15. Tan, J., Cooke, J., Clarke, N. and Tannock, G.A. (2008) Optimization of methods for the isolation of Marek's disease viruses in primary chicken cell cultures. *J. Virol. Methods*, 147: 312-318.

16. Schat, K.A. (1987) Marek's disease: A model for protection against herpesvirus induced tumours. *Cancer Surv.*, 6: 1-37.

17. Liu, J.L., Ye, Y., Lee, L.F. and Kung, H.J. (1998) Transforming potential of the herpesvirus oncoprotein MEQ: Morphological transformation, serum-independent growth, and inhibition of apoptosis. *J. Virol.*, 72: 388-395.

18. Chang, K.S., Ohashi, K. and Onuma, M. (2002) Diversity (polymorphism) of the MEQ gene in the attenuated Marek's disease virus (MDV) serotype one an MDV-transformed cell lines. *J. Vet. Med. Sci.*, 64: 1097-1101.

19. Brown, A.C., Baigent, S.J., Smith, L.P., Chattoo, J.P., Petherbridge, L.J., Hawes, P., Allday, M.J. and Nair, V. (2006) Interaction of MEQ protein and C-terminal-binding protein is critical for induction of lymphomas by Marek's disease virus. *Proc. Natl. Acad. Sci. USA.*, 103: 1687-1692.

20. Maotani, K., Kanamori, A., Ikuta, K., Ueda, S., Kato, S. and Hirai, K. (1986) Amplification of a tandem direct repeat within inverted repeats of Marek's disease virus DNA

during serial *in vitro* passage. *J. Virol.,* 58: 657-660.

21. Shamblin, C.E., Greene, N., Arumugaswami, V., Dienglewicz, R.L. and Parcells, M.S. (2004) Comparative analysis of Marek's disease virus (MDV) glycoprotein-lytic antigen pp38-and transformation antigen MEQ-encoding genes: Association of MEQ mutations with MDVs of high virulence. *Vet. Microbiol.,* 102: 147-167.

22. Lee, S., Takagi, M., Ohashi, K., Sugimoto, C. and Onuma, M. (2000) Difference in the MEQ Gene between oncogenic and attenuated strain of Marek's disease virus serotype 1. *J. Vet. Med. Sci.,* 62(3): 287-292.

23. Frank, F. (2001) Marek's disease: History, actual and future perspectives. *Lohmann Inform.,* 25: 1-5.

24. Balachandran, K., Pazhanivel, N., Vairamuthu, S. and Murali Manohar, B. (2009) Marek's disease and lymphoid leukosis in chicken - a histopathological survey. *Tamil Nadu J. Vet. Anim. Sci.* 5: 167-170.

25. Hablolvarid, M. (2011) Investigation on incidence of Marek's disease in broiler flocks of some regions in Tehran province, Iran. *Arch. Razi Inst.,* 66(2): 109-114.

26. Musa, I.W., Bisalla, M., Mohammed, B., Sa'idu, L. and Abdu, P.A. (2013) Retrospective and clinical studies of Marek's disease in Zaria, Nigeria. *J. Bacteriol. Res.,* 5(2): 13-21.

27. OIE. (2012) Manual of Diagnostic Tests and Vaccines for Terrestrial Animals. Ch. 2. 3. 13. World Organization for Animal Health, Paris. p545-554.

28. Murata, S., Hayashi, Y., Kato, A., Isezaki, M., Takasaki, S., Onuma, M., Osa, Y., Asakawa, M., Konnai, S. and Ohashi, K. (2012) Surveillance of Marek's disease virus in migratory and sedentary birds in Hokkaido, Japan. *Vet. J.,* 192(3): 538-540.

29. Van Iddekinge, B.J., Stenzler, L., Schat, K.A., Boerrigter, H. and Koch, G. (1999) Genome analysis of Marek's disease virus strain CVI-988: Effect of cell culture passage on the inverted repeat regions. *Avian Dis.,* 43(2): 182-188.

30. Tian, M.X., Deng, R., Cao, S.J., Wen, X.T., Zou, N.L., Liu, P. and Huang, Y. (2010) Isolation of a field Marek's disease virus with acute oncogenicity from Tibetan chickens in China and sequence analysis of oncogenic genes. In: Proceedings of 2010 First International Conference on Cellular, Molecular Biology, Biophysics and Bioengineering. p259-263.

31. Tian, M., Zhao, Y., Lin, Y., Zou, N., Liu, C., Liu, P., Cao, S., Wen, X. and Huang, Y. (2011) Comparative analysis of oncogenic genes revealed unique evolutionary features of field Marek's disease virus prevalent in recent years in China. *Virology,* 8: 121.

32. Hassanin, O., Abdallah, F. and EL-Araby, I.E. (2013) Molecular characterization and phylogenetic analysis of Marek's disease virus from clinical cases of Marek's disease in Egypt. *Avian Dis.,* 57: 555-561.

23

Age-specific changes in electrocardiographic parameters in bipolar limb leads of conscious female native cats of Odisha

Subhashree Sarangi, A. P. K. Mahapatra, S. Mohapatra and A. K. Kundu

Department of Veterinary Physiology, College of Veterinary Science & Animal Husbandry, Odisha University of Agriculture & Technology, Bhubaneswar - 751 003, Odisha, India.
Corresponding author: Subhashree Sarangi, e-mail: subhashreesarangi2010@gmail.com,
APKM: ambika28@hotmail.com, SM: swagat.physiology@gmail.com, AKK: kunduakk@yahoo.in

Abstract

Aim: To study and compare the age-specific changes in electrocardiographic (ECG) parameters in bipolar limb leads of conscious female native cats of Odisha.

Materials and Methods: 20 healthy female native cats aged between 4 and 36 months of age were selected for the study. These queens were divided into two groups of 10 animals each. Group 1 constituted the queens aged 4-10 months (before puberty) with a mean weight of 2.28 kg (±0.4 standard error [SE]), and those aged 11-36 months (after puberty) with a mean weight of 3.72 kg (±0.6 SE) were in Group 2. The ECG was recorded with a 12-lead standard ECG recorder, Cardiart 108 T-MK VII-BPL (India) in the Leads I, II, and III.

Results: The mean heart rates were 160.73 (±7.83) beats/min and 139.09 (±2.72) beats/min in the cats aged 4-10 months and 11-36 months, respectively. Significant differences existed among Q- and R-wave amplitudes and duration of QT-interval in Lead I. In Lead II, duration of QT and RR intervals, duration of ST-segment and amplitudes of P- and R-waves varied significantly. Significant differences were also observed in the P- and R-wave amplitudes in Lead III. The mean electrical axis was 63.11 (±1.98°) and 50.03 (±4.86°) in the cats aged 4-10 months and 11-36 months, respectively.

Conclusion: Since the ECG studies on conscious cats are scanty, and the number of native cats being presented in veterinary hospitals and clinics has increased drastically, there is a need to establish the reference values for ECG parameters in conscious native cats so that the cardiovascular abnormalities can be predicted.

Keywords: age-specific, conscious cat, electrocardiogram, mean electrical axis, native.

Introduction

The domestic cat has a long history as a research subject; stray cats were used as research subjects by Claude Bernard and others during the early years of experimental medicine, their small size and availability making them popular candidates for both medical and surgical explorations. These have been used extensively for neurological research, brain and vision studies as well as for toxicology and endocrinology experiments. Moreover, these animals serve as excellent companion animals and are susceptible to many diseases, of both infectious and non-infectious origin.

Prediction and evaluation of cardiac diseases, particularly in small animals, is vital and this is possible with the use of an electrocardiograph. Electrocardiogram (ECG) is the recording of the potentials generated by the electrical current due to the passage of cardiac impulses through the heart. The ECG studies on cats are scanty, and those made earlier

have focused mainly on anesthetic protocols [1] and a recent one on breed [2]. Some studies have also been reported on breed and age in dogs [3,4], goats [5], and sheep [6], the relation between ECG parameters and ion channels in dogs and rabbits [7,8], asphyxic episodes in rats [9], and anesthetic protocols in dogs [10].

Previous studies have been centered on the Lead II parameters only, and the purpose of this study was to expand the knowledge on the Leads I and III also. Few studies have revealed that the cardiac physiology of cats during the early life differs from that of adults [4,11], which might be due to differences in autonomic innervations of the heart and vasculature, resulting in marked differences in baroreflex control of circulation [12].

ECG parameters are not affected by gender difference [13], and puberty generally occurs between 5 and 9 months in queens [14]. Therefore, the aim of our experiment was to study and compare the age-specific changes in ECG parameters in Leads I, II, and III of conscious female native cats of the region.

Materials and Methods

Ethical approval

The experiments were conducted as per the guidelines laid down by the Institutional Ethical Committee and in accordance with the country law.

The ECG was recorded as per standard procedure without causing any discomfort to animals.

Animal groups

20 healthy female native cats aged between 4 and 36 months of age were selected for the study. The animals were judged healthy on the basis of history, physical examination, and ECG. These queens were divided into two groups of 10 animals each. Group 1 constituted the queens aged 4-10 months (before puberty) with a mean weight of 2.28 kg (±0.4 SE), and those aged 11-36 months (after puberty) with a mean weight of 3.72 kg (±0.6 SE) were in Group 2.

Study method

The ECG was recorded with a 12-lead standard ECG recorder, Cardiart 108 T-MK VII-BPL (India) in the Leads I, II and III. The ECG was set for a paper speed of 25 mm/s and sensitivity of 1 (1 cm=1 mV) with the filter (50 Hz) turned "on." The ECG was recorded with the cat in standard body position; restrained in right lateral recumbency (Figure-1). The right forelimb and left forelimb electrodes were placed proximal to the olecranon on the caudal aspect of the respective forelimbs while the right hind limb and left hind limb electrodes were placed over the patellar ligament on the anterior aspect of the respective hind limbs using alligator clips after applying a little cardiac gel [15].

Statistical analysis

The data obtained for each parameter in both the groups were tabulated and analyzed statistically by t-test to find out the mean and SE. A significance level of 5% (P<0.05) was adopted to compare the mean values of both the groups. The results are presented in table.

Results

The ECG was recorded with the typical P-QRS-T-waves each time (Figure-2). P-wave represents the depolarization of atrial muscle. Depolarization of the ventricles is represented by the QRS complex, which is followed by repolarization of the ventricles, represented by the T-wave. ECG intervals are clinically very useful. The P-R interval, measured from the beginning of the P-wave to the beginning of the QRS complex, represents the time required for the

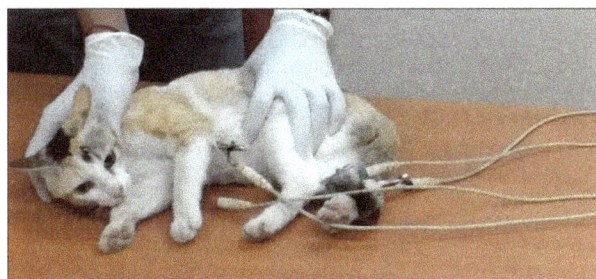

Figure-1: Position while recording of the electrocardiogram in a conscious female native cat of Odisha.

wave of excitation to travel from the sinoatrial node to the ramifications of the His–Purkinje system. The duration of the QRS complex represents the spread of impulses throughout ventricular muscle and is a measure of the intraventricular conduction time. The Q-T interval, measured from the beginning of the Q to the end of the T-wave, reflects the approximate duration of ventricular systole and the ventricular refractory period. The P-R, S-T, and T-P segments are periods of electrical inactivity during which no deflections are observed with respect to the baseline; however, P-R and S-T segments are clinically important since they occur between the waves of a single cardiac cycle. The dominant direction of electrical forces is given by the mean electrical axis (MEA).

The reference values (mean ± SE) of ECG parameters varying significantly (P<0.05) in Leads I, II, and III are shown in Table-1. The mean heart rates were 160.73 (±7.83 SE) beats/min and 139.09 (±2.72 SE) beats/min in the cats aged 4-10 months and 11-36 months respectively. Significant differences existed among Q- and R-wave amplitudes and duration of QT-interval in Lead I. In Lead II, duration of QT and RR intervals, duration of ST-segment and amplitudes of P- and R-waves varied significantly. Significant differences were also observed in the P- and R-wave amplitudes in Lead III. The MEA was 63.11 (±1.98 SE)° and 50.03 (±4.86 SE)° in the cats aged 4-10 months and 11-36 months, respectively.

Discussion

Previous studies have reported that heart rate values range from 160 to 240 beats/min in normal healthy cats [16]. The parasympathetic system is predominant in adults resulting in a lower heart rate than the younger ones who possess a dominant sympathetic system [15]. Again, puberty generally occurs between 5 and 9 months for queens [14]. Cardiovascular activities are reported to be affected by different levels of sex hormones such as estradiol and dihydrotestosterone [7]. Therefore, it may be concluded that the heart rate is higher in cats aged 11-36 months due to increased estrogen levels, and this is in agreement with an experiment on dogs where heart rate decreased in the absence of sex hormones [8].

QT-interval results obtained in the Leads I and II are compatible with a study on rabbits which suggests that estrogen lengthens the Q-T interval in sexually mature female dogs [8]. R-R interval was found to be greater in adult cats which may be due to changes in QT-RR relationships from young to adult stages [17]. No literature was available on the duration of S-T segment and amplitudes of P-, Q-, and R-waves. However, the MEA values were quite lower than those reported in kitten and adult Angora cats [3], which might be due to differences in breed characteristics, i.e., shape and size of the heart.

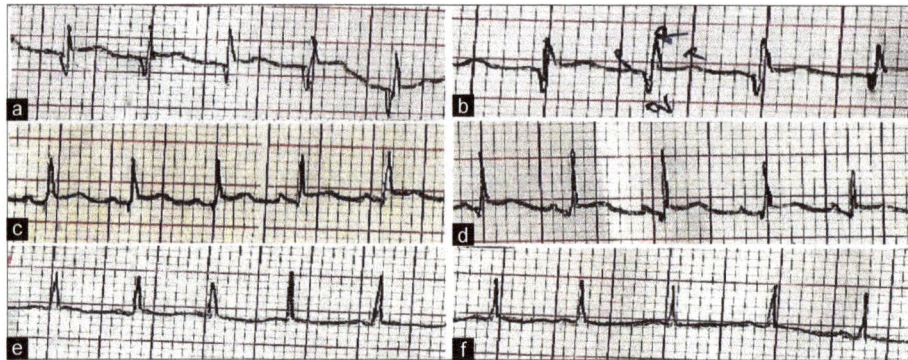

Figure-2: Electrocardiograms recorded in bipolar limb leads of conscious female native cats of Odisha, (a) 4-10 mon, L-I, (b) 11-36 mon, L-I, (c) 4-10 mon, L-II, (d) 11-36 mon, L-II, (e) 4-10 mon, L-III and (f) 11-36 mon, L-III.

Table-1: Reference values (mean±SE) of electrocardiographic parameters varying significantly (P<0.05) in bipolar limb leads of conscious female native cats of Odisha (rest are not significant).

Parameters	Group 1	Group 2
Lead I		
Duration (s)		
QT interval	0.11±0.014	0.16±0.014
Amplitude (mV)		
Q-wave	0.3±0.031	0.18±0.037
R-wave	0.54±0.024	0.66±0.05
Lead II		
Duration (s)		
QT interval	0.15±0.014	0.2±0.012
RR interval	0.39±0.008	0.44±0.0001
ST segment	0.03±0.014	0.08±0.012
Amplitude (mV)		
P-wave	0.18±0.02	0.12±0.02
R-wave	0.62±0.048	0.44±0.024
Lead III		
Amplitude (mV)		
P-wave	0.12±0.013	0.17±0.015
R-wave	0.46±0.081	0.22±0.037
Heart rate (beats/min)	160.73±7.83	139.09±2.72
MEA (°)	63.11±1.98	50.03±4.86

MEA=Mean electrical axis, SE=Standard error

Conclusion

Since the ECG studies on conscious cats are scanty, and the number of native cats being presented in veterinary hospitals and clinics has increased drastically, there is a need to establish the reference values for ECG parameters in conscious native cats. ECG is an important diagnostic tool to detect and evaluate many kinds of cardiovascular abnormalities or arrhythmias such as atrial fibrillation, ventricular tachycardia, conduction block, and premature atrial and ventricular complexes, and diagnosis would be possible only if the normal values are established for the breed.

Authors' Contributions

This study was planned by SS and AKK. SS carried out the research under the guidance of APKM and SM. All the authors participated in draft and revision of the manuscript. All the authors read and approved the final manuscript.

Acknowledgments

The authors are thankful to the Director, Teaching Veterinary Clinical Complex for providing facilities to carry out the research and Department of Veterinary Physiology, College of Veterinary Science and Animal Husbandry, OUAT, Bhubaneswar, India for generation of funds for the present study.

Competing Interests

The authors declare that they have no competing interests.

References

1. Kanda, T. and Hikasa, Y. (2008) Neurohormonal and metabolic effects of medetomidine compared with xylazine in healthy cats. *Can. J. Vet. Res.*, 72(3): 278-286.
2. Atmaca, N., Simsek, O., Arikan, S. and Kabakci, R. (2014) Evaluation of some electrocardiographic parameters of kitten and adult angora cats. *Res. J. Vet. Pract.*, 2(6): 113-116.
3. Atmaca, N. and Emre, B. (2010) Some electrocardiographic parameters of the Kangal dogs. *J. Anim. Vet. Adv.*, 9: 949-953.
4. Mohapatra, S., Mahapatra, A.P.K., Pradhan, S.R. and Kundu, A.K. (2015) Electrocardiographic changes in Labrador dogs with age. *Ind. J. Vet. Sci. Biotech.*, 10(4): 19-22.
5. Atmaca, N., Simsek, O. and Emre, B. (2014) Some electrocardiographic values of Angora goats. *Ankara Univ. Vet. Fak Derg.*, 61: 15-19.
6. Mohapatra, S., Dwivedy, S., Mohapatra, S.S., Mahapatra, A.P.K. and Kundu, A.K. (2015) Comparison of electrocardiogram between young and adult male Ganjam sheep of Odisha. *Ind. Vet. J.*, 92(6): 66-68.
7. Drici, M.D., Burklow, T.R., Haridasse, V., Glazer, R.I. and Woosley, R.L. (1996) Sex hormones prolong the QT interval and downregulate potassium channel expression in the rabbit heart. *Circulation*, 94: 1471-1474.
8. Fülöp, L., Bányász, T., Szabó, G., Tóth, I.B., Bíró, T., Lôrincz, I., Balogh, Á., Petô, K., Mikó, I. and Nánási, P.P. (2006) Effects of sex hormones on ECG parameters and expression of cardiac ion channels in dogs. *Acta Physiol.*, 188: 163-171.
9. Bacova, I., Scorc, P. Jr and Bracokova, I. (2010) Chronophysiologic aspects of ECG changes during a systemic asphyxic episode and subsequent reoxygenation in an experimental rat model. *Bratisl. Lek. Listy.*, 111(3): 121-125.
10. Khurana, A., Kumar, A., Sharma, S.K. and Kumar, A. (2014) Electrocardiographic and haemato-biochemical effects of two balanced anesthetic protocols in dogs. *Vet. World*, 7(10): 835-841.

11. Gomes Lourenco, M.L. and Ferreira, H. (2003) Electrocardiographic evolution in cats from birth to 30 days of age. *Can. Vet. J.*, 44: 914-917.

12. Papaioannou, V.E. (2007) Heart rate variability, baroreflex function and heart rate turbulence: Possible origin and implications. *Hell. J. Cardiol.*, 48: 278-289.

13. Kilicalp, D. and Cinar, A. (2003) Investigation of the effects of age, sex and season on electrocardiographs (ECG values) and heart radiographs of healthy van cats. *Turk. J. Vet. Anim. Sci.*, 27: 101-107.

14. Little, S.E. (2011) Female reproduction. In: Little SE, editor. The Cat: Clinical Medicine and Management. 1st ed.

Elsevier Saunders, St. Louis, MO, USA. pp 1195-1227.

15. Tilley, L.P. (1992) Essentials of Canine and Feline Electrocardiography - Interpretation and Treatment. 3rd ed. Lea and Febiger, Philadelphia, USA.

16. Gordon, S.G. and Estrada, A.H. (2013) The ABCDs of Small Animal Cardiology: A Practical Manual. 1st ed. Life Learn Inc., Guelph, Canada.

17. Drici, M.D., Arrighi, I., Chouabe, C., Mann, J.R., Lazdunski, M., Romey, G. and Barhanin, J. (1998) Involvement of is K-associated K1 channel in heart rate control of repolarization in a murine engineered model of Jervell and Lange-Nielsen syndrome. *Circ. Res.*, 83: 95-102.

24

Genetic structure of *Mugil cephalus* L. populations from the northern coast of Egypt

Mahmoud Magdy[1], Mariam Gergis Eshak[2] and Mohamed Abdel-Salam Rashed[2]

1. Department of Genetics, Faculty of Agriculture, Ain Shams University, 68 Hadayek Shubra, 11241 Cairo, Egypt;
2. Department of Cell Biology, National Research Centre, Dokki, Giza, Egypt.
Corresponding author: Mariam Gergis Eshak, e-mail: mgergis@yahoo.com, MM: m.elmosallamy@agr.asu.edu.eg, MAR: rashed50@yahoo.com

Abstract

Aim: The gray mullet, *Mugil cephalus*, has been farmed in semi-intensive ponds with tilapia and carps in Egypt for years. The current study used the fluorescent amplified fragment length polymorphism (F-AFLP) technique to search for genetic differences between the populations of *M. cephalus* in the northern region of Egypt and to detect the gene flow between sampled locations and the homogeneity within *M. cephalus* genetic pool in Egypt.

Materials and Methods: To fulfill the study objectives 60 (15/location) samples were collected from four northern coast governorates of Egypt (Alexandria "sea," Kafr El-Sheikh "farm," Damietta "farm" and Port Said "sea"). Three replicates of bulked DNA (5 samples/replicate) for each location were successfully amplified using the standard AFLP protocol using fluorescent primers. DNA polymorphism, genetic diversity, and population structure were assessed while positive outlier loci were successfully detected among the sampled locations. Based on the geographical distribution of sampling sites, the gene flow, the genetic differentiation, and correlations to sampling locations were estimated.

Results: A total of 1890 polymorphic bands were scored for all locations, where 765, 1054, 673, and 751 polymorphic bands were scored between samples from Alexandria, Kafr El-Sheikh, Damietta and Port Said, respectively. The effective number of alleles (n_e) for all bulked samples combined together was 1.42. The expected heterozygosity under Hardy–Weinberg assumption (H_e) for all bulked samples combined together was 0.28. Bulked samples from Damietta yielded the lowest n_e (1.35) and the lowest H_e (0.23) when inbreeding coefficient (F_{IS}) = 1. Bulked samples from Kafr El-Sheikh scored the highest n_e (1.55) and the highest H_e (0.37). Bulked samples from Alexandria scored 1.40 for n_e and 0.26 for H_e, while bulked samples from Port Said scored 1.39 for n_e and 0.26 for H_e. The observed bulked samples formed three sub-population groups, where none is limited to a certain sampling location. A high differentiation among locations was detected, however, is not fully isolating the locations. Gene flow was 0.58. Positive outliers loci (117) were detected among the four sampled locations while weak significant correlation (r=0.15, p=0.03) was found for the distance between them.

Conclusion: Even though this species is cultivated in Egypt, the wild population is still present and by the current study a flow of its genes is still exchanged through the northern coast of Egypt. Which contribute to the cultivated populations leading to heterogeneity in its genetic pool and consequently affects the production consistency of *M. cephalus* in Egypt.

Keywords: fluorescent amplified fragment length polymorphism, isolation by distance, Mantel test, marine fish, *Mugil cephalus*, natural selection pressure, population structure.

Introduction

The gray mullet, *Mugil cephalus* Linnaeus, is commonly referred to as the striped, gray, or black mullet [1]. The gray mullet has been farmed for centuries in extensive and semi-intensive ponds in many countries. Traditional aquaculture methods employed for raising mullet are now advanced, especially in Italy. Flathead gray mullet is a very important aquaculture species in Egypt, where its farming has been traditional in the "hosha" system in the delta region for centuries. Since the early 1960s, flathead gray mullet has also been cultured in semi-intensive ponds with tilapia and carps in Egypt [2].

Mugil cephalus is cosmopolitan in the coastal waters of most tropical and subtropical zones and it is commonly found between 42° N and 42° S [3]. It is catadromous, frequently found coastally in estuaries and freshwater environments. Adult mullet have been found in waters ranging from zero salinity to 75% while juveniles can only tolerate such wide salinity ranges after they reach lengths of 4-7 cm. Flathead gray mullet is a diurnal feeder, consuming mainly zooplankton, dead plant matter, and detritus. Mullet have thick-walled gizzard-like segments in their stomach along with a long gastrointestinal tract that enables them to feed on detritus. Trials on the artificial propagation of flathead gray mullet have been carried out, but most of the commercial aquaculture production of flathead gray mullet still depends on fry collected from the wild, which is cheaper.

Several population genetic studies targeted the gray Mullet habitat in the Mediterranean Sea, Atlantic Ocean and, to a lesser extent, East Pacific and Indian Oceans, as a model of study in order to obtain more information for the biodiversity conservation and fishery management. These studies included allozyme analysis, biochemical markers and mitochondrial DNA sequences [4-12], and more recently, the amplified fragment length polymorphism (AFLP) [13].

The AFLP technique is widely used in phylogenetic and population genomics studies, particularly in non-model organisms for which no prior DNA sequence information is available [14]. Wide multi-locus screening (also known as genome scan) of the locus-specific signature can reflect efficiently the 'adaptive divergence and genetic differentiation within a population [15]. AFLP-based genome scans have been used successfully to detect genetic differentiation due to adaptation to altitude, adaptation to soil type, insecticide resistance or ecotype divergence [16-22]. The most studies using population genomics approaches conclude that a substantial proportion of the genomes analyzed shows potential signatures of selection (about 5% of the analyzed *loci*; Nosil *et al.* [23]).

The objectives of this study were to use fluorescent AFLP based genome scanning to search for genetic differences within and between the sampled populations of *M. cephalus* and; to detect the gene flow between sampled locations and the homogeneity within *M. cephalus* genetic pool in the northern region of Egypt.

Materials and Methods

Ethical approval

The catching of the fish material used in the current study was permitted by the General Authority for Fish Resources Development, Ministry of Agriculture, Egypt and the Animal research ethics approval sub-committee of the Genetics department committee, Faculty of Agriculture, Ain Shams University, Egypt.

Sampling and DNA extraction

Fish samples were gathered from four locations along the northern coast governorates of Egypt (Location 1: Alexandria, sea "latitude: 31.200 and longitude: 29.919," Location 2: Kafr El-Sheikh, farm "latitude: 31.106 and longitude: 30.942," Location 3: Damietta, farm "latitude: 30.046 and longitude: 31.254" and Location 4: Port Said, sea "latitude: 31.418 and longitude: 31.814"; Figure-1). The DNA extractions were carried out from fins of 60 collected fish samples (15/location) using Wizard® Genomic DNA Purification Kit (PROMEGA, USA) by following the manufacturer's manual. DNA quality was then tested using agrose gel electrophoresis (1%) contain 1 μl of ethidium bromide (100 mg/ml), and electrophoresed for 1 h (4V/cm). When successful, DNA was bulked in three replicates (5 samples/replicate), that lead to 12 bulked samples (3-bulked sample/location).

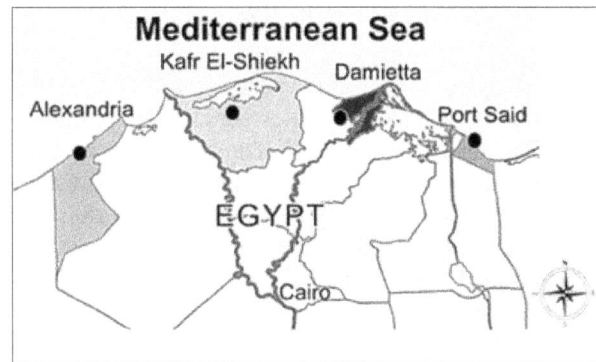

Figure-1: Sampling location along the northern coast governorates of Egypt (Alexandria "sea," Kafr El-Sheikh "farm," Damietta "farm" and Port Said "sea").

AFLP-polymerase chain reaction (PCR)

The original protocol of Vos *et al.* [14] was followed using fluorescent primers instead of radioactive agents. All primers and adaptors were synthesized (Invitrogen, UK) and prepared as recommended (Table-1). Six different selective PCR combinations (3 Eco+NNN × 2 Mse+NNN primers) were amplified using the original PCR program. Private Service was contracted to visualize the amplified products using ABI3730 DNA analyzer (Applied Biosystems, USA) with a size standard GS500-LIZ (Macrogen Genescan Service, Korea).

Data analysis
Band scoring

Automated AFLP scoring was performed using two programs Peak Scanner™ (Applied Biosystems, USA) for peak calling and Rawgeno V2 for automated scoring, according to the software's manuals. The analysis of the AFLP data was based on the band-binary criterion (i.e. codifying the detected bands to, 1 when the presence and 0 when absent) and processed according to Bonin *et al.* [24].

Genetic diversity and population structure

To investigate the genetic structure, Bayesian clustering method was applied by using Structure V2.2 [25]. Triple independent simulations were performed per each assumed number of sub-populations K (K=1 to 6). Parameters were set as the following burn-in period of 10,000 out of 100,000 MCMC iterations, and admixture ancestry model was set on.

Outlier loci detection

This procedure identifies *loci* which exhibit higher or a lower fixation index (F_{ST}) values than the great majority of neutral markers. Mcheza software [26] was used to detect positive outliers considering only polymorphic *loci*. Under the default parameters, Mcheza was run five times with 100,000 simulations at 100% confidence limit. *Loci* that constantly appeared to be an outlier in each run were included in the genetic differentiation analyses.

Genetic differentiation, gene flow and geographical influence

Analysis of molecular variance (AMOVA) was performed to test the population genetic differentiation by using Arlequin V3.5 [27]. The significance of F_{ST} was tested with 10000 permutations for the detected AFLP *loci*. Gene flow (Nm) based on F_{ST} value was estimated using AFLP-Surv [28]. The effect of the geographical distance between sampled locations on the distribution of the genotypes of *M. cephalus* was tested using Mantel test (to measure the association between two matrices) implemented in GenAlEx V6 [29]. The genetic distance and log (genetic distance) matrices of AFLP all loci and AFLP positive outlier *loci* were tested against the geographical distance and the log (geographical distance). Data and log data were used to find which were the most appropriate to represent a better correlation using Mantel test [30]. The significance of the correlation value was tested with 10,000 permutations.

Results

Fragment analysis and band scoring

PCR amplification was successful for six pairs of AFLP selective primers. Band scoring for each primer pair gathered bands between 50 and 650 bp (Figure-2). A total of 1890 polymorphic bands were scored from all primer pairs for all the 12 bulked samples. Polymorphic bands for each location were 765, 1054, 673 and 751 for Alexandria, Kafr El-Sheikh, Damietta and Port Said, respectively. The mean band presence was ~799 while the mean fragment size was ~360 bp with a standard deviation of ~160 bp. A weak significant negative correlation was found between fragment sizes and frequencies (r=−0.19; p<0.00).

Genetic diversity and population structure

The effective number of alleles (n_e) for all bulked samples combined was 1.42. The expected heterozygosity under Hardy–Weinberg assumption (H_e) for all bulked samples combined together was 0.28. Bulked samples from Damietta yielded the lowest n_e (1.35) and the lowest H_e (0.23) when F_{IS}=1. Bulked samples from Kafr El-Sheikh scored the highest n_e (1.55) and the highest H_e (0.37). Bulked samples from Alexandria scored 1.40 for n_e and 0.26 for H_e, while bulked samples from Port Said scored 1.39 for n_e and 0.26 for H_e (Table-2).

The highest average of "estimated Ln probability score" with the lowest variance, sub-population number estimated by the Bayesian inference was K=3, indicating that the observed bulked samples most probably originated from three sub-populations (groups; Figure-3).

Group 1 possesses the highest number of individuals (8) regardless of its geographical location. These are bulked samples number 1 and 2 (Alexandria), 5 and 6 (Kafr El-Sheikh), 8 (Damietta) and 10, 11 and 12 (Port Said). Group 2 consists of a unique bulked sample number 4 from Kafr El-Sheikh location. Group 3 consists of three bulked samples that are number 3 (Alexandria) and 7 and 9 (Damietta). The only homogeneous location that belongs to a certain group was Port Said sampling location (Figure-4).

Detection of positive selection *loci*

The AFLP data set were analyzed for outlier *loci* detection by using the Mcheza software between

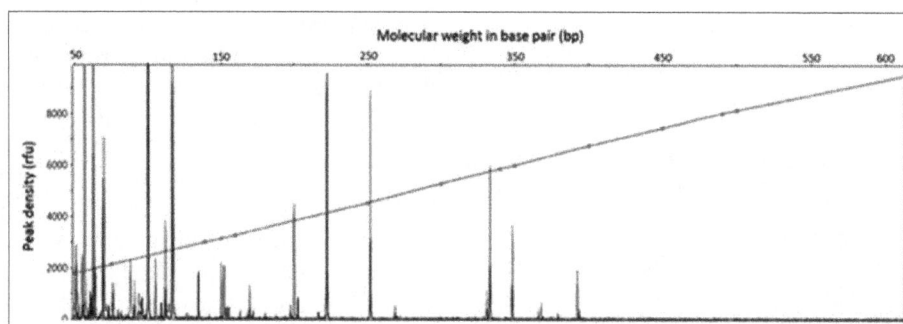

Figure-2: Fragment analysis chromatogram example of bulked sample no. 1 from Alexandria. Multiplexed selective amplified fragment length polymorphism-polymerase chain reaction of: FAM-Eco-ACA × Mse-CAA (blue peaks), HEX-Eco-AGG × Mse-CAA (green peaks) and CY3-Eco-ATA × Mse-CAA (black peaks), are shown. Only peaks within 50-600 bp were considered.

Table-1: Sequence 5′- 3′ of primers and adaptors used to establish the AFLP-PCR technique according to the original protocol of Vos *et al.* [14].

Oligo	5′ - sequence - 3′	Oligo	5′ - sequence - 3′
MseI-Adap1	GACGATGAGTCCTGAG	EcoRI-Adap1	CTCGTAGACTGCGTACC
MseI-Adap2	TACTCAGGACTCAT	EcoRI-Adap2	AATTGGTACGCAGTC
Mse-C	GATGAGTCCTGAGTAA**C**	Eco-A	GACTGCGTACCAATTC**A**
Mse-CAA	GATGAGTCCTGAGTAA**CAA**	Eco-ACA	*FAM*-GACTGCGTACCAATTC**ACA**
Mse-CTC	GATGAGTCCTGAGTAA**CTC**	Eco-AGG	*HEX*-GACTGCGTACCAATTC**AGG**
		Eco-ATA	*CY3*-GACTGCGTACCAATTC**ATA**

Selective nucleotide are in bold. AFLP=Amplified fragment length polymorphism, PCR=Polymerase chain reaction

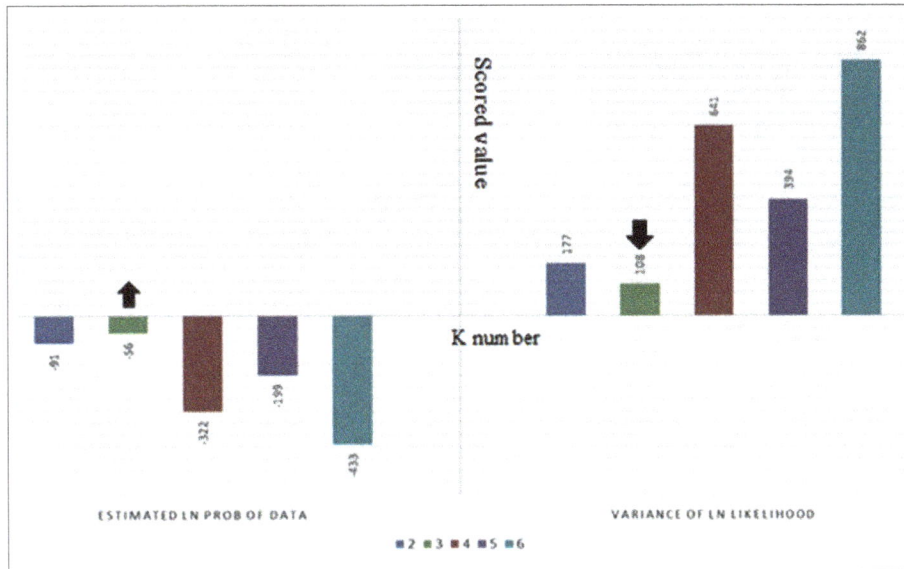

Figure-3: Graphical plotting of structure software output scores based on amplified fragment length polymorphism *loci*. Estimated *ln* probability (LnP) and variance of *ln* likelihood (VLn) for K=[2-6], are shown. K=3 shows the lowest VLn and highest LnP.

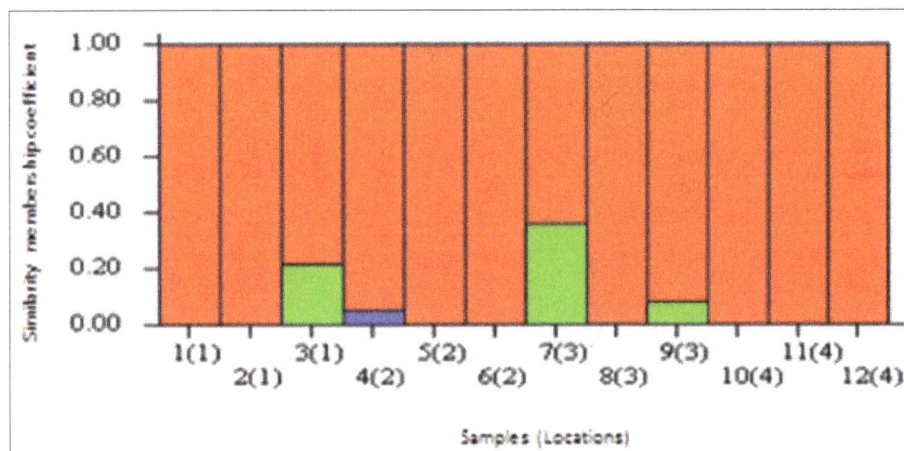

Figure-4: Amplified fragment length polymorphism marker-based structure bar plot graph of K=3, for 12 samples in 4 locations. Samples are ordered by group assignment and locations are indicated between brackets.

Table-2: Genetic diversity and DNA polymorphism based on AFLP bands.

Parameter/location	Alexandria	Kafr El-Sheikh	Damietta	Port said	All samples
Number of polymorphic bands	765	1054	673	751	1890
Mean heterozygosity (H_e)	0.26	0.37	0.23	0.26	0.28
Standard deviation (H_e)	0.32	0.33	0.31	0.32	0.32
Mean effective number of alleles (n_e)	1.40	1.55	1.35	1.39	1.42
Standard deviation (n_e)	0.49	0.49	0.47	0.48	0.48

AFLP=Amplified fragment length polymorphism

the four locations. Across the 16 pairwise analyses between the four groups, 117 out of 1890 polymorphic *loci* (6.19%) were identified as outlier *loci* under directional selection at the 99.5% confidence level (Figure-5). The 117 *loci* appeared constantly as outlier *loci* among the four geographical locations in each run.

Genetic differentiation, gene flow and geographical influence

An AMOVA test was used to measure the changes in the pairwise differentiation of the F_{ST} for the AFLP dataset. F_{ST} of 0.46 (p<0.00), partitioned into a major genetic variation originated within locations, accounting for 53% of the total variations, while 47% of the genetic variation occurred among locations (Table-3). Gene flow (N_m) was estimated of 0.58 based on Wright's fixation index (F_{ST}=0.46), where "N_m=[(1/F_{ST})−1]/2."

Partial Mantel test between the geographical distance and AFLP all loci data set for both data and log data showed no significant correlation, along

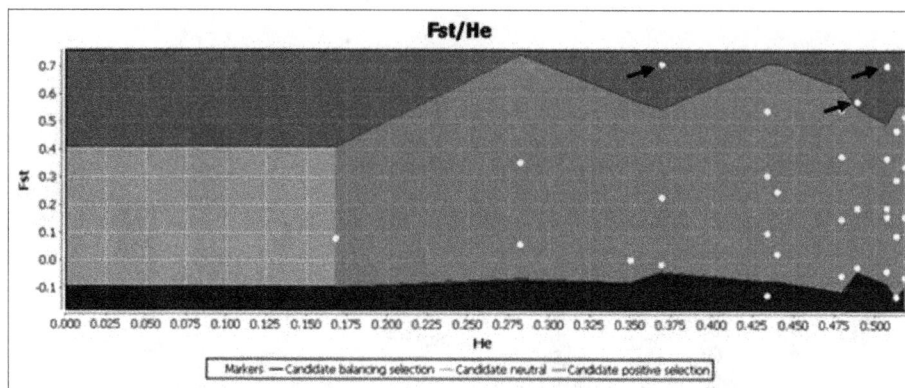

Figure-5: Graphical plot produced by Mcheza software of F_{ST} values against heterozygosity (H_e) for each of the 1890 amplified fragment length polymorphism (AFLP) *loci*. The lower and higher zones represent the 0.5% and 99.5% confidence intervals, respectively. *Loci* in the semi-dark gray zone above the 99.5% are regarded as positive outlier *loci*. Each dot indicates an AFLP *locus*, loci scored the same value appears as one dot.

Table-3: Genetic differentiation through AMOVA of *M. cephalus* based on the AFLP *loci* dataset.

Source of variance	df	SS	Variance components	Percentage of variation
Among locations	3	2395.58	193.09	47
Within locations	8	1754	219.25	53
Total	11	4149.58	412.34	

F_{ST}=0.46 (p<0.00). The source of variance (among and within locations), the degree of freedom (df), the SS, the variance components and the percentage of variation, are shown. SS=Sum of squares, AMOVA=Analysis of molecular variance, *M. cephalus*=*Mugil cephalus*, AFLP=Amplified fragment length polymorphism

with the AFLP outlier data against the geographical data. However, weak significant correlation (r=0.15, p=0.03) was found between log (AFLP outlier) matrix against geographical distance matrix.

Discussion

In Egypt, mullet fish especially *M. cephalus* is economically a very important fish because it has high market value and has been cultivated successfully by fish farmers [31]. Several studies targeted the species *M. cephalus* with many aims, however, less were concerned by its population structure and genetic diversity as it is mainly farmed. Even though, wild populations are still present and by the current study, a flow of its genes are still exchanged through the northern coast of Egypt, thus contribute to the cultivated populations.

The AFLP technique permits a genome-wide scan of the genetic variability with a high number of variable markers. Therefore, there is a relative good chance to detect markers under selection either directly or because they are located near a gene under selection. The high reading output and the extensive statistical refining were expected to reflect more clearly the genetic variability of the studied samples. The mean expected heterozygosity under Hardy–Weinberg assumption (H_e) was 0.28, which reflects the low diversity level of *M. cephalus* genetic pool from the sampled locations. The structure program implements a model-based clustering method for inferring

population structure using molecular data consisting of unlinked markers. The method was introduced by Pritchard *et al.* [32] and extended in sequels by Falush *et al.* [33,34]. The method application is to detect the population structure, identifying distinct genetic groups, assigning samples to sub-populations, and identifying migrants in admixed samples. The bulked samples of Groups 2 and 3 showed mixed portions of Group 1 (inferred by color), which deduce a weak attachment to its assigned cluster, and that they might be grouped to such cluster only when the information about the sampling locations was included. Samples that are genetically related are from different geographical locations, had exactly the same similarity membership coefficient (i.e., a value in which a sample is assigned to a certain group) although they originate from distant locations. Thus, multiple introductions are inferred among sampled locations of *M. cephalus* in the northern coast of Egypt. Such conclusion was further tested and proved by AMOVA.

Currently, there is increasing interest in identifying genes or outlier *loci* that underlie adaptations to different factors in several species [18,35,36]. Outlier *loci* are revealed by unusually high levels of population differentiation at specific marker *loci* [15,37,38]. Those *loci* that are involved in adaptation to local environmental conditions are indeed expected to exhibit increased differentiation among locations along with a decreased diversity within locations [18].

For example, the study of the genetic frame of adaptation to a gradient of altitude in the common frog (*Rana temporaria* L.) by Bonin *et al.* [18] showed that approximately 2% of the AFLP *loci* they screened exhibited elevated altitudinal differentiation. Another recent example was presented by Magdy *et al.* [39] on the cord moss (*Funaria hygrometrica* Hedw.) in which the genome scanning successfully detected loci under selection that were strongly correlated with the gradient of environmental factors in Sierra Nevada mountains. Because local adaptation and directional selection should have *locus*-specific effects of reducing genetic variability within populations and increasing differentiation between populations, *loci* that are outliers for these characteristics are strong candidate regions for involvement in adaptation to the certain environment.

This study is the first report on the detection of candidate *loci* under selection by a genome scan in the *M. cephalus* in the northern coast of Egypt. The AFLP genome scan analysis revealed 117 *loci* as under selection among a total of 1890 *loci* scored in this study. Meyer *et al.* [20] noted that the power of the analysis is directly associated with the genome coverage. These 117 *loci* possess a high credibility because, they were picked up by an exhaustive method (Dfdist embedded in Mcheza software), a very stringent significance criterion of 99.5% was applied, and simulations were set up to the maximum number allowed by the program. Since a high number of reasonable size bands between 150 and 600 bp were found, the *loci* under selection detected here should prove to have a good reliability.

The AMOVA produces estimates of variance components and F-statistics analogs [40]. In our case, AMOVA results were significant; reflect an approximate level of differentiation among sampled locations and within each location (47% and 53%, respectively). Gene flow (N_m) is a major factor influencing the genetic structure and differentiation among populations. Gene flow was 0.58, the detection of gene flow shows that the genetic differentiation among locations is not absolute. In other words, a complete reproductive isolation between the sampled locations is not the case. Wright [41] proposed that when the gene flow among the locations $N_m > 1$, the homogenization is the result. When $N_m < 1$, the locations can be strongly differentiated. According to these criteria, strong genetic differentiation exists among the studied locations.

To elucidate the genetic bases of adaptation to different environments represents a goal of central importance and interest in evolutionary biology [15]. Testing the correlation between the differences in geographic distance among sampled location and the genetic diversity of each sampled location would greatly indicate the geographic influence on the gene flow and further the population structure. Such test is usually known as isolation by distance and was extensively reported during the last decade [42]. The presence of a correlation between the genetic variation and the geographic distance (even though it is weak) along with the detected gene flow between the studied locations, it supports the presence of a certain gene flow limited by the distance between the sampling locations due to some environmental obstacles more than biological reasons. The outliers contribute to such assumption, as it raise the presence of selection mechanism based on the location conditions. However, it is not absolute that wild populations might decrease the isolation level through the gene flow caused by its movement along the northern coast attracted by the zooplankton, dead plant matter, and detritus near the shore, and being used as fries for cultivation [2].

As the detected AFLP *loci* are likely located in non-coding DNA, some of the outlier *loci* may only exhibit the signature of selection because they are linked to the actual target [43]. Although it is difficult to know the location and function of the detected outlier *loci*, the genome scan of *M. cephalus* still offers a window to unravel the genetic basis of fish adaptation without known phenotypes and whole genome sequences. Nowadays, the AFLP primers that were used to amplify the identified outlier *loci* can be used to construct a reduced representation library of the *M. cephalus* genome using next-generation sequencing technology [44].

Authors' Contributions

MM has carried out the experimental work in the MAR laboratory and then he prepared the manuscript, while ME has checked the manuscript and polished English language. All authors read and approved the final manuscript.

Acknowledgments

The authors kindly acknowledge Prof. Dr. Farid Estino for his critical reviewing of the article. The current research was co-funded by the internal fund provided by the Genetics department, Faculty of Agriculture, Ain Shams University, Egypt.

Competing Interests

The authors declare that they have no competing interests.

References

1. Nelson, J.S., Crossman, E.J., Espinosa-Pérez, H., Findley, L.T., Gilbert, C.R., Lea, R.N. and Williams, J.D. (2004) Common and scientific names of fishes from the United States, Canada and Mexico. American Fisheries Society, Bethesda, Maryland.

2. FAO. (2015) Aquaculture feed and fertilizers resources information system, special profiles: Flathead grey mullet – *Mugil cephalus*. Available from: http://www.fao.org/fishery/culturedspecies/Mugil_cephalus/en. Accessed on 11-01-2015.

3. Thomson, J.M. (1963) Synopsis of Biological Data on the Grey Mullet: Mugil Cephalus Linnaeus 1758. Division of Fisheries and Oceanography. CSIRO, Australia. p78.

4. Crosetti, D., Avise, J.C., Placidi, F., Rossi, A.R. and Sola, L. (1993) Geographic variability in the grey mullet *Mugil cephalus*: Preliminary results of mtDNA and chromosome analyses. *Aquaculture*, 111(1): 95-101.

5. Crosetti, D., Nelson, W.S. and Avise, J.C. (1994) Pronounced genetic structure of mitochondrial DNA among populations of the circumglobally distributed grey mullet (*Mugil cephalus*). *J. Fish Biol.*, 44(1): 47-58.

6. Corti, M. and Crosetti, D. (1996) Geographic variation in the grey mullet: A geometric morphometric analysis using partial warp scores. *J. Fish Biol.*, 48(2): 255-269.

7. Rossi, A.R., Capula, M., Crosetti, D., Sola, L. and Campton, D.E. (1998a) Allozyme variation in global populations of striped mullet, *Mugil cephalus* (Pisces: Mugilidae). *Mar Biol*, 131(2): 203-212.

8. Rossi, A.R., Capula, M., Crosetti, D., Campton, D.E., and Sola, L. (1998b) Genetic divergence and phylogenetic inferences in five species of Mugilidae (Pisces: Perciformes). *Mar Biol*, 131(2): 213-218.

9. Rocha-Olivares, A., Garber, N.M. and Stuck, K.C. (2000)

High genetic diversity, large inter-oceanic divergence and historical demography of the striped mullet. *J. Fish Biol.*, 57(5): 1134-1149.

10. Huang, C., Weng, C. and Lee, S. (2001) Distinguishing two types of gray mullet, *Mugil cephalus* L. (Mugiliformes: Mugilidae), by using glucose-6-phosphate isomerase (GPI) allozymes with special reference to enzyme activities. *J. Comp. Physiol. B.*, 171(5): 387-394.

11. Shen, K.N., Jamandre, B.W., Hsu, C.C., Tzeng, W.N. and Durand, J.D. (2011) Plio-Pleistocene sea level and temperature fluctuations in the northwestern Pacific promoted speciation in the globally- distributed flathead mullet *Mugil cephalus*. *BMC Evol. Biol.*, 11(1): 83.

12. Durand, J.D., Blel, H., Shen, K.N., Koutrakis, E.T., and Guinand, B. (2013) Population genetic structure of *Mugil cephalus* in the mediterranean and Black Seas: A single mitochondrial clade and many nuclear barriers. *Mar. Ecol. Prog. Ser.*, 474: 243-61.

13. Liu, J.Y., Lun, Z.R., Zhang, J.B. and Yang, T.B. (2009) Population genetic structure of striped mullet, *Mugil cephalus*, along the coast of China, inferred by AFLP fingerprinting. *Biochem. Syst. Ecol.*, 37(4): 266-274.

14. Vos, P., Hogers, R., Bleeker, M., Reijans, M., Van de Lee, T., Hornes, M., Friters, A., Pot, J., Paleman, J., Kuiper, M. and Zabeau, M. (1995) AFLP: A new technique for DNA fingerprinting. *Nuc. Acids Res.*, 23(21): 4407-4414.

15. Storz, J.F. (2005) Using genome scans of DNA polymorphism to infer adaptive population divergence. *Mol. Ecol.*, 14(3): 671-688.

16. Wilding, C.S., Butlin, R.K. and Grahame, J. (2001) Differential gene exchange between parapatric morphs of *Littorina saxatilis* detected using AFLP markers. *J. Evol. Biol.*, 14(4): 611-619.

17. Campbell, D. and Bernatchez, L. (2004) Generic scan using AFLP markers as a means to assess the role of directional selection in the divergence of sympatric whitefish ecotypes. *Mol. Biol. Evol.*, 21(5): 945-956.

18. Bonin, A., Taberlet, P., Miaud, C. and Pompanon, F. (2006) Explorative genome scan to detect candidate loci for adaptation along a gradient of altitude in the common frog (*Rana temporaria*). *Mol. Biol. Evol.*, 23(4): 773-783.

19. Savolainen, V., Anstett, M.C., Lexer, C., Hutton, I., Clarkson, J.J., Norup, M.V., Powell, M.P., Springate, D., Salamin, N. Baker, W.J. (2006) Sympatric speciation in palms on an oceanic island. *Nature*, 441(7090): 210-213.

20. Meyer, C.L., Vitalis, R., Saumitou-Laprade, P. and Castric, V. (2009) Genomic pattern of adaptive divergence in *Arabidopsis halleri*, a model species for tolerance to heavy metal. *Mol. Ecol.*, 18(9): 2050-2062.

21. Paris, M., Boyer, S., Bonin, A., Collado, A., David, J.P. and Despres, L. (2010) Genome scan in the mosquito *Aedes rusticus*: Population structure and detection of positive selection after insecticide treatment. *Mol. Ecol.*, 19(2): 325-337.

22. Poncet, B.N., Herrmann, D., Gugerli, F., Taberlet, P., Holderegger, R., Gielly, L., Rioux, D., Thuiller, W., Aubert, S. and Manel, S. (2010) Tracking genes of ecological relevance using a genome scan in two independent regional population samples of *Arabis alpina*. *Mol. Ecol.*, 19(14): 2896-2907.

23. Nosil, P., Funk, D.J. and Ortiz-Barrientos, D. (2009) Divergent selection and heterogeneous genomic divergence. *Mol. Ecol.*, 18(3): 375-402.

24. Bonin, A., Ehrich, D. and Manel, S. (2007) Statistical analysis of amplified fragment length polymorphism data: A toolbox for molecular ecologists and evolutionists. *Mol. Ecol.*, 16(18): 3737-3758.

25. Hubisz, M.J., Falush, D., Stephens, M. and Pritchard, J.K. (2009) Inferring weak population structure with the assistance of sample group information. *Mol. Ecol. Resour.*, 9(5): 1322-1332.

26. Antao, T. and Beaumont, M.A. (2011) Mcheza: A workbench to detect selection using dominant markers. *Bioinformatics*, 27(12): 1717-1718.

27. Excoffier, L. and Lischer, H.E. (2010) Arlequin suite ver 3.5: A new series of programs to perform population genetics analyses under Linux and Windows. *Mol. Ecol. Resour.*, 10(3): 564-567.

28. Vekemans, X., Beauwens, T., Lemaire, M. and Roldán-Ruiz, I. (2002) Data from amplified fragment length polymorphism (AFLP) markers show indication of size homoplasy and of a relationship between degree of homoplasy and fragment size. *Mol. Ecol.*, 11(1): 139-151.

29. Peakall, R. and Smouse, P.E. (2012) Gen Al Ex 6.5: Genetic analysis in excel. Population genetic software for teaching and research-an update. *Bioinformatics*, 28(19): 2537-2539.

30. Bohonak, A.J. (2002) IBD (Isolation by Distance): A program for analyses of isolation by distance. *J. Hered.*, 93(2): 153-154.

31. Bahnasawy, M., Khidr, A.A. and Dheina, N. (2009) Seasonal variations of heavy metals concentrations in mullet, *Mugil cephalus* and *Liza ramada* (Mugilidae) from Lake Manzala, Egypt *J. Aquat. Biol. & Fish*, 13(2): 81-100.

32. Pritchard, J.K., Stephens, M. and Donnelly, P. (2000) Inference of population structure using multilocus genotype data. *Genetics*, 155(2): 945-959.

33. Falush, D., Stephens, M. and Pritchard, J.K. (2003) Inference of population structure using multilocus genotype data: Linked loci and correlated allele frequencies. *Genetics*, 164(4): 1567-1587.

34. Falush, D., Stephens, M. and Pritchard, J.K. (2007) Inference of population structure using multilocus genotype data: Dominant markers and null alleles. *Mol. Ecol. Notes*, 7(4): 574-578.

35. Nosil, P., Egan, S.P. and Funk, D.J. (2008) Heterogeneous genomic differentiation between walking-stick ecotypes: "Isolation by adaptation" and multiple roles for divergent selection. *Evolution*, 62(2): 316-336.

36. Manel, S., Joost, S., Epperson, B.K., Holderegger, R., Storfer, A., Rosenberg, M.S., Scribner, K.T., Bonin, A. and Fortin, M.J. (2010) Perspectives on the use of landscape genetics to detect genetic adaptive variation in the field. *Mol. Ecol.*, 19(17): 3760-3772.

37. Black IV, W.C., Baer, C.F., Antolin, M.F. and DuTeau, N.M. (2001) Population genomics: Genome-wide sampling of insect populations. *Annu. Rev. Entomol.*, 46(1): 441-469.

38. Luikart, G., England, P.R., Tallmon, D., Jordan, S. and Taberlet, P. (2003) The power and promise of population genomics: From genotyping to genome typing. *Nat. Rev. Genet.*, 4(12): 981-994.

39. Magdy, M., Werner, O., McDaniel, S.F., Goffinet, B. and Ros, R.M. (2015) Genomic scanning using AFLP to detect loci under selection in the moss *Funaria hygrometrica* along a climate gradient in the Sierra Nevada Mountains, Spain. *Plant Biol.*, doi: 10.1111/plb.12381.

40. Excoffier, L., Smouse, P.E. and Quattro, J.M. (1992) Analysis of molecular variance inferred from metric distances among DNA haplotypes: Application to human mitochondrial DNA restriction data. *Genetics*, 131(2): 479-491.

41. Wright, S. (1931) Evolution in Mendelian populations. *Genetics*, 16(2): 97.

42. Jensen, J.L., Bohonak, A.J. and Kelley, S.T. (2005) Isolation by distance, web service. *BMC Genet.*, 6(1): 13.

43. Schlötterer, C. (2003) Hitchhiking mapping–functional genomics from the population genetics perspective. *Trends Genet.*, 19(1): 32-38.

44. Hohenlohe, P.A., Catchen, J., Cresko, W.A. (2012) Population genomic analysis of model and non model organisms using sequenced RAD tags. In: Pompanon, F., Bonin, A., editors. Data Production and Analysis in Population Genomics. Humana Press, New York, U.S.A. p235-260.

25

Effect of feeding cottonseed meal on some hematological and serum biochemical parameters in broiler birds

G. Thirumalaisamy[1], M. R. Purushothaman[2], P. Vasantha Kumar[2] and P. Selvaraj[3]

1. Division of Animal Nutrition, ICAR – National Dairy Research Institute, Karnal - 132 001, Haryana, India;
2. Department of Animal Nutrition, Veterinary College and Research Institute, Tamil Nadu Veterinary and Animal Sciences University, Namakkal - 637 002, Tamil Nadu, India; 3. Department of Veterinary Physiology, Veterinary College and Research Institute, Tamil Nadu Veterinary and Animal Sciences University, Namakkal - 637 002, Tamil Nadu, India.
Corresponding author: G. Thirumalaisamy, e-mail: nutritionthirumalai@gmail.com,
MRP: mrpurushothaman@yahoo.com, PVK: drpvknkl@gmail.com, PS: pselvaraj67@yahoo.com

Abstract

Aim: The study was undertaken to find out the effect of feeding cottonseed meal (CSM) on performance of hematological and serum biochemical parameters in broiler birds.

Materials and Methods: A 6-week biological trial was carried out with 432-day-old Cobb 400 broiler chicks distributed to nine experimental diets with six replicates, each containing eight chicks. The experimental diets were formulated based on total amino acids (BTAA) or based on digestible amino acids (BDAA) with or without iron supplementation with two levels of CSM (2% and 4%) and control diet based on maize – soybean. The whole blood was subjected to hematological studies. The serum samples were analyzed for protein fractions and lipid profiles.

Results: The packed cell volume (PCV) value, red blood cell (RBC) numbers, and hemoglobin (Hb) were lower in iron unsupplemented CSM BTAA or BDAA diets than the control (33.86-35.54 vs. 36.41%, 2.78-2.87 vs. 2.98 × 10⁶/µl, and 10.30-10.70 vs. 10.88%). Supplementation of iron in CSM diets improved the PCV, RBC numbers, and Hb, and the values were comparable to the control. White blood cell numbers, mean corpuscular volume, mean corpuscular Hb (MCH), and MCH concentration values were comparable to the control. The erythrocyte osmotic fragility (EOF) was poor in birds fed diets containing up to 4% CSM BTAA or CSM BDAA without iron supplementation (32.02-32.57 vs. 28.77%). Supplementation of iron improved the EOF. The serum cholesterol level did not change with or without iron supplementation.

Conclusion: This study suggested that feeding of CSM BTAA or BDAA up to 4% level voiding iron supplementation lowers the hematological parameters, whereas supplementation of iron did not alter serum protein fractions and cholesterol profile; however, it had lowered some hematological parameters, which was rectified by iron supplementation.

Keywords: broiler, cottonseed meal, hematological and serum parameters, iron supplementation.

Introduction

In recent years, the cost of conventional protein source for broilers, *viz.*, soybean meal has increased by 60%. This increase has resulted in increased cost of broiler meat production. Hence, alternative cheap protein source needs to be evaluated and incorporated in broiler rations to reduce the cost of broiler meat production [1]. The poultry feed industry and nutritional researchers are in search of alternative protein sources which not only supports the highest performance and efficiency but also safeguard the health of the bird and safety of the product.

Cottonseed meal (CSM) has been promising plant protein replacer of the conventional protein meals such as soybean meal and groundnut cake [2].

India is the second largest producer of cottonseed next to China. The production of cottonseed in India was 12.29 MMT in 2013 [3]. For every 1 kg of cotton (*Gossypium* sp.) lint produced, there is an availability of 1.65 kg of cotton seed [4]. The unit (g) price of soybean and CSM protein is 9.3 (42/kg for 450 g of protein) and 5.4 (21/kg for 390 g of protein) paise, respectively. Even a 1% replacement of soybean protein with CSM protein will result in savings of 390/ton of broiler feed.

Modern cottonseed processing industries are equipped to decorticate cotton seed, and hence, the meals obtained are higher in protein and lesser in fiber than the undecorticated CSM. Similarly, the advancement made in the solvent extraction technology has resulted in low oil content [5]. The above two processes in modern cottonseed industry have provided an opportunity to incorporate the decorticated deoiled CSM in the poultry feed.

However, the main problem that has limited its utilization in animal feeding thus far is the presence of gossypol, a toxic polyphenolic compound that naturally found in the pigment glands of the cottonseed [6], and this is present in free and bound forms. The free form is more toxic to monogastric animals. It can negatively affect animal growth, digestive health, and reproduction [7-10]. The free gossypol is higher in direct solvent extracted than mechanical extruded CSM [11]. The cottonseed oil extraction industry employs initially mechanical and subsequently solvent extracted. Hence, the CSM available locally contains low free gossypol due to the destruction of gossypol by heat and pressure [12].

Gossypol readily binds with a free epsilon amino group of lysine during processing, thereby reducing proteolytic action [13]. In addition, gossypol has direct inhibiting action on intestinal enzymes, and it combines with iron thereby reduces hemoglobin (Hb) synthesis and activity of respiratory enzymes. Hence, the use of this CSM is limited. Supplementation of lysine and iron are likely to ameliorate the negative effect of the toxic principle [14]. The objective of the present study was to evaluate the hematological and serum characters of the broiler birds fed CSM based on total amino acids (BTAA) or based on digestible amino acids (BDAAs) with or without iron supplementation.

Materials and Methods

Ethical approval

The study was conducted following approved guidelines with the Institutional Animal Ethics Committee and conformed to the "Guidelines for the Care and Use of Animals in Research."

Location of study and period

All procedures in the experiment were carried out in the Department of Animal Nutrition, Veterinary College and Research Institute, Namakkal, Tamil Nadu Veterinary and Animal Sciences University (TANUVAS), during the month of November 2014 to January 2015.

Biological experiment

The experimental broiler pre-starter, starter, and finisher diets were formulated by the inclusion of CSM at varying levels (0%, 2%, and 4% of feed). The various experimental diets are as follows:

- T1 - Standard broiler diet BTAA (control)
- T2 - 2% CSM inclusion BTAA
- T3 - 4% CSM inclusion BTAA
- T4 - 2% CSM inclusion BDAA
- T5 - 4% CSM inclusion BDAA
- T6-T2 with supplementation of ferrous sulfate 1:1 ratio ($FeSO_4$: Free gossypol), i.e., 0.4 g of Fe/kg of the diet
- T7-T3 with supplementation of ferrous sulfate 1:1 ratio ($FeSO_4$: Free gossypol), i.e., 0.8 g of Fe/kg of the diet
- T8-T4 with supplementation of ferrous sulfate 1:1 ratio ($FeSO_4$: Free gossypol), i.e., 0.4 g of Fe/kg of the diet
- T9-T5 with supplementation of ferrous sulfate 1:1 ratio ($FeSO_4$: Free gossypol), i.e., 0.8 g of Fe/kg of the diet.

The Treatments 1, 2, and 3 were formulated with the total (reported analytical) amino acids content of the ingredients and the total (reported analytical) amino acid requirement of the birds, i.e., total amino acid indicates both the digested and undigested amino acid component. The Treatments 4 and 5 were formulated with the digestible (reported available) amino acids content of the ingredients and the digestible (reported available) amino acid requirement of the birds, i.e., digestible amino acid indicates the available amino acid component.

The ingredients and nutrient composition of broiler pre-starter, starter, and finisher diets are presented in Table-1. The pre-starter, starter, and finisher diets were fed to birds from 1 to 14, 15 to 28, and 29 to 42 days of age, respectively. The biological experiment was conducted with 432-day-old Cobb 400 broiler chicks. The chicks were wing banded, weighed individually, and assigned randomly to nine experimental diets with six replicates for each diet, and each had eight chicks. Completely randomized design was followed.

Analytical methods
Chemical analysis and assay of gossypol

The CSM and the experimental diets were analyzed for proximate principles, calcium, and total phosphorus as per the protocol suggested by AOAC [15]. The total gossypol and free gossypol content of the CSM were analyzed as per AOCS [16,17]. The proximate principles and gossypol content of experiment CSM are presented in Table-2.

Blood, serum sample collection and analysis

The experimental birds were slaughtered at the end of the trial (42nd day); the blood samples were collected and subjected to hematological studies. After blood collection, the serum samples were harvested and stored at −20°C until further analysis. Total erythrocyte and leukocyte counts were estimated on the same day of blood collection. Hb was estimated by Drabkin and Austin [18] method and packed cell volume (PCV) by microhematocrit centrifugation [19] in the whole blood. Total protein, albumin, globulin, and cholesterol in serum samples were estimated using standard diagnostic kits (Span Diagnostics Ltd., Surat, India).

Table-1: Proximate principles (percent on DM basis), mineral and gossypol content of experiment CSM.

Compositions	Experiment CSM (%)
DM	89.86
Crude protein	39.02
Crude fiber	11.92
Ether extract	3.07
Total ash	7.15
Nitrogen free extract	38.84
Calcium	0.22
Total phosphorus	1.16
Total gossypol	2.62
Free gossypol	0.40

CSM=Cottonseed meal

Erythrocyte fragility was measured as percentage hemolysis using 0.65% buffered saline solution [20].

Statistical analyses

The data generated from the experimental study were subjected to statistical analysis by following the standard procedures of Snedecor and Cochran [21] with the help of IBM SPSS [22] version 20.0 software package. Comparison between groups was made by one-way ANOVA, and the data on hematological and serum parameters were analyzed in repeated measures ANOVA. Results were presented as means and standard error of means. The significance of the difference between means was compared using Duncan's multiple range test.

Results and Discussion

Hematological parameters

The hematological parameters of broilers fed CSM are presented in Table-3. Inclusion of CSM BTAA or BDAA without iron supplementation up to 4% level showed lower PCV value, red blood cell (RBC) numbers, and Hb over the control (33.86-35.54 vs. 36.41%, 2.78-2.87 vs. 2.98 × 10^6/µl, and 10.30-10.70 vs. 10.88%). This suggests that a negative influence on blood hemopoiesis. Supplementation of iron up to 4% level CSM BTAA or BDAA diet had comparable PCV, RBC numbers, and Hb to the control. In earlier, worker also confirmed that significant reduction in PCV, RBC, and Hb at 30% level of CSM

fed birds [23]. Apata [24] suggested that the significant reductions in RBC, RBC, and Hb may be results of factors acting together in an antinutrient containing dietary ingredient to induce inhibition of hemopoiesis, or a combined toxic factor-induced RBC hemolysis leading to an increase in plasma volume. This work was consistent with observations of Reddy and Salunkhe [25] and Kannan et al. [26], who stated that dietary antinutrients form a complex with dietary irons at intestinal or tissue level which, in turn, results in the diminished oxygen carrying capacity of blood. The antinutrient iron complex, in turn, reduces the amount of iron required for the functioning and regeneration of RBC, which is reflected in Hb.

White blood cell numbers, mean corpuscular volume, mean corpuscular Hb (MCH), and MCH concentration (MCHC) values were not significantly alter whether diet is formulated CSM BTAA or BDAA with or without iron supplementation when compared to the control.

The erythrocyte osmotic fragility (EOF) was increased when diet included at 4% CSM BTAA or CSM BDAA without iron supplementation compared to the control (31.98-32.89 vs. 28.77%). However, supplementation of iron up to 4% level in CSM BTAA or BDAA had observed comparable EOF to the control diet. Osmotic fragility of erythrocytes measures the ability of erythrocytes to resist osmotic stresses. Reyes et al. [27] observed that gossypol binds strongly

Table-2: Ingredients (as such basis) and nutrients composition (percent DM) of broiler pre-starter, starter, and finisher diet.

Ingredients (percent)	Pre-starter					Starter					Finisher				
	T1	T2	T3	T4	T5	T1	T2	T3	T4	T5	T1	T2	T3	T4	T5
Maize	61.85	61.33	60.82	61.44	60.95	63.67	63.15	62.64	63.27	62.78	61.30	60.91	60.52	60.70	60.33
Soybean meal	33.83	32.26	30.68	32.11	30.50	32.73	31.16	29.58	31.00	29.39	31.37	29.67	27.98	29.69	27.96
Rice bran oil	1.13	1.21	1.30	1.19	1.27	0.81	0.90	0.98	0.87	0.95	4.21	4.28	4.35	4.35	4.42
Calcite	1.96	1.98	2.01	1.98	2.01	2.03	2.05	2.08	2.05	2.08	2.03	2.05	2.07	2.05	2.07
Dicalcium phosphate	0.75	0.72	0.70	0.72	0.70	0.45	0.42	0.39	0.42	0.40	0.47	0.45	0.42	0.45	0.42
Methionine	0.176	0.178	0.181	0.179	0.183	0.140	0.142	0.144	0.143	0.145	0.228	0.230	0.238	0.231	0.239
Lysine	0.229	0.234	0.240	0.296	0.315	0.095	0.100	0.105	0.167	0.187	0.318	0.324	0.330	0.336	0.356
Cottonseed meal	0.00	2.00	4.00	2.00	4.00	0.00	2.00	4.00	2.00	4.00	0.00	2.00	4.00	2.00	4.00
Nutrients* (%)															
Crude protein	22.17	22.08	22.27	22.28	22.25	21.61	21.62	21.54	21.63	21.51	20.32	20.17	20.04	20.27	20.02
Crude fiber	3.94	4.09	4.28	4.10	4.28	3.89	4.00	4.15	4.10	4.17	3.74	3.90	4.24	3.94	4.18
Ether extract	2.83	2.87	2.79	3.30	3.27	4.93	5.08	5.13	5.06	5.10	5.97	6.06	6.15	6.03	5.99
Total ash	6.50	7.68	7.61	6.85	7.12	7.40	6.57	5.96	6.07	5.64	6.25	6.09	6.33	6.90	6.45
Nitrogen free extract	64.56	63.28	63.05	63.48	63.09	62.17	62.74	63.22	63.15	63.59	63.72	63.78	63.24	62.86	63.36
Calcium	1.09	1.10	1.19	1.08	1.06	0.99	1.06	0.97	0.99	0.96	0.96	0.97	0.97	0.99	0.98
Available phosphorus*	0.45	0.45	0.45	0.45	0.45	0.40	0.40	0.40	0.40	0.40	0.40	0.40	0.40	0.40	0.40
Lysine*	1.20	1.20	1.20	1.24	1.26	1.07	1.07	1.07	1.12	1.13	1.16	1.16	1.16	1.17	1.18
Methionine*	0.52	0.52	0.52	0.52	0.52	0.48	0.48	0.48	0.48	0.48	0.54	0.54	0.54	0.54	0.54
Metabolisable energy (Kcal/kg)*	3.00	3.00	3.00	3.00	3.00	3.05	3.05	3.05	3.05	3.05	3.20	3.20	3.20	3.20	3.20

Treatments 6 and 8 are the same as Treatments 2 and 4 with addition of iron sulfate at 0.4 g/kg of feed, and Treatments 7 and 9 are the same as Treatments 3 and 5 with addition of iron sulfate at 0.8 g/kg of feed. Supplied per kg of diet: Vitamin A–16,500 IU, vitamin B$_2$–10 mg, vitamin D$_3$–3200 IU and vitamin K–2 mg. Supplied per kg of diet: Thiamin–4 mg, pyridoxine–8 mg, cyanocobalamin–40 mcg, vitamin E–40 mg, niacin–60 mg, calcium D pantothenate–40 mg, and folic acid–4 mg. Coccidiostat added at 0.5 g/kg of feed supplied 125 mg of di-nitro-ortho-toluamide. Supplied per kg of diet: Manganese–54 mg, zinc–52 mg, iron–20 mg, iodine–2 mg, copper–2 mg, cobalt–1 mg. *Calculated value. DM=Dry matter

Table-3: Effect of feeding CSM on hematological parameters in broilers.

Treatments	PCV (%)	RBC (10⁶/µl)	WBC (10³/µl)	Hb (g/dl)	MCV (fl)	MCH (pg)	MCHC (%)	EOF (%)
T1	35.93^b±0.28	2.95^c±0.05	3.23±0.07	10.88^c±0.15	122.21±1.95	36.96±0.56	30.27±0.34	28.77^a±0.60
T2	33.98^a±0.15	2.81^{ab}±0.03	3.29±0.03	10.47^{ab}±0.06	121.24±1.14	37.34±0.36	30.81±0.25	32.27^c±0.66
T3	33.68^a±0.40	2.76^a±0.03	3.26±0.05	10.30^a±0.07	122.25±1.70	37.38±0.36	30.63±0.45	32.57^c±1.17
T4	34.29^a±0.16	2.82^{ab}±0.06	3.33±0.04	10.50^{ab}±0.07	121.91±1.64	37.32±0.48	30.63±0.28	32.02^{bc}±1.13
T5	34.07^a±0.15	2.80^{ab}±0.04	3.32±0.04	10.43^{ab}±0.13	121.84±1.09	37.29±0.60	30.59±0.28	32.41^c±0.66
T6	35.54^b±0.23	2.88^{abc}±0.03	3.30±0.08	10.66^{bc}±0.10	123.61±1.12	37.06±0.36	30.01±0.40	30.33^{abc}±1.19
T7	35.40^b±0.26	2.84^{abc}±0.04	3.26±0.07	10.62^{abc}±0.12	124.77±1.55	37.40±0.44	30.00±0.33	30.96^{abc}±1.07
T8	35.86^b±0.14	2.92^{bc}±0.03	3.16±0.05	10.70^{bc}±0.11	122.94±0.87	36.69±0.45	29.85±0.38	29.12^{ab}±0.99
T9	35.31^b±0.21	2.90^{bc}±0.04	3.11±0.04	10.63^{abc}±0.11	121.99±1.23	36.71±0.47	30.09±0.18	29.67^{abc}±0.88

Each value is the mean of 12 observations. Mean with at least one common superscript in a column do not differ significantly (p>0.05). MCV=Mean corpuscular volume, PCV=Packed cell volume, RBC=Red blood cell, Hb=Hemoglobin, WBC=White blood cell, MCH=Mean corpuscular hemoglobin, MCHC=Mean corpuscular hemoglobin concentration, EOF=Erythrocyte osmotic fragility, CSM=Cottonseed meal

Table-4: Effect of feeding CSM on serum protein fractions in broilers.

Treatments	Total protein (g/dl)	Albumin (g/dl)	Globulin (g/dl)	A/G ratio
T1	4.12±0.07	1.79±0.03	2.34±0.07	0.77±0.03
T2	4.10±0.08	1.71±0.03	2.39±0.07	0.72±0.02
T3	4.08±0.07	1.79±0.03	2.29±0.09	0.80±0.04
T4	4.10±0.07	1.70±0.02	2.40±0.05	0.71±0.02
T5	3.93±0.09	1.74±0.03	2.19±0.09	0.81±0.04
T6	3.87±0.08	1.71±0.03	2.16±0.09	0.81±0.04
T7	4.01±0.07	1.75±0.03	2.26±0.07	0.78±0.03
T8	4.03±0.07	1.73±0.02	2.31±0.06	0.76±0.02
T9	3.90±0.06	1.76±0.02	2.14±0.07	0.84±0.03

Each value is the mean of 12 observations. CSM=Cottonseed meal

Table-5: Effect of feeding CSM on serum cholesterol in broilers.

Treatments	Total cholesterol (mg/dl)	HDL (mg/dl)	LDL (mg/dl)	Triglycerides (mg/dl)
T1	204.58±1.80	98.16±1.09	88.15±2.59	91.37±1.71
T2	205.52±1.96	97.31±0.79	89.75±2.08	92.29±1.43
T3	202.64±2.11	99.18±1.07	84.97±2.41	92.43±1.43
T4	201.24±1.78	95.06±0.72	87.53±1.75	93.27±1.06
T5	205.32±1.12	95.65±1.39	89.84±2.77	94.15±0.83
T6	205.24±1.25	98.20±1.16	88.14±1.29	94.52±1.12
T7	205.94±2.43	98.37±0.73	88.91±2.30	93.36±0.84
T8	202.72±2.11	99.22±1.51	84.85±2.94	93.22±1.07
T9	200.86±1.56	97.55±1.24	84.54±1.64	93.83±1.20

Each value is the mean of 12 observations. HDL=High-density lipoprotein, LDL=Low-density lipoprotein, CSM=Cottonseed meal

to lipid bilayers and induces an electrical conductance that is accompanied by an increase in proton permeability. This affects the fluidity of membranes. In the present study, EOF was affected by treatment suggesting alteration of membrane integrity due to iron addition to the diet which may also explain the changes in Hb and MCHC values among treatments. Iron in the diet, on the other hand, was able to eliminate some of the negative effects of gossypol in CSM.

Serum parameters

The results of the biochemical estimation of serum protein fractions are presented in Table-4. The serum protein fractions in terms of total protein, albumin, globulin, and albumin globulin ratio did not significantly influence between the all dietary treatments.

Serum cholesterol values are presented in Table-5. The serum cholesterol in terms of total

cholesterol HDL, LDL, and triglycerides did not statistically significant between the dietary treatments. The present study clearly indicates that all the diets supported normal balance between the anabolism and catabolism of body proteins. It concurs with previous workers reported inclusion of CSM at 10% in broilers [28], 20% in lambs [26], and complete replacement of low gossypol CSM in laying hens [29] were not affecting the serum protein fractions and cholesterol values.

Conclusions

CSM BTAA or BDAA up to 4% level without iron supplementation had lowered hematological parameters, whereas supplementation of iron in CSM BTAA or BDAA had enhanced the hematological parameters. The serum protein and cholesterol parameters did not significantly influence when the diet formulated CSM BTAA or BDAA up to 4% level.

Authors' Contributions

This study was a part of M.V.S.c. thesis of the first author GT, who carried out the research under the guidance of Professor and Head MRP. PVK and PS helped during trial and laboratory analyses. The article was drafted by GT and MRP. The revision was made by GT and MRP. All authors have read and approved the final version of the manuscript.

Acknowledgments

The authors are highly thankful to TANUVAS, for providing necessary funds to carry out the work.

Competing Interests

The authors declare that they have no competing interests.

References

1. Sun, H., Tang, J.W., Yao, X.H., Wu, Y.F., Wang, X. and Feng, J. (2013) Effects of dietary inclusion of fermented cottonseed meal on growth, cecal microbial population, small intestinal morphology, and digestive enzyme activity of broilers. *Trop. Anim. Health Prod.*, 45: 987-993.

2. Abdulrashid, M., Joseph, Z.O., Mohammed, A. and Adamu, H.Y. (2013) Response of broiler chickens fed cottonseed meal based diets. *Int. J. Adv. Agric. Res.*, 1: 62-65.

3. Food and Agricultural Organization, (FAO). (2014) Cottonseed Production in India. Available from: http://www.faostat3.fao.org/. Accessed on 16-03-2015.

4. Sunilkumar, G., Campbell, L.M., Puckhaber, L., Stipanovic, R.D. and Rathore, K.S. (2006) Engineering cottonseed for use in human nutrition by tissue-specific reduction of toxic gossypol. *Proc. Nat. Acad. Sci.*, 103: 18054-18059.

5. Saxena, D.K., Sharma, S.K. and Sambi, S.S. (2012) Kinetics and thermodynamics of gossypol extraction from defatted cottonseed meal by ethanol. *Pol. J. Chem. Technol.*, 14(2): 29-34.

6. Zotte, A.D., Brand, T.S., Hoffman, L.C., Schoon, K., Cullere, M. and Swart, R. (2013) Effect of cottonseed oil-cake inclusion on ostrich growth performance and meat chemical composition. *Meat Sci.*, 93: 194-200.

7. Cai, C., Li, E., Ye, Y., Krogdahl, A., Jiang, G., Wang, Y. and Chen, L. (2011) Effect of dietary graded levels of cottonseed meal and gossypol on growth performance, body composition and health aspects of allogynogenetic silver crucian carp, *Carassius auratus gibelio*♀ × *Cyprinus carpio*♂. *Aquac. Nutr.*, 17(4): 353-360.

8. El-Saidy, D.M.S. and Saad, A.S. (2011) Effects of partial and complete replacement of soybean meal with cottonseed meal on growth, feed utilization and haematological indexes for mono-sex male Nile tilapia, *Oreochromis niloticus* (L.) Fingerlings. *Aquac. Res.*, 42(3): 351-359.

9. Özdoğan, M., Wellmann, K. and Paksuz, E. (2012) Effect of gossypol on blood serum parameters and small intestinal morphology of male broilers. *J. Anim. Physiol. Anim. Nutr.*, 96(1): 95-101.

10. Zheng, Q.M., Wen, X.B., Han, C.Y. and Li, H.B. (2012) Effect of replacing soybean meal with cottonseed meal on growth, hematology, antioxidant enzymes activity and expression for juvenile grass carp, *Ctenopharyngodon*

11. idellus. *Fish Physiol. Biochem.*, 38: 1059-1069.

11. Calhoun, M.C., Huston, J.E., Kuhlmann, S.W., Baldwin, B.C.J., Engdahl, B.S. and Bales, K.W. (1989) Comparative Toxicity of Gossypol Acetic Acid and Free Gossypol in Cottonseed Meal and Pima Cottonseed to Lambs. Progress Report 4779. Texas Agricultural Experiment Station, College Station, TX.

12. Jones, L.A. (1981) Nutritional values for cottonseed meal. *Feedstuffs*, 53(52): 19.

13. Phelps, R.A. (1966) Cottonseed meal for poultry: From research to practical application. *World Poult. Sci. J.*, 22: 86-112.

14. Boling, S.D., Edwards, H.M., Emmert, J.L., Biehl, R.R. and Baker, D.H. (1998) Bioavailability of iron in cottonseed meal, ferric sulfate, and two ferrous sulfate by-products of the galvanizing industry. *Poult. Sci.*, 77: 1388-1392.

15. AOAC. (1995) Official Methods of Analysis Association of Official Analytical Chemists. 16th ed. Association of Official Analytical Chemists, Washington, DC, USA.

16. AOCS. (1985b) Determination of total gossypol. Official method Ba. 8-78. Official and Tentative Methods of Analysis. 3rd ed. American Oil Chemists Society, Chicago.

17. AOCS. (1985a) Determination of free gossypol. Official method Ba. 7 – 58. Official and Tentative Methods of Analysis. 3rd ed. American Oil Chemists Society, Chicago.

18. Drabkin, D.L. and Austin, J.M. (1932) Spectrophotometric studies, spectrophotometric constants for common haemoglobin derivatives in human, dog and rabbit blood. *J. Biochem.*, 98: 719-773.

19. Jain, N.C. (1986) Hematologic technique – Hematocrit or packed cell volume. In: Schalm's Veterinary Hematology. 4th ed. Lea and Febiger, Philadelphia, PA. p36-41.

20. Buffenstein, R., McCarron, H.C.K. and Dawson, T.J. (2001) Erythrocyte osmotic fragility of red (*Macropus rufus*) and grey (*Macropus fuliginosus* and *Macropus giganteus*) kangaroos and free-ranging sheep of the arid region of Australia. *J. Comp. Physiol. B.*, 171: 41-47.

21. Snedecor, G.W. and Cochran, W.G. (1989) Statistical Methods. 9th ed. Oxford and IBH Pub., Co., New Delhi.

22. IBM SPSS. (2011) IBM SPSS Statistics for Windows, Version 20.0. IBM Corp, Armonk, NY.

23. Adeyemo, G.O. (2010) Effects of exposure duration to cottonseed cake based diets on broiler performance. *Int. J. Poult. Sci.*, 9(2): 162-166.

24. Apata, D.F. (1990) Biochemical, Nutritional and Toxicological Assessment of Some Tropical Legume Seeds. Ph.D. Thesis, University of Ibadan.

25. Reddy, N.R. and Salunkhe, D.K. (1982) Phytates in legumes and cereals. *Rev. Adv. Food Res.*, 28: 1-8.

26. Kannan, A., Sastry, V.R.B., Agarwal, D.K. and Kumar, A. (2013) Effect of feeding of calcium hydroxide-treated or vitamin E-supplemented cottonseed meal on plasma gossypol levels, blood parameters, and performance of Bikaneri lambs. *Trop. Anim. Health Prod.*, 45: 1289-1295.

27. Reyes, J., Allen, J., Tanphaichir, N., Belleve, A.R. and Benos, D.J. (1984) Molecular mechanism of gossypol action on lipid membranes. *J. Biol. Chem.*, 259: 9607-9615.

28. Mandal, A.B., Elangovan, A.V., Shrivastav, A.K., Johri, A.K., Kaur, S. and Johri, T.S. (2004) Comparison of broiler chicken performance when fed diets containing meals of Bollgard II hybrid cotton containing Cry-X gene (Cry1Ac and Cry2Ab gene), parental line or commercial cotton. *Br. Poult. Sci.*, 45: 657-663.

29. He, T., Zhang, J., Wang, J., Wu, S.G., Yu, H.Y. and Qi, G.H. (2015) Application of low gossypol cottonseed meal in laying hens' diet. *Poult. Sci.*, 94(10):2456-63.

26

New insights on ill-thriftiness in early-weaned buffalo calves

Nasr-Eldin M. Aref[1], Ali El-Sebaie[1] and Hammad Zaghloul Hammad[2]

1. Department of Animal Medicine, Faculty of Veterinary Medicine, Assiut University, Assiut, Egypt; 2. Animal Health Research Institute, Sohag, Egypt.
Corresponding author: Nasr-Eldin M. Aref, e-mail: nasreldeen.aref@vet.au.edu.eg,
AE: sebaie-ah@vet.au.edu.eg, HZH: azazy699@yahoo.com

Abstract

Aim: The present study was designed to: (1) Investigate the effect of weaning time on various metabolic indices and growth pattern in buffalo calves compared to cow calves under field condition and (2) Shed light on the potential relationship between early weaning, growth metabolites, and suboptimal growth (ill-thrift) in buffalo calves.

Materials and Methods: A total number of 18 neonatal calves of both sexes and species (cattle and buffalo) were included in the study. Animals were divided into three groups according to their age at weaning as following: Cow calves (n=8) weaned at 4.5 months, buffalo calves (n=6) weaned at 3.5 months (early-weaned), and buffalo calves (n=4) weaned at 5.5 months (late-weaned). Morphological traits, growth metabolites, and hormonal profile were measured at monthly interval over the period of the study and around the time of weaning (2 weeks pre- and post-weaning).

Results: The obtained results showed that the trend of growth pattern was significantly increased in a linear pattern in cow calves and late-weaned buffalo calves, whereas early-weaned buffalo calves showed sharp decline in their body weight (BW) post-weaning. By the end of the study, early-weaned buffalo calves showed the lowest BW gain (ill-thrift). There is a positive association between the morphological traits and various growth metabolites and hormonal indices. A significant decrease (p<0.05) in the concentrations of growth hormones (insulin-like growth factor-1 [IGF-1] and insulin) and other metabolites were reported in early-weaned buffalo calves compared to other animals. There is no association between stress indices (cortisol level and neutrophil to lymphocyte ratio) and growth rate.

Conclusion: Suboptimal growth rate (ill-thriftiness) is common in early-weaned buffalo calves and is attributed to low blood levels of growth metabolites, in particularly, IGF-1. In addition, the strong positive associations between concentrations of IGF-1 and morphological characters of growth suggest that IGF-1 is a reliable indicator for assessing metabolic status of individual calves.

Keywords: calves, growth, hormone, insulin, insulin-like growth factor-1, weaning.

Introduction

Livestock production is an important part of the national economy and is an integral component of sustainable food production. However, there are several challenges to achieve an efficient production system and consequently good livestock profitability. One of the most important production challenges for the livestock industry is to maintain a normal growth rate throughout the animal's life [1].

Growth is a dynamic process which is regulated by several factors including metabolic hormones (growth hormone [GH], thyroid hormones, insulin, and leptin), nutritionally-related metabolites (protein, glucose, lipid, minerals, and vitamins), and growth factors (insulin-like growth factor-1 [IGF-1]) [2]. The changes in circulating concentrations of these metabolites are important signals of the metabolic status of growing animals [3]. The somatotropic axis is the most important hormonal system for growth, which primarily consists of GH, IGF-1, and their carrier proteins and receptors [4,5].

Suboptimal growth or ill-thrift is a common problem for many of livestock producers. While there are several risk factors associated with ill-thrift in calves, the transition period of weaning is considered an important factor for poor growth rate especially for early-weaned animals [6]. Weaning is a multifactorial stress or in which socio-psychologic, nutritional, and physical stressors are combined. Psychological stress is present in the form of maternal separation and social disruption, whereas physical and nutritional stressors are often present in the introduction of/and adaptation to a new diet and a new environment [7].

Comparing to cow calves, buffalo calves may struggle to accomplish a successful weaning transition. Therefore, slaughtering of recently-weaned buffalo calves is a common trend in Egypt to avoid the cost of management and delayed marketing.

Following earlier studies on cow calves, the transitional period of weaned buffalo calves needs an in-depth exploration to elucidate the different factors that contribute to growth retardation. The analysis of growth indicators is a reliable method for the evaluation of growth pattern [8]. In addition, using of growth biomarkers may offer predictive value for suboptimal growth (ill-thrift). Our hypothesis proposed that early-weaned buffalo calves experience different concentrations of growth metabolites than late-weaned buffalo and cow calves.

Therefore, the present study was carried out to: (1) Determine the morphological characters of growth (body weight [BW], height, girth, crown ramp length (CRL), and average daily change [ADC]) in weaned buffalo and cow calves, (2) Evaluate the indices of growth metabolites (glucose, total protein [TP], urea, insulin, and IGF-1) and stress (cortisol, albumin/globulin [A/G] ratio, white blood cells [WBCs], and neutrophil to lymphocyte ratio [N/L] ratio) in weaned buffalo and cow calves, and (3) Determine the relationship between the morphological characters of growth and blood biomarkers of growth metabolites and stress in weaned buffalo and cow calves.

Materials and Methods

Ethical approval

The present study was approved by the Institutional Animal Ethics Committee of The Faculty of Veterinary Medicine at Assiut University.

Animals farm and weaning strategy

A total number of 18 neonatal calves of both sexes and species (cattle and buffalo) were included in the study. Animals were divided into three groups according to their age at-weaning time as following: Cow calves (n=8) weaned at 4.5 months, buffalo calves (n=6) weaned at 3.5 months (early-weaned), and buffalo calves (n=4) weaned at 5.5 months (late-weaned). These animals were belonging to a private commercial feedlot farm located 10 km north to Sohag city-Egypt. Farm adopted traditional weaning method. Briefly, calves present together with their dams suckling whole milk *ad libitum*. No milk replacer provided to calves. At the time of weaning, calves were separated from their dams and moved into a dry lot pen with feed bunks and water troughs. Calves were fed on straw mixture (wheat straw, alfalfa hay, caraway hay, cumin hay, and fenugreek hay) as roughage components and concentrate mixture to meet their nutrient requirement for a daily gain. Concentrate mixture consisted of soybean cake and cottonseed meal (25%), maize crushed (40%), wheat bran (32%), mineral mixture (2%), and common salt (1%). High-quality green fodders offered *ad libitum* to calves with clean drinking water. No changes in the aspects of calf's management over the period of study.

Determination of morphological characters of growth

All calves were subjected to assessment of BW and the body morphological measurements including: Heart girth, height at withers, and CRL. Initial BWs and body morphological measurements of the animals were recorded at the start of the study, monthly over the period of the study, and around the time of weaning (2 weeks pre- and post-weaning). BW (BW/Kg) was measured using a portable weight platform; heart girth (G/cm) and CRL (CRL/cm) were measured using a tape measure; height at withers (HT/cm) was measured using a height stick. All characteristics were measured by the same person. The ADC of the morphological characters of growth (weight, height, girth, and CRL) was calculated pre-weaning, post-weaning, and all over the study period for each calf. The total ADC was determined mathematically by subtraction the starting measurements from the end measurement and divided by the number of days between the two time points, to give the total ADC in each morphological characters of growth over the study period. Pre-weaning ADC was calculated subtracting start measurements from the weaning day measurements and divided by the number of days between the two time points to give the ADC in each parameter. Post-weaning ADC was similarly calculated by subtracting weaning day measurements from the end measurements and divided by the number of days between the two time points to give the ADC in each parameter.

Clinical examination

The health status of the studied animals was monitored through careful clinical examination according to Cockcroft [9].

Blood sampling, timing, and assays methods

Blood and serum samples were collected according to Otter [10]. Whole blood samples were used for CBC, whereas serum samples were used for determination of TP (g/L), albumin (g/L), urea (mmol/L), insulin (μIU/mL), IGF-1 (ng/mL), and cortisol (ng/mL). Samples were collected at a monthly interval from the start to the end of the study. Additional samples were collected around the times of weaning (2 weeks pre- and 2 weeks post-weaning) at weakly interval to elucidate the impact of weaning on growth and stress parameters.

Total leukocytic count ($\times 10^6$/L), neutrophils (%), and lymphocytes (%) were determined using an automated hematology analyzer (ADVIA 2120, Bayer Healthcare, Siemens, UK) equipped with software for bovine blood. N/L ratio was calculated by dividing the percent of neutrophils by percent of lymphocytes for each sample.

Serum biochemical analysis including TP (g/L), albumin concentration (g/L), serum glucose level (mmol/L), and serum urea (mmol/L) were determined spectrophotometrically using diagnostic test kits (Gesellschaft für Biochemica und Diagnostica GmbH, Germany). Serum globulin level (g/L) was determined mathematically by subtraction of the serum albumin level (g/L) from the serum TP level (g/L). A/G ratio was calculated by dividing the values of serum albumin by serum globulin.

IGF-1 (ng/mL) and cortisol concentrations (ng/mL) were measured by DRG IGF-1 600 enzyme-linked immunosorbent assay (ELISA) kit (EIA-4140) and DRG cortisol ELISA Kit (EIA-1887), respectively (DRG Diagnostics, GmbH, Germany, Division of DRG International, Inc.). Both tests are solid phase ELISA for quantitative *in vitro* diagnostic measurement of IGF-1 and cortisol based on the principle of competitive binding. The intensity of color developed is reverse proportional to the concentration of hormone in the sample. All technical procedures described by the manufacturer were followed.

Estimation of insulin level (μIU/mL) was performed using DRG Insulin ELISA kit (EIA-2935) (DRG Diagnostics, GmbH, Germany, Division of DRG International, Inc.). The DRG Insulin ELISA kit is a solid phase ELISA based on the sandwich principle. The intensity of color developed is proportional to the concentration of insulin in the sample. All technical procedures described by the manufacturer were followed.

A microtiter plate reader (Stat Fax - 2100, Awareness, Technology Inc., USA) provided with printer EPSON-LX 300+ was used to read the ELISA plate.

Statistical analysis

Data were analyzed using the packaged SPSS program for Windows version 10.0.1 (SPSS Inc., Chicago, IL, USA). Differences between groups were determined by the one-way analysis of variance followed by the Student's *t*-test or the pairwise multiple comparison procedures (when significant *F*-test was found) using Duncan's new multiple range test. Data were presented as mean ± standard error (Standard error of the mean). Pearson correlation coefficients (r) were determined between paired variables for individual animals for cow calves (n=8) and buffalo calves (n=10). The significance level was set at $p \leq 0.05$.

Results

Growth curve

Time-course evaluation of growth patterns of calves over the studied period is shown in Figure-1. Both cow and late-weaned buffalo calves groups showed a consistent gain of BW as indicated by an increasing linearity of growth curve (Figure-1a and b) while early-weaned buffalo calves experienced a marked drop in the BW post-weaning

(Figure-1c) and could not achieve the same BW of the other 2 groups at the end of the study.

BW (BW/kg)

BW (kg) showed significant differences between groups over the period of the study (Figure-2). The prominent feature was a significant decrease in the BW in early-weaned buffalo calves compared with cow and late-weaned buffalo calves. The ADCs of BW (kg/day) at pre-weaning period of cow calves, early-weaned buffalo calves, and late-weaned buffalo calves were 0.65±0.04, 0.75±0.05, and 0.88±0.06 kg/day, respectively, while in the post-weaning period were 0.55±0.06, 0.30±0.1, and 0.48±0.03, respectively. The results showed a significant decrease in ADC of BW in early weaned buffalo calves compared with the other two groups over period of the study. Within the same group, there were no significant differences in the ADC of BW between the pre-weaning and post-weaning periods in cow calves while there was significantly decrease in the ADC of BW in both early- and late-weaned buffalo calves at post-weaning compared with the pre-weaning period.

Height (cm)

There were significant differences in height (cm) between all groups over the period of the study (Figure-2). At the pre-weaning time, there were significant increases in the height of late-weaned buffalo calves compared with other two groups. Within the same group, all calves showed significantly increase in the heights at post-weaning compared with pre-weaning time. There were significant differences in ADC of height (cm/day) between the three groups over the period of the study. Late-weaned buffalo calves showed significantly higher ADC of height (cm/day) than the other two groups. Within the same group, ADC of height (cm/day) was significantly decreased in all groups at post-weaning compared with the pre-weaning period.

Girth (cm)

There were significant differences in girth and ADC of girth between all groups of the study (Figure-2). For cow calves, early- and late-weaned buffalo calves, the mean values of girth at pre-weaning were 108.75±2.43, 102.33±2.08, and 123.75±3.54, respectively, whereas at post-weaning were 121.12±1.96, 105.67±1.89, and 135.25±3.09,

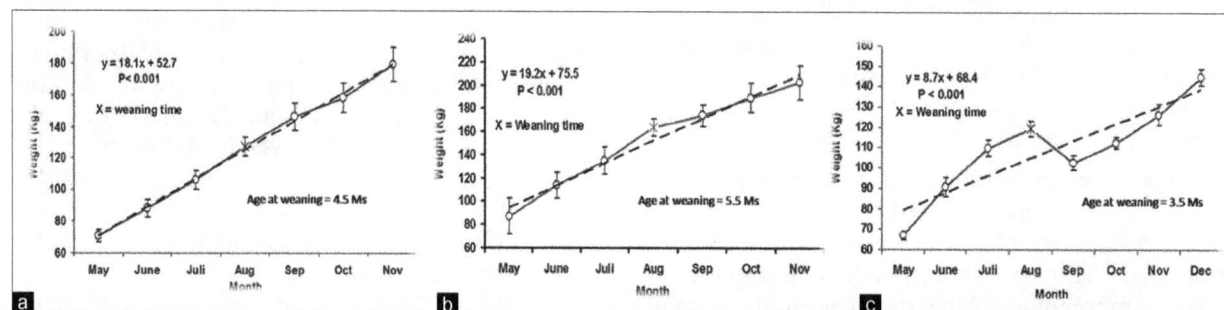

Figure-1: Pattern of growth curve of cow calves (a), late-weaned (b), and early-weaned buffalo calves (c) group.

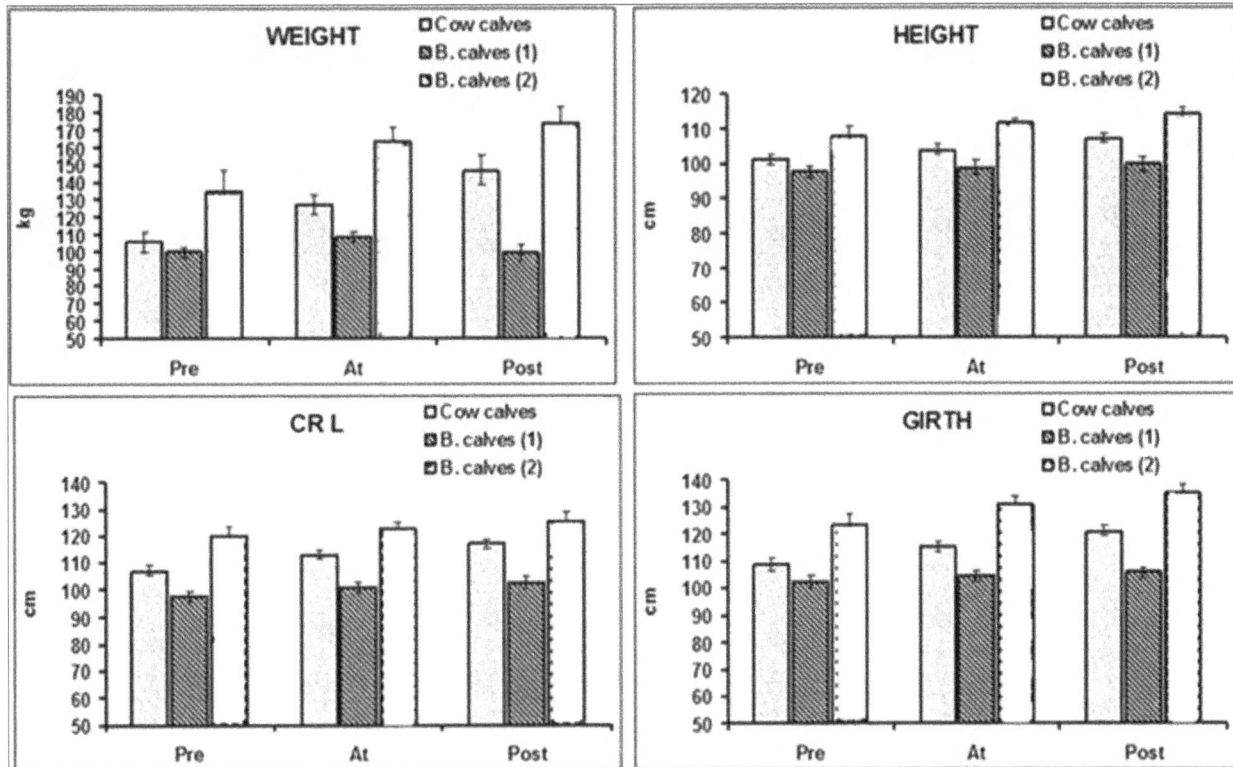

Figure-2: Time-course evaluation (mean±standard error) of morphological traits of cow calves, late- and early-weaned buffalo calves group.

respectively. Late-weaned buffalo calves showed significant higher girth than other groups over the period of the study. Within the same group, cow calves showed significantly increase girth (cm) post-weaning, whereas other two groups of buffalo calves showed no significant differences in girth. The ADC of girth (cm/day) in cow calves was significantly higher than buffalo calves groups at post-weaning period. Within the same group, the ADC of girth was significantly lower in early-weaned buffalo calves at post-weaning compared with pre-weaning periods.

CRL (CRL/cm)

CRL (cm) showed significant differences between all groups over the period of the study (Figure-2). Within the same group, CRL (cm) was significantly increase in cow calves at-weaning time and post-weaning period compared to the pre-weaning period of the study. The ADC of CRL (cm/day) in early-weaned buffalo calves was significantly lower compared with the other two groups over the period of the study. Within the same group, post-weaning period the ADC of CRL (cm/day) was significantly lower than pre-weaning times in all groups.

Clinical observation

Abnormal clinical signs were observed in only two calves of early-weaned group in the form of diarrhea (3-6 days post-weaning) and spontaneously resolved within 2 days without treatment. The animals of this group showed signs of ill-thriftiness in the form of stunting or delayed growth with alopecia,

rough hair, poor body condition, emaciation, and pale mucous membrane.

Metabolic and stress indices

The analysis of biochemical, hormonal, and stress indices including serum glucose, urea, TP, albumin, insulin, IGF-1, and cortisol were presented in Figure-3.

Relationships between metabolic variables with the growth rates

The correlation coefficient between the morphological characters of growth and various metabolites of the cow and buffalo calves was presented in Table-1. Obtained data showed strong positive correlations between IGF-1 and all morphological characters of growth. There were also positive correlations between insulin and height and girth. Glucose level was found to be associated with height, girth, and CRL. The urea concentration showed significant relationships with height, girth, and CRL in buffalo calves while it is associated with girth and CRL in cow calves. There was also an association between protein profile and morphological characters of growth. There was no correlation between cortisol level and morphological characters of growth.

Discussion

Morphological characters of growth

Screening of the collected data about the BW and its ADC showed that early-weaned buffalo group suffered from a drop in weight gain post-weaning for 2 weeks after weaning. This finding was in agreement with Ali et al. [6] and Phillips et al. [11]. The authors concluded that poor growth rate in early

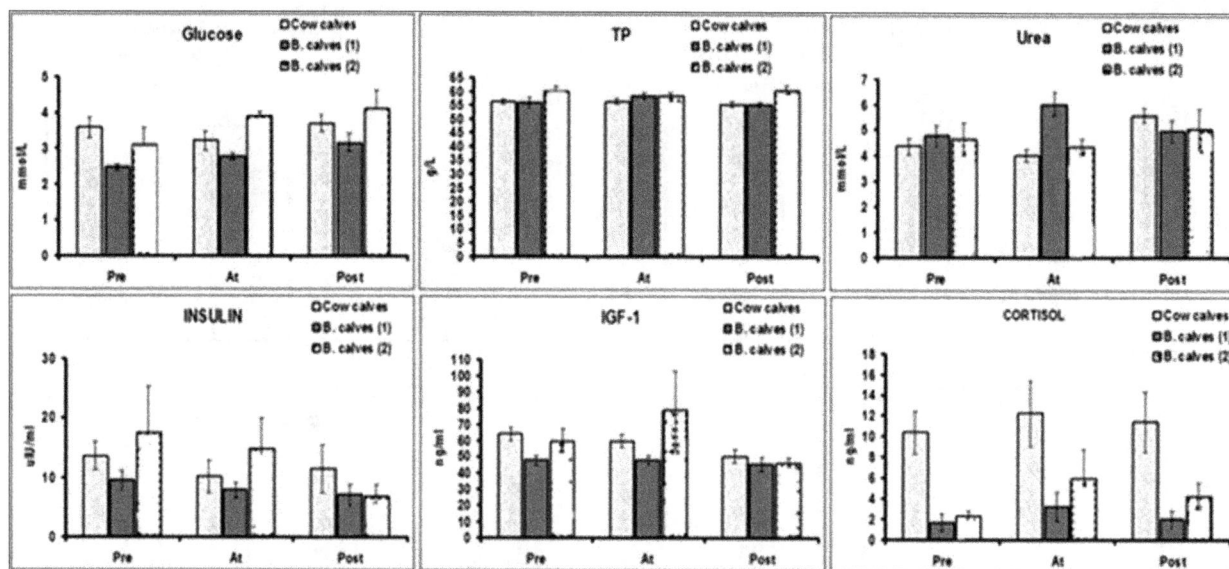

Figure-3: Time-course evaluation (mean±standard error) of biochemical, hormonal, and stress indices of cow calves, late- and early-weaned buffalo calves group.

Table-1: Pearson correlation coefficients (r) between biochemical, hormonal, and physical indices in cow and buffalo calves.

Parameter	Glucose	TP	Albumin	Globulin	Urea	Insulin	IGF-1	Cortisol
Height								
Cow calves								
r	0.331	0.366	0.134	0.355	0.229	0.289	0.598	0.022
P	0.009	0.003	0.298	0.003	0.061	0.019	0.000	0.851
Buffalo calves								
r	0.386	0.425	0.175	0.402	0.301	0.355	0.688	0.031
P	0.008	0.002	0.256	0.002	0.048	0.019	0.000	0.765
Weight								
Cow calves								
r	0.133	0.158	0.101	0.276	0.016	0.189	0.328	0.218
P	0.296	0.199	0.410	0.029	0.865	0.127	0.007	0.081
Buffalo calves								
r	0.186	0.213	0.154	0.344	0.022	0.256	0.394	0.264
P	0.205	0.198	0.372	0.021	0.788	0.102	0.006	0.079
Girth								
Cow calves								
r	0.401	0.458	0.278	0.375	0.318	0.426	0.579	0.109
P	0.002	0.000	0.018	0.003	0.013	0.001	0.000	0.364
Buffalo calves								
r	0.453	0.499	0.352	0.452	0.354	0.468	0.644	0.156
P	0.001	0.000	0.012	0.002	0.009	0.000	0.000	0.325
CRL								
Cow calves								
r	0.627	0.276	0.187	0.207	0.264	0.204	0.428	0.138
P	0.000	0.024	0.121	0.097	0.044	0.113	0.001	0.246
Buffalo calves								
r	0.686	0.344	0.251	0.246	0.302	0.255	0.493	0.170
P	0.246	0.024	0.121	0.097	0.044	0.113	0.001	0.000

Correlation is significant at p<0.05. IGF-1=Insulin-like growth factor-1, CRL=Crown-ramp length, TP=Total protein

45-day-old weaned buffalo calves accompanied by a parallel depression in the rumen total volatile fatty acid concentration; the addition of mixture of acetic and propionic acids to stimuli rumen condition did not produce any improvement in growth. Decreased ADC in early-weaned buffalo calves post-weaning could be attributed down-regulation of IGF-1 production [12,13] due to poor post-weaning adaptation and incomplete rumenal development. On contrary,

Pasha [14] stated that buffalo calves can be successfully weaned as early as 8 weeks of age without negatively affecting growth performance. The obtained results of height and ADC of height, girth, and ADC of girth were similar to that reported by Swali *et al.* [15] and Brickell *et al.* [16], respectively; however, screening the collected data of CRL and ADC of CRL (cm/day) showed lower values than that estimated by these authors.

Clinical observations

Screening the collected data about weaning associated clinical signs suggested that ill-thriftiness was present in the early-weaned buffalo calves. Diarrhea was observed in only 2 out of 6 animals in early-weaned buffalo calves. Poor ruminal adaptation with subsequent nutrients deficiency is most likely cause of suboptimal growth in these calves. Our finding agreed with that reported by Abou El-Amaiem [17], who found that there were significant correlations between ill-thrift and young aged buffalo calves as well as diarrheic animals.

Metabolic indices

Glucose

Glucose concentration is an indication of the energy status of individual animals. Reduced nutrient intake, periods of fasting and stress can cause reduction in blood glucose concentrations [18]. The highest blood glucose concentrations in both cow and late-weaned buffalo calves reflect the association between energy intake and growth in these groups. This finding is in accordance with previous studies in Holstein calves [19-21]. While late-weaned buffalo calves attained similar BW and blood glucose level to cow calves, the finding of the currect study may suggest that cow calves are superior to buffaloes in their growth rate. Furthermore, early-weaned buffalo calves had the lowest blood glucose level and growth rate and more likely to be culled, primarily due to ill-thriftiness. The positive link between blood glucose concentrations and time of weaning in buffalo calves may raise the question of how long farmers could keep buffalo calves with their dams, on the expense of their profitability from milk production.

Urea

In the present study, the blood urea level was positively correlated with CRL and girth while it showed weak and no positive association with height and weight, respectively. These results were in agreement with Swali et al., [15]. Data showed temporary increase in blood urea level at weaning in early-weaned buffalo calves which could be attributed to the shortfall in energy during this times. This shortfall in energy could be met by the catabolism of body protein, which results in an increased blood urea concentration [22]. On the other hand, blood urea level showed significant increase in cow and late-weaned buffalo calves post-weaning compared with pre- and at-weaning times. It is known that urea may be elevated due to either a high protein intake from the initial diet or following catabolism of body protein reserves when energy intake is restricted [23].

Insulin

The obtained values of insulin level in the present study showed significant increase in all groups at pre-weaning time, however the highest insulin levels were present in late-weaned buffalo calves. By increasing the age of the calves, insulin levels decrease to normal. Higher insulin concentrations during pre-weaning time were associated with greater height and girth. A similar finding was reported by Swali et al. [15] which suggests that high insulin is associated with an alteration in body proportion.

IGF-1

IGF-1 regulates both skeletal and muscle development in growing cattle [24]. In the present study, IGF-1 concentration was positively associated with growth in all size parameters, reinforcing the important role of IGF-1 in the control of body growth. This is in accordance with previous findings that reported similar correlations between IGF-1 concentration at birth and subsequent growth in bull calves [25], lambs [22], and pigs [26]. We found that early-weaned buffalo calves had the lowest IGF-1 concentrations, and lowest body weight gain (ill-thrift) while cow and late-weaned buffalo calves had higher growth rate and higher levels of IGF-1. The positive association between growth and IGF-1 concentration reported in the current study is thought to reflect the association between energy intake and growth in these groups. IGF-1 is considered a suitable index of metabolic status as its concentration does not change in relation to time of feeding [27]. In milk-fed calves, insulin and glucose concentrations increase within 30 min, taking 4-6 h to return to basal concentrations post-prandially [27]. As it was not possible to be certain of the interval between feeding and blood sampling in this on-farm trial, IGF-1 concentration was considered as a reliable indicator for assessing the metabolic status of individual calves [16] and its association with growth.

Stress indices

Cortisol

Several studies assessed the level of cortisol in calves; however, there is wide variation in its value. In the present study, cortisol levels fall within the range reported by Aggarwal and Singh [18] and Hickey et al. [28]. The current study showed no significantly differences in cow calves group over the period of study suggesting that weaning is not a stressor in this animals or cortisol is not a reliable index for assessing stress. In contrast to that, the obtained data of cortisol levels showed slight increase at weaning in both groups of buffalo calves. These findings were in agreement with that reported by Kim et al. [19] suggesting that buffalo calves may be more vulnerable to stress than cow calves because they are highly social animals with strong instincts and closely bonded with their dams [20]. Although buffalo calves may subject to stress of weaning, cortisol level showed no association with growth parameters in the present study.

Protein profile

Collected data about protein profile were similar to that reported by El-Bahr and El-Deeb [20]. The significant increase of the level of TP, albumin and globulin in late-weaned buffalo calves group strongly suggests that these animals are well adapted to weaning compared with the other two groups. Increase in TP values with increase in age has been reported by other workers [11]. Data showed no significant difference in the A/G ratio among the studied groups during preweaning time while it significantly decrease in buffalo groups compared with cow calves postweaning.

WBCs picture

Total leukocytic count, neutrophil %, lymphocyte %, and N/L ratio showed no significant changes among groups in the present study. Similar finding was reported by Earley et al. [29]. Within the same group, early-weaned buffalo calves showed significant increase in N/L ratio at pre-weaning and at-weaning periods. This finding was in agreement with Kim et al. [19]. The authors suggested that weaning affects leukocyte level and that the N/L ratio may be effective biomarker of stress responses. Lynch et al. [30] suggested that the glucocorticoids are a main contributing factor to the alteration of N/L ratio. Therefore, changes in the N/L ratio are thought to be a potential biological indicator of stress and disease susceptibility.

Conclusion

Suboptimal growth rate (ill-thrift) in early-weaned buffalo calves is attributed to low blood levels of growth metabolites, in particularly, IGF-1. In addition, the strong positive associations between concentrations of IGF-1 and morphological characters of growth suggest that IGF-1 is a reliable test for assessing metabolic status of individual calves. This may be diagnostically useful as it is often not possible to obtain accurate information on nutrient intakes or disease at a farm level.

Authors' Contributions

NMA and AES have formulated the research plan. HZH conducted clinical examination and collected samples. NMA analyzed samples. AES and HZH drafted the manuscript and NMA revised and submitted it. All authors read and approved the final manuscript.

Acknowledgments

We are grateful to the Farm Director and Head Department of Animal Medicine at Assiut University, for helping us gain access to the facilities needed to conduct this study. We are also thankful to Dr. Mostafa Saleh at Animal Health Research Institute-New Valley Branch for helping us in data analysis.

Competing Interests

The authors declare that they have no competing interest.

References

1. Weary, D.M., Jasper, J. and Hötzel, M.J. (2008) Understanding weaning distress. *Appl. Anim. Behav. Sci.,* 110: 24-41.

2. Ingole, S.D., Deshmukh, B.T., Nagvekar, A.S. and Bharucha, S.V. (2012) Serum profile of thyroid hormones from birth to puberty in buffalo calves and heifers. *J. Buffalo Sci.,* 1: 39-49.

3. Damptey, J., Obese, F., Aboagye, G. and Ayizanga, R. (2013) Correlations among concentrations of some metabolic hormones and nutritionally-related metabolites in beef cows. *Open J. Anim. Sci.,* 3: 176-180.

4. Govoni, K.E., Hoagland, T.A. and Zinn, S.A. (2004) The ontogeny of the somatotropic axis in Hereford calves from birth to one year of age and its responses to administration of exogenous bovine somatotropin. *J. Anim. Sci.,* 82: 1646-1655.

5. Agudelo-Gómez, D., Lugo, N.A. and Muñoz, M.F. (2009) Growth curves and genetic parameters in Colombian buffaloes (*Bubalus bubalis* Artiodactyla, *Bovidae*). *Rev. Colomb. Cien. Pecu,* 22: 178-188.

6. Ali, M.A., El-khodery, S.A. and El-said, W.E. (2015) Potential risk factors associated with ill-thrift in buffalo calves (*Bubalus bubalis*) raised at smallholder farms in Egypt. *J. Adv. Res.,* 4: 601-607.

7. Veissier, I. and Le Neindre, P. (1989) Weaning in calves: Its effect on social organization. *Appl. Anim. Behav. Sci.,* 24: 43-54.

8. Herosimczyk, A., Lepczyński, A., Dratwa-Chałupnik, A., Kurpińska, A., Klonowska, A. and Skrzypczak, W.F. (2011) Age-related changes of selected blood biochemical indicators in dairy calves during their first week of life. *Folia Biol. Krak.,* 59: 25-30.

9. Cockcroft, P. (2015) Diagnosis and clinical reasoning in cattle practice. In: Bovine Medicine. 3rd ed. John Wiley & Sons, Ltd., New Jersey. p124-132.

10. Otter, A. (2013) Diagnostic blood biochemistry and haematology in cattle. *BVA Pract.,* 35: 17-16.

11. Phillips, W.A., Juniewicz, P.E., Zavy, M.T. and Von Tungel, D.L. (1989) The effect of the stress of weaning and transport on white blood cell patterns and fibrinogen concentration of beef calves of different genotypes. *Can. J. Anim. Sci.,* 69: 333-340.

12. Hammon, H.M., Schiessler, G., Nussbaum, A. and Blum, J.W. (2002) Feed intake patterns, growth performance, and metabolic and endocrine traits in calves fed unlimited amounts of colostrum and milk by automate, starting in the neonatal period. *J. Dairy Sci.,* 85: 3352-3362.

13. Haley, D.B., Bailey, D.W. and Stookey, J.M. (2005) The effects of weaning beef calves in two stages on their behavior and growth rate. *J. Anim. Sci.,* 83: 2205-2214.

14. Pasha, T.N. (2013) Prospect of nutrition and feeding for sustainable buffalo production. *Buffalo Bull.,* 32: 91-110.

15. Swali, A., Cheng, Z., Bourne, N. and Wathes, D.C. (2008) Metabolic traits affecting growth rates of pre-pubertal calves and their relationship with subsequent survival. *Domest. Anim. Endocrinol.,* 35: 300-313.

16. Brickell, J.S., McGowan, M.M. and Wathes, D.C. (2009) Effect of management factors and blood metabolites during the rearing period on growth in dairy heifers on UK farms. *Domest. Anim. Endocrinol.,* 36: 67-81.

17. Abou El-Amaiem, W.E. (2012) Some Studies On Ill-thriftiness in Buffalo Calves with Special Reference to Participatory Epidemiology. PhD. Thesis - Mansoura University-Egypt.

18. Aggarwal, A. and Singh, M. (2010) Hormonal changes in heat stressed Murrah buffaloes under two different cooling systems. *Buffalo Bull.,* 29: 1-6.

19. Kim, M.H., Yang, J.Y., Upadhaya, S.D., Lee, H.J, Yun, C.H. and Ha, J.K. (2011) The stress of weaning influences serum levels of acute-phase proteins iron-binding proteins, inflammatory cytokines, cortisol, and leukocyte subsets in Holstein calves. *J. Vet. Sci.,* 2: 151-157.

20. Mustafa, M.U., Shahid, M. and Mehmood, B. (2010) Management practices and health care of buffalo calves in

Sheikhupura district, Pakistan. *Buffalo Bull.,* 3: 217-224.

21. El-Bahr, S.M. and El-Deeb, W.M. (2013) Acute phase proteins, lipid profile and proinflammatory cytokines in healthy and bronchopneumonic water buffalo calves. *Am. J. Biochem. Biotechnol.,* 1: 34-40.

22. Greenwood, P.L., Hunt, A.S., Slepetis, R.M., Finnerty, K.D., Alston, C., Beermann, D.H. and Bell, A.W. (2002) Effects of birth weight and postnatal nutrition on neonatal sheep. III. Regulation of energy metabolism. *J. Anim. Sci.,* 80: 2850-2861.

23. Terré, M., Devant, M. and Bach, A. (2006) Performance and nitrogen metabolism of calves fed conventionally or following an enhanced-growth feeding program during the preweaning period. *Livest. Sci.,* 105: 109-119.

24. Bass, J., Oldham, J., Sharma, M. and Kambadur, R. (1999) Growth factors controlling muscle development. *Domest. Anim. Endocrinol.,* 17: 191-197.

25. Smith, J.M., Van Amburgh, M.E., Diaz, M.C., Lucy, M.C. and Bauman, D.E. (2002) Effect of nutrient intake on the development of the somatotropic axis and its responsiveness to GH in Holstein bull calves. *J. Anim. Sci.,* 80: 1528-1537.

26. Carroll, J.A., Veum, T.L. and Matteri, R.L. (1998) Endocrine responses to weaning and changes in post-weaning diet in the young pig. *Domest. Anim. Endocrinol.,* 15: 183-194.

27. Vicari, T., van den Borne, J.C., Gerrits, W.J., Zbinden, Y. and Blum, J.W. (2008) Postprandial blood hormone and metabolite concentrations influenced by feeding frequency and feeding level in veal calves. *Domest. Anim. Endocrinol.,* 34: 74-88.

28. Hickey, M.C., Drennan, M. and Earley, B. (2003) The effect of abrupt weaning of suckler calves on the plasma concentrations of cortisol, catecholamines, leukocytes, acute-phase proteins and *in vitro* interferon-gamma production. *J. Anim. Sci.,* 81: 2847-2855.

29. Earley, B., Buckham-Sporer, K., Gupta, S., Pang, W. and Ting, S. (2010) Biologic response of animals to husbandry stress with implications for biomedical models. *Open Access Anim. Physiol.,* 2: 25-42.

30. Lynch, E.M., Earley, B., McGee, M. and Doyle, S. (2010) Effect of abrupt weaning at housing on leukocyte distribution, functional activity of neutrophils, and acute phase protein response of beef calves. *BMC Vet. Res.,* 6: 39-48.

27

A comparison of titers of anti-*Brucella* antibodies of naturally infected and healthy vaccinated cattle by standard tube agglutination test, microtiter plate agglutination test, indirect hemagglutination assay, and indirect enzyme-linked immunosorbent assay

Anju Mohan[1], Hari Mohan Saxena[1] and Puneet Malhotra[2]

1. Department of Veterinary Microbiology, College of Veterinary Science, Guru Angad Dev Veterinary and Animal Sciences University, Ludhiana - 141 004, Punjab, India; 2. Department of Animal Genetics and Breeding, College of Veterinary Science, Guru Angad Dev Veterinary and Animal Sciences University, Ludhiana - 141 004, Punjab, India.
Corresponding author: Hari Mohan Saxena, e-mail: hmsaxena@yahoo.com, AM: anz089@gmail.com, PM: dr.puneetmalhotra@rediffmail.com

Abstract

Aim: We determined the antibody response in cattle naturally infected with brucellosis and normal healthy adult cattle vaccinated during calf hood with strain 19.

Materials and Methods: The antibody titers were measured by standard tube agglutination test (STAT), microtiter plate agglutination test (MAT), indirect hemagglutination assay (IHA), and indirect enzyme-linked immunosorbent assay (iELISA) as per standard protocols.

Results: The mean STAT titers were 1.963±0.345 in infected cattle and 1.200±0.155 in healthy vaccinated cattle. The difference was extremely significant (p<0.0001). The mean MAT titers were 2.244±0.727 in infected cattle and 1.200±0.155 in healthy vaccinated cattle. The difference was very significant (p<0.005). The mean IHA titers in infected cattle were 2.284±0.574, and those in healthy vaccinated cattle were 1.200±0.155. The difference was extremely significant (p=0.0002). However, the difference in mean iELISA titers of infected cattle (1.3678±0.014) and healthy vaccinated cattle (1.367±0.014) was non-significant. The infected animals showed very high titers of agglutinating antibodies compared to the vaccinated animals. However, it cannot be ascertained whether these antibodies are due to vaccine or response to infection. Since the infected animals had been vaccinated earlier, the current infection may suggest that vaccination was unable to induce protective levels of antibody. The heightened antibody response after infection may also indicate a secondary immune response to the antigens common to the vaccine strain and wild *Brucella* organisms.

Conclusion: The brucellosis infected animals showed very high titers of agglutinating antibodies compared to the vaccinated animals.

Keywords: antibody titers, *Brucella,* brucellosis, *Brucella abortus* S19 vaccine, bovine brucellosis.

Introduction

Brucellosis is a major bacterial zoonosis of global importance. Brucellosis occurs worldwide but is much controlled in developed countries by routine screening of domestic animals and vaccination program. Clinical disease is still common in Middle East, Asia, Africa, South and Central America, the Mediterranean Basin, and the Caribbean. About 500,000 cases of human brucellosis are estimated to occur worldwide every year. It causes heavy economic loss to the animal industry through abortion, delayed conception, and temporary or permanent infertility in the affected animals [1].

Bovine brucellosis is endemic in all states of India. In India, the occurrence of brucellosis is to the extent of 10% in the marginal herds and 50% in organized farms, and the socio-economic impact of the disease was estimated to run over Rs. 500 crores annually. In Punjab, overall 17.7% prevalence of brucellosis was reported in cattle and buffaloes [2,3]. Brucellosis in animals is clinically characterized by late-term abortions and retention of placenta in females and orchitis and epididymitis in males, with excretion of organisms in semen, uterine discharges, and in milk [4]. Once infected, the animal may continue to shed bacteria and remains a source of infection to others for long period [3]. Mass vaccination is crucial for the control and eradication of bovine brucellosis. The widely used vaccine against brucellosis is derived from the smooth live vaccine strain (S19) for cattle. Although it has some undesirable traits, it has proven to be very useful under most conditions [5-7]. *Brucella abortus* S19 has been effective for the control of brucellosis in adult bovines and preventing abortion as well as decreasing the prevalence in herds [8].

The antibodies induced by vaccination interfere in serological diagnosis of brucellosis. Little data are available in the published literature on comparison of antibody titers due to vaccination and those due to natural infection in cattle. The present study was, therefore, undertaken to explore this aspect of serology of bovine brucellosis.

Materials and Methods

Ethical approval

All the experimental protocols performed on cattle were approved by the Institutional Animal Ethics Committee (IAEC). Animals were kept in IAEC approved facilities and received feed and water *ad libitum*.

Infected and vaccinated cattle

A total of 15 naturally infected brucellosis positive adult cattle, which were vaccinated during calf hood with *B. abortus* strain 19 vaccine (Bruvax; Indian Immunologicals), and 6 normal healthy calf hood vaccinated Holstein-Friesian crossbred adult cattle maintained at the University Dairy Farm were included in the study.

B. abortus strain 19 (vaccine strain)

The standard vaccine strain *B. abortus* strain 19, procured from the Biological Standardization Division, IVRI, Izatnagar, was used in the present study.

Collection of serum

Blood samples were collected from cattle through jugular vein for obtaining sera for studying the humoral immune response of the animals. Sera were separated and stored at $-20°C$ until further use.

Analysis of immune responses

Rose Bengal plate agglutination test (RBPT)

Equal volumes (10 µl each) of RBPT colored antigen (Punjab Veterinary Vaccine Institute, Ludhiana) and test serum were mixed on a clean glass slide [9] with the help of a sterilized toothpick. The slide was observed for 4 min for the formation of clumps. The formation of clumps was considered a positive test, whereas the absence of clear clumps was considered a negative reaction.

Estimation of antibody titers by standard tube agglutination test (STAT)

The standard OIE method [10] was followed (Table-1). The highest serum dilution showing 50% agglutination was taken as the end point for the titer. A titer of 1:40 or above was considered positive.

Controls

1: Tube No. 08 - 25% agglutination
2: Tube No. 09 - 50% agglutination
3: Tube No. 10 - 75% agglutination.

Microtiter plate agglutination test (MAT)

MAT was performed as per the method reported earlier [11].

Procedure

a. Serum samples were serially diluted two-fold in a final volume of 100 µl in 96 well U-bottom microtiter plate (Tarsons)

b. Equal volume of 100 µl *B. abortus* plain antigen (Punjab Veterinary Vaccine Institute, Ludhiana) was added to each well. Negative control well containing 100 µl of sterilized normal saline solution (NSS) and 100 µl of the antigen was also kept

c. The plate was covered with a lid and incubated at 37°C for 24 h followed by incubation at 4°C for 1 h

d. The formation of matt signified agglutination while button formation was indicative of a negative reaction. Titers ($\log_{10}$ values) were recorded as the reciprocal of the highest dilution of the serum giving at least 50% agglutination.

Indirect hemagglutination assay (IHA)

The method reported earlier [12] was followed with minor modifications.

Fixation of sheep red blood cells (sRBCs)

Sheep blood was collected aseptically by jugular vein puncture into Alsever's solution (1:1) and kept at 4°C for 7 days before further processing. The

Table-1: STAT protocol.

Tube No.	Carbol saline (in ml)	Test serum (in ml)	*B. abortus* plain antigen (in ml)	Final dilution
1	0.8	0.2	0.5	1:10
2	0.5	Serial dilution was performed after thorough mixing. 0.5 ml of the contents was transferred from tube No. 1 to the next tube up to tube No. 7. Finally, 0.5 ml of the contents was discarded from tube No. 7	0.5	1:20
3	0.5		0.5	1:40
4	0.5		0.5	1:80
5	0.5		0.5	1:160
6	0.5		0.5	1:320
7	0.5		0.5	1:640
8	1.25		0.75	
9	1.50		0.50	
10	1.75		0.25	

STAT=Standard tube agglutination test, *B. abortus=Brucella abortus*

blood was then centrifuged at 1500 rpm for 10 min to pack the erythrocytes. The packed RBCs were washed three times with 5-6 volumes of chilled NSS by centrifugation. Finally, a 10% (v/v) suspension of RBCs was prepared in chilled NSS and stored at 4°C.

Fixation and treatment of sRBCs with tannic acid

a. A 1% v/v solution of glutaraldehyde was prepared in NSS and stored at 4°C. Equal volumes of chilled glutaraldehyde solution and 10% washed sRBC suspension were mixed and allowed to stand at 4°C for 30 min with intermittent gentle stirring.

b. The sensitized sRBCs were packed by centrifugation at 1500 rpm for 10 min at room temperature followed by three washes in NSS to remove free glutaraldehyde and resuspended in the same buffer containing 0.1% sodium azide to yield a 10% suspension of sRBCs. The glutaraldehyde fixed sRBCs (G-sRBCs) were then stored at 4°C.

c. A 10% suspension of G-sRBCs was mixed with an equal volume of phosphate-buffered saline (PBS) containing 0.005% tannic acid (w/v) and incubated at 37°C with occasional shaking. The tanned G-sRBCs (TG-sRBCs) were pelleted by centrifugation at 650 $\times g$ for 10 min at room temperature and washed three times with PBS to yield a 10% suspension.

Preparation of antigen

The antigen prepared as described earlier was heated at 56°C for 30 min in a water bath with frequent shaking. Heat treated suspension was then centrifuged at 8000 rpm for 15 min at 4°C. The clear supernatant was separated and stored at −20°C until use.

Sensitization of TG-sRBCs with antigen

a. One volume of packed RBCs and 15 volumes of the antigen were mixed and incubated for 1-2 h at 37°C in a water bath with frequent shaking

b. The sensitized cells thus prepared were washed 3 times with NSS by centrifugation at 2000 rpm for 5 min. After the final wash, packed cells were resuspended in chilled NSS to obtain 1% suspension.

Adsorption of serum samples

a. To remove the heterophile antibodies, all the test serum samples (3 volumes) were adsorbed with packed sRBCs (1 volume) for 2 h at 37°C with periodic shaking before the test proper. The RBCs were removed by centrifugation

b. The suspension was centrifuged at 600 $\times g$ for 15 min at 4°C in a refrigerated centrifuge. The supernatant was collected and used for the test.

Test protocol for IHA

a. PBS (160 µl) and inactivated adsorbed serum (40 µl) were added to the first well (1 in 4 dilution), and 100 µl of PBS was added to all the other wells of a 96 well U-bottom microtiter plate (Tarsons). Two-fold serial dilutions of serum were made in a final volume of 100 µl

b. An equal volume (100 µl) of the 0.5% sensitized RBC suspension was added to all the wells. The plates were shaken and left at room temperature for 2 h.

Coarse agglutination of RBCs (matt formation) indicated a positive result and formation of a small button of deposited cells was considered as a negative result.

Controls

The following three controls were included with each test:
*   Antigen control: 100 µl of sensitized and adsorbed RBCs
*   RBC control: 100 µl of 1:4 dilution of serum and 100 µl of sensitized RBCs
*   Serum control: 100 µl of untreated erythrocytes and 100 µl of test sera.

Enzyme-linked immunosorbent assay (ELISA)

The serum samples of cattle were tested using Brucellosis Serum ELISA test kit (Idexx). The kit is based on indirect ELISA (iELISA) using inactivated antigen of *B. abortus*. The binding of the antibodies in cattle serum samples with precoated inactivated antigen on microtiter plate is detected by peroxidase-labeled anti-ruminant immunoglobulin G (IgG). The degree of the color that develops (optical density [OD] measured at 450 nm) is directly proportional to the amount of antibody specific for *B. abortus* present in the sample. The diagnostic relevance of the result is obtained by comparing the OD in wells containing the samples with the OD from wells containing the positive control. Antibody titers were calculated using an equation of regression.

Procedure

All reagents were thawed to 25°C and mixed by gentle vortexing before use.

a. Dispensed 90 µl of diluted wash solution (1:10) into each well of the microtiter plate

b. Added 10 µl of the undiluted serum samples and controls into the appropriate wells of the microtiter plate making the final dilution 1:10

c. Mixed the contents within each well by gently shaking the microtiter plate

d. Covered the microtiter plate with a lid and incubated for 60 min at 37°C in a humid chamber

e. Washed each well with approximately 300 µl wash solution 3 times. Aspirated liquid contents of all the wells after each wash. Following the final aspiration, firmly tapped the residual wash fluid from each plate onto absorbent material. Drying of plate between washes and before the addition of the next reagent was avoided

f. Dispensed 100 µl conjugate into each well

g. Covered and incubated the microtiter plate for 60 min at 37°C in a humid chamber

h. Washed each well and aspirated the liquid contents of all the wells after each wash

i. Dispensed 100 μl of 3,3',5,5'-Tetramethylbenzidine substrate into each well and incubated the substrate at 18-26°C for 15 min
j. Stopped the color reaction by adding 100 μl of stop solution per well
k. The OD was recorded in an ELISA reader at a wavelength of 450 nm.

Calculation of antibody titers

Antibody titer (Log_{10}) $Y = a + bx$

Where, constant $a = 1.35$; constant $b = 0.05$; $X = $ OD value of a test well/Mean $+3$ standard deviation value of negative control wells. The standard error of the Y estimate (antibody titer) was $+0.19$ $\log_{10}$.

Statistical analysis of data

Data pertaining to antibody titers by STAT, MAT, IHA, and iELISA were statistically analyzed by analysis of variance and t-test.

Results and Discussion

Antibody titers of infected or vaccinated cattle were estimated by STAT, MAT, IHA, and iELISA (Tables-2 and 3, Figure-1). STAT revealed the mean titers in infected cattle to be 1.963 ± 0.345, and the corresponding values in healthy vaccinated cattle were 1.200 ± 0.155. The difference was extremely significant $(p<0.0001)$. The mean MAT titers in infected cattle were 2.244 ± 0.727, and the corresponding values in healthy vaccinated cattle were 1.200 ± 0.155. The difference was very significant $(p<0.005)$. IHA revealed the mean titers in infected cattle to be 2.284 ± 0.574, and the corresponding values in healthy vaccinated cattle were 1.200 ± 0.155. The difference was extremely significant $(p=0.0002)$. Interestingly, the difference between the mean iELISA titers of infected cattle (1.3678 ± 0.014) and healthy vaccinated cattle (1.367 ± 0.014) was non-significant.

Even though a number of antigenic components of Brucella have been characterized, the antigen that dominates the antibody response is the lipopolysaccharide (LPS). Numerous outer and inner membrane, cytoplasmic, and periplasmic protein antigens have also been characterized. Some are recognized by the immune system during infection and are potentially useful in diagnostic tests. The L7/L12 ribosomal proteins are important in stimulating cell-mediated responses [13].

Immune response of host to Brucella infection is mediated through both humoral and cell-mediated immunity [14]. The role of humoral immunity against intracellular bacterial infections is limited and not protective. Antibody-mediated opsonization by Igs (IgM, IgG1, IgG2a, and IgG3) enhances phagocytic uptake of bacteria, limiting the level of initial infection with Brucella but has little effect on the intracellular course of Brucella infection [15,16].

B. abortus strain 19 is used as a live vaccine and is normally given to female calves aged between 3 and 6 months as a single subcutaneous dose of $5\text{-}8 \times 10^{10}$ viable organisms. It is believed to induce protective

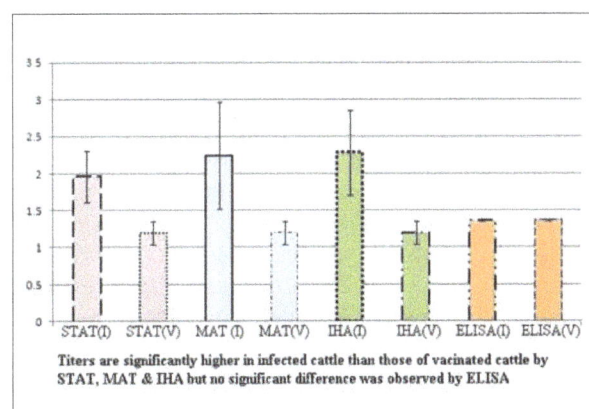

Titers are significantly higher in infected cattle than those of vaccinated cattle by STAT, MAT & IHA but no significant difference was observed by ELISA

Figure-1: Antibody titers in brucellosis infected or vaccinated cattle by standard tube agglutination test, microtiter plate agglutination test, indirect hemagglutination assay test, and indirect enzyme-linked immunosorbent assay.

Table-2: Antibody titers of cattle naturally infected with brucellosis.

S. No.	Antibody titers $(\log_{10})$			
	STAT	MAT	IHA	iELISA
1	1.903	2.204	2.204	1.4259
2	2.204	3.107	3.408	1.4328
3	1.602	3.408	2.505	1.4296
4	1.903	3.107	3.107	1.4264
5	1.602	1.602	1.602	1.3615
6	2.204	1.602	1.903	1.4226
7	2.806	3.709	3.107	1.4243
8	1.903	2.204	2.505	1.4251
9	1.602	1.903	1.602	1.3878
10	2.204	1.602	2.505	1.4539
11	1.602	1.903	1.903	0.6101
12	1.602	1.602	1.602	1.2935
13	2.204	1.602	1.903	0.4963
14	1.903	1.903	2.204	1.4084
15	2.204	2.204	2.204	1.4732
Mean±SD	1.963±0.345	2.244±0.727	2.284±0.574	1.3678±0.014

SD=Standard deviation, STAT=Standard tube agglutination test, MAT=Microtiter plate agglutination test, IHA=Indirect hemagglutination assay test, iELISA=Indirect enzyme-linked immunosorbent assay

Table-3: Antibody titers of healthy cattle vaccinated with *B. abortus* strain 19 vaccine.

S. No.	Antibody titers (log_{10})			
	STAT	**MAT**	**IHA**	**iELISA**
1	1.301	1.301	1.301	1.361
2	1.301	1.301	1.301	1.361
3	1.301	1.301	1.301	1.361
4	1.000	1.000	1.000	1.361
5	1.000	1.000	1.000	1.367
6	1.301	1.301	1.301	1.396
Mean±SD	1.200±0.155	1.200±0.155	1.200±0.155	1.367±0.014

SD=Standard deviation, STAT=Standard tube agglutination test, MAT=Microtiter plate agglutination test, IHA=Indirect hemagglutination assay test, iELISA=Indirect enzyme-linked immunosorbent assay

immunity against *B. abortus* in cattle [17]. However, the effectiveness of this vaccine varies with the age of vaccination, dose, route, and prevalence of brucellosis in the herd [18]. *B. abortus* strain 19 vaccine remains a reference vaccine to which any other vaccine is compared. Persistent antibodies could be detected up to 10-11 months post-vaccination [19].

As evident from our present data, infected animals have very high titers of antibodies compared to the vaccinated animals. However, the high titers do not indicate whether these are protective antibodies due to vaccine or acute response to infection in the absence of a differentiation of infected from vaccinated animals (DIVA) assay or whether they are of any relevance to prognosis. Since the infected animals were the ones who had already been vaccinated during calf hood, the infection in these animals may suggest that the vaccine was unable to induce protective levels of antibody. Second, the heightened antibody response after infection may indicate a secondary immune response to the genus-specific antigens of *Brucella*.

The different titers observed in the same animals by agglutination assays (STAT, MAT, and IHA) and iELISA can be reconciled with the fact that these assays target antigens of different nature, i.e., agglutination assays are directed toward particulate antigens, whereas ELISA detects immune response to soluble antigens. ELISA is generally used to detect IgG antibodies [20]. In brucellosis, specific IgM antibodies dominate during the acute phase of the disease [21]. Specific IgG antibodies are present in the serum of patients at later stages of the illness and in the serum of relapsing patients [22]. ELISA is used to discriminate between the presence of specific IgM and IgG antibodies and to roughly assess the stage of illness [23].

In many countries, STAT is the routine diagnostic test for human and animal brucellosis. It has been reported [24] that STAT has a greater accuracy than that of the RBPT (93.3% and 76.6%, respectively). In a study [25], *Brucella* antibodies were investigated in bovine sera by RBPT, serum agglutination test, MAT, and 2-mercaptoethanol MAT, and MAT was determined as a fast, reliable, and economic test. On evaluation of canine brucellosis by MAT, it was shown [26] that MAT was more sensitive, simpler to perform, and easier than tube agglutination test.

A study [27] has shown that the use of sheep erythrocytes sensitized with a specific LPS antigen in the IHA test provided a specific method, which is more sensitive than the agglutination test. A study [28] was carried out to compare the efficacy of RBPT, STAT, and DotELISA in immunological detection of antibodies to *B. abortus* in sera. The study revealed that DotELISA was the most sensitive of the three tests used. In a study by Ghodasara *et al.* [29], STAT and iELISA were compared for detection of *Brucella* antibodies in cows and buffaloes. The seropositivity was found highest by iELISA (25%) followed by STAT (14.45%). iELISA, RBPT, MAT, and PCR were evaluated [30] for diagnosis of brucellosis in buffaloes, and it was concluded that iELISA detected more samples as positive among these tests. Currently, no DIVA vaccine against brucellosis is available in the market. Identification of extracellular proteins from *Brucella* may aid in discovery of better vaccines or diagnostic molecules [31].

Since cell-mediated immunity is known to play an important role in brucellosis, it would be pertinent to incorporate antigens and adjuvants in the vaccine which could generate cellular immunity of a high protective level to be effective in control of brucellosis.

Conclusion

We determined the antibody titers by STAT, MAT, IHA, and ELISA in cattle naturally infected with brucellosis and normal healthy adult cattle vaccinated during calf hood with strain 19. The differences between the mean STAT, MAT, and IHA titers of infected cattle and healthy vaccinated cattle were highly significant (p<0.0001, p<0.005, and p=0.0002, respectively). However, the difference in mean iELISA titers of infected cattle and healthy vaccinated cattle was non-significant. The infected animals showed very high titers of agglutinating antibodies compared to the vaccinated animals.

Authors' Contributions

AM did the experiments; HMS conceived the idea, planned the study, and wrote manuscript; PM maintained the animals in the farm. Both authors read and approved the final manuscript.

Acknowledgment

Dr. Parkash Singh Brar, Director, Livestock Farms, Guru Angad Dev Veterinary and Animal Sciences University permitted us to carry out the study on cattle maintained in the University Dairy Farm and Dr. Mayank Rawat, Principal Scientist, Indian Veterinary Research Institute discussed with Hari Mohan Saxena about post vaccinal antibody titers in case of S-19 vaccine.

Competing Interest

The authors declare that they have no competing interests.

References

1. Kollannur, J.D., Rathore, R. and Chauhan, R.S. (2007) Epidemiology and economics of brucellosis in animals and its zoonotic significance. Proceedings of XIII International Congress in Animal Hygiene. International Society for Animal Hygiene. p466-468.
2. Jain, U., Bisht, B., Sahzad, P.ragati. and Dwivedi, K. (2013) Outbreak of brucellosis in buffaloes aborted in a village Mahuan, district Mainpuri, UP, India - A case report. *Vet. World*, 6(1): 51-52.
3. Pandeya, Y.R., Joshi, D.D., Dhakal, S., Ghimire, L., Mahato, B.R., Chaulagain, S., Satyal, R.C. and Sah, S.K. (2013) Seroprevalence of brucellosis in different animal species of Kailali district Nepal. *Int. J. Infect. Microbiol.*, 2(1): 22-25.
4. Godfroid, J., Garin-Bastuji, B., Saegerman, C. and Blasco, J.M. (2013) Brucellosis in terrestrial wildlife. *Sci. Tech. Rev. Off. Int. Epiz.*, 32(1): 27-42.
5. Moriyon, I., Grillo, M.J., Monreal, D., Gonzalez, D., Marin, C., Lopez-Goni, I., Mainar-Jaime, R.C., Moreno, E. and Blasco, J.M. (2004) Rough vaccines in animal brucellosis: Structural and genetic basis and present status. *Vet. Res.*, 35(1): 1-38.
6. Schuurman, H.J. (1983) The serological response of adult cattle to vaccination with reduced dose *Brucella abortus* S19, a trial under Zambian conditions. *Vet. Q.*, 5: 94-96.
7. Schurig, G.G., Sriranganathan, N. and Corbel, M.J. (2002) Brucellosis vaccines: Past, present and future. *Vet. Microbiol.*, 90: 479-496.
8. Avila-Calderón, E.D., Lopez-Merino, A., Sriranganathan, N., Boyle, S.M. and Contreras-Rodríguez, A. (2013) A History of the development of *Brucella* vaccines. *BioMed. Res. Int.*, 2013: Article ID: 743509.
9. Morgan, W.J., Mackinnon, D.T., Gill, K.P.W., Gower, S.G.M. and Norris, P.I.W. (1978) Brucellosis Diagnosis: Standard Laboratory Techniques Report Series No. 1. MAFF, Weybridge, England.
10. OIE Terrestrial Manual. (2009) Brucellosis. OIE, Paris Ch. 2.4.3. p1-35.
11. Williams, J.E. and Whittemore, A.D. (1971) Serological diagnosis of pullorum disease with the microagglutination system. *Appl. Microbiol.*, 21: 392-399.
12. Sawada, T., Rimler, R.B. and Rhoades, K.R. (1982) Indirect haemagglutination test that uses glutaraldehyde fixed sheep erythrocytes sensitized with extract antigens for detection of *Pasteurella* antibody. *J. Clin. Microbiol.*, 15(5): 752-756.
13. Oliveira, S.C. and Splitter, G.A. (1994) Subcloning and expression of *Brucella abortus* L7/L12 ribosomal gene and T-lymphocyte recognition of the recombinant protein. *Infect. Immun.*, 62: 5201-5204.
14. Skendros, P. and Boura, P. (2013) Immunity to brucellosis. *Sci. Tech. Rev. Off. Int. Epiz.*, 32(1): 137-147.
15. Bellaire, B.H., Roop, R.M. 2nd. and Cardelli, J.A. (2005) Opsonized virulent *Brucella abortus* replicates within nonacidic, endoplasmic reticulum-negative, LAMP-1-positive phagosomes in human monocytes. *Infect. Immun.*, 73: 3702-3713.
16. Baldwin, C.L. and Goenka, R. (2006) Host immune responses to the intracellular bacterium *Brucella*: Does the bacterium instruct the host to facilitate chronic infection? *Crit. Rev. Immunol.*, 26: 407-442.
17. Buck, J.M. (1930) Studies of vaccination during calfhood to prevent bovine infectious abortion. *J. Agric. Res.*, 41: 667-689.
18. Rahman, H. (2012) National Control Program on Brucellosis: Aims and Strategies. *Tech. Bull.* PD-ADMAS, India (15).
19. Nielsen, K. and Duncan, J.R. (1988) Antibody isotype response in adult cattle vaccinated with *Brucella abortus* strain 19. *Vet. Immunol. Immunopathol.*, 19: 205-214.
20. Long, G.Y., Liang, H.Z. and Liu, J.S. (1986) Immunization of rabbits against pasteurellosis. *Chin. J. Vet. Sci. Technol.*, 2: 3-7.
21. Smits, H.L., Abdoel, T.H., Solera, J., Clavijo, E. and Diaz, R. (2003) Immunochromatographic *Brucella*-specific immunoglobulin M and G lateral flow assays for rapid sero-diagnosis of human brucellosis. *Clin. Diag. Lab. Immunol.*, 10: 1141-1146.
22. Ariza, J., Pellicer, T., Pallares, R., Foz, A. and Gudiol, F. (1992) Specific antibody profile in human brucellosis. *Clin. Infect. Dis.*, 14: 131-140.
23. Smits, H.L. and Kadri, S.M. (2005) Brucellosis in India: A deceptive infectious disease. *Indian J. Med. Res.*, 122(5): 375-384.
24. Hassanain, N.A. and Ahmed, W.M. (2012) Efficacy of sero-logical tests in comparison with PCR for diagnosis of brucellosis. *World J. Med. Sci.*, 7(4): 243-247.
25. Sareyyupoglu, B., Cantekin, Z. and Mustak, H.K. (2010) Investigation of *Brucella* antibodies in bovine sera by rose Bengal plate test (RBPT), serum agglutination test (SAT), microagglutination test (MAT) and 2-mercaptoethanol - microagglutination (2-ME-MAT) test. *Ankara Univ. Vet. Fak. Derg.*, 57: 157-160.
26. Kimura, M., Imaoka, K., Suzuki, M., Kamiyama, T. and Yamada, M. (2008) Evaluation of a microplate agglutination test (MAT) for serological diagnosis of canine brucellosis. *J. Vet. Med. Sci.*, 70(7): 707-709.
27. Versilova, P.A., Cernyseva, M.I., Aslanjan, R.G. and Knjazeva, E.N. (1974) Diagnosis of human and animal brucellosis by the indirect haemagglutination test. *Bull. World Health Organ.*, 51: 191-197.
28. Chachra, D., Kaur, H., Chandra, M. and Saxena, H.M. (2012) Isolation, electron microscopy and physicochemical characterization of a brucella phage against *Brucella abortus* vaccine strain S19. *Internet J. Microbiol.*, 10(2). DOI: 10.5580/2c47.
29. Ghodasara, S., Roy, A., Rank, D.N. and Bhander, B.B. (2010) Identification of *Brucella* species from animals with reproductive disorders by polymerase chain reaction assay. *Buffalo Bull.*, 29(2): 98-108.
30. Malik, R., Gupta, M.P., Sidhu, P.K., Filia, G., Saxena, H.M. and Shafi, T.A. (2013) Comparative evaluation of indirect enzyme linked immunosorbent assay, rose Bengal plate test, microagglutination test and polymerase chain reaction for diagnosis of brucellosis in buffaloes. *Turk. J. Vet. Anim. Sci.*, 37: 306-310.
31. Jain, S., Kumar, S., Dohre, S., Afley, P., Sengupta, N. and Alam, S.I. (2014) Identification of a protective protein from stationary-phase exoproteome of *Brucella abortus*. *Pathog. Dis.*, 70: 75-83.

28

Effect of curing ingredients and vacuum packaging on the physico-chemical and storage quality of ready-to-eat *Vawksa rep* (smoked pork product) during refrigerated storage

Deepshikha Deuri[1], Pragati Hazarika[1], Tarun Pal Singh[2], Lalchamliani Chhangte[2], Parminder Singh[3] and Suman Talukder[2]

1. Division of Livestock Products Technology, College of Veterinary Sciences and Animal Husbandry, CAU, Selesih, Aizawl, Mizoram, India; 2. Division of Livestock Products Technology, Indian Veterinary Research Institute, Izzatnagar, Bareilly, Uttar Pradesh, India; 3. Veterinary Officer, Department of Animal Husbandry, Government of Punjab, Amritsar, Punjab, India.
Corresponding author: Deepshikha Deuri, e-mail: drdeuri10@gmail.com,
PH: pragati.h@rediffmail.com, TPS: tarunsingh835@gmail.com, LC: drchami17@gmail.com,
PS: pssandhulpt@gmail.com, ST: drttalukder@gmail.com

Abstract

Aim: The present study was conducted for the development of ready-to-eat *Vawksa rep* (smoked pork product) and to study the synergistic effect of curing ingredients and vacuum packaging on the physico-chemical and storage quality during refrigerated storage at ($4°C\pm1°C$) for 15 days.

Materials and Methods: Four different batches of *Vawksa rep* samples were prepared, i.e., T-1 (uncured, first cooked at 121°C for 15 min, and then smoked at 120°C for 30 min), T-2 (uncured, cooked, and smoked simultaneously at 120°C for 45 min), T-3 (cured, first cooked at 121°C for 15 min, and then smoked at 120°C for 30 min), and T-4 (cured, cooked, and smoked simultaneously at 120°C for 45 min).

Results: Cooking yield was significantly higher ($p<0.05$) for the T-4. The pH of T-3 and T-4 samples was significantly higher ($p<0.05$) on day 15. The tyrosine value of all the samples increased significantly ($p<0.05$) among the different days of analysis. Thiobarbituric acid value was significantly ($p<0.05$) lower in T-3 sample both at the beginning and at the end of storage period. In microbiological profile, total plate count was lower in T-3 and T-4 than T-1 and T-2. However, *Escherichia coli* count was negative for T-3 and T-4 samples throughout the storage period. Among sensory attributes, T-3 and T-4 samples registered superior scores for color, flavor, texture, juiciness, and overall acceptability.

Conclusion: Furthermore, *Vawksa rep* (smoked pork product) could be prepared easily with little technology up-gradation and with a negligible escalation of production cost.

Keywords: curing, smoking, storage quality, vacuum packaging, *Vawksa rep.*

Introduction

Meat is a highly perishable commodity due to a rich source of nutrients. Color, microbial growth, and lipid oxidation are considered important factors for limiting the shelf-life and consumer acceptance of meat and meat products [1]. Thus for extending the shelf-life, the use of a combination technology of different processing, packaging, and preservation conditions is a need of the hour.

Smoking is one of the oldest food processing technologies which not only improve the sensory quality but also inactivates a number of enzymes and microflora [2]. The active components of smoking which produce these activities are phenols, carbonyls, acids, alcohols, esters, lactones, polycyclic aromatic hydrocarbons, pyrazines, pyrrole, and furan derivatives [3]. It mainly improves color, odor and texture (firmness/hardness), physico-chemical, and microbial quality. However, smoking is often coupled with curing, salting, packaging, and chilling techniques to produce synergistic effects toward spoilage micro-organisms and to increase the shelf-life [4]. Vacuum packaging of meat is meant to retard or completely check the oxidative reactions and inhibit the microbial growth by reducing the amount of oxygen in contact with the product. Vacuum packaging preserves the natural flavor of the product, in addition to a number of advantages including such as saving of space and energy during storage, transport and distribution, reduction in weight loss, better-keeping qualities, and better display of the product [5].

Ready-to-eat food products form an important part of the diet in our day-to-day life. *Vawksa rep*, not ready-to-eat but a ready-to-cook smoked pork product, is one of the most popular traditional meat products of Mizoram. *"Sa-rep"* means *"smoked meat"* (where *"Sa"* stands for meat and *"rep"* means dehydrated or dry ones in Mizo language) is prepared locally in Mizoram and is preferred and widely consumed by the majority of middle-class income Mizo people [6]. It is prepared by mild smoking (2-3 h) of pork chunks of almost uniform size. The problem associated with *Vawksa rep* is that it has a short shelf-life because pork is highly prone to lipid oxidation due to the presence of excessive amounts of fat in it, and second, no other processing and preservation (except smoking) treatments are applied to this product for prolonging its shelf-life. Moreover, the product is sold without proper packaging, thereby increasing the chances of physical, chemical, and microbial contamination, in addition to fat oxidation. Keeping in view of the above-mentioned problems, the present study was undertaken for the development of ready-to-eat *Vawksa rep* and to study the synergistic effect of curing, smoking, and vacuum packaging on the physico-chemical, sensory, and microbial quality during refrigerated storage conditions.

Materials and Methods

Preparation of *Vawksa rep* meat samples

Raw pork cuts (hams) were purchased from the freshly slaughtered Yorkshire pig carcasses of about 8 months to 1 year of age from local market. In the laboratory, these were cut into small pieces of uniform size (3″×3″) with the help of a knife. Traditional *Vawksa rep* was prepared by piercing the pork chunks to the wooden stick and then placing the meat chunks 30 cm above the fire for 45 min. Hardwood was used for smoking of meat. Uncured pork chunks were first pressure cooked at 121°C for 15 min and subsequently smoked (CS) in the smoke unit (Kerres Showsmoker CS 350 EL) for 30 min at 120°C (T-1); cooked and smoked simultaneously (Directly smoked, DS) in the smoke unit at 120°C for 60 min (T-2). The pork chunks of uniform sizes (3″×3″) were cured for 24 h using curing mixture (Table-1). Cured pork chunks were pressure cooked at 121°C for 15 min and subsequently smoked in the smoke unit for 30 min at 120°C (T-3); cooked and smoked simultaneously in the smoke unit at 120°C for 45 min (T-4). These treatments were packed and sealed using the vacuum packaging machine in high-density polyethylene (HDPE, 3 Mil) bags and kept at refrigeration temperature (4°C±1°C) for 15 days. The samples were analyzed for different physico-chemical, sensory, and microbiological quality parameters at 1, 5, 10, and 15 days.

Table-1: Formulation for marination of pork chunks.

Ingredients	Quantity
Salt	1.5%
Sodium nitrate (NaNO$_3$)	200 mg/kg
Sodium nitrite (NaNO$_2$)	150 mg/kg
Spice-mix	2%
Sodium tripolyphosphate	0.5%
Yoghurt	10%
Sugar	1.5%

Physico-chemical quality parameters
Cooking yield

Cooking yield was calculated by dividing the weights of raw and cooked sample before with that of after cooking, multiplied by 100.

Cooking loss

Cooking loss was calculated by subtracting weight of the cooked product from the weight of the raw pork chunks.

pH

The pH of the sample was determined using a pH meter (Cyberscan 1000 Euteoh Instruments) and by following the methods as described by Bendall [7].

Texture analysis

Texture of the samples was analyzed using food texture analyzer (TA HD- Plus) with a load cell of 250 kg on different days of analysis. Measurements were taken at room temperature with a sample size of 2×2 cm^3. Data collection and analysis were performed using the Texture Expert Stable Micro Systems computer program, version 1.16.

Tyrosine value (TV) and thiobarbituric acid value (TBA)

TV and TBA were determined as per the standard methods proposed by Pearson [8] and Witte *et al.* [9], respectively.

Microbiological quality parameters

Total plate count (TPC), coli titer count, and *E. coli* counts of the samples were performed following the methods as described by APHA [10]. The average number of colonies was multiplied by the reciprocal of the dilution and expressed as $\log_{10}$ cfu/g.

Organoleptic quality parameters
Assessment of odor

All the *Vawksa rep* meat samples were assessed by a semi-trained panel of 25-30 judges by using a 10 point hedonic scorecard scale [8] on day 1st and thereafter, on 5th, 10th, and 15th days of storage.

Sensory evaluation

A six member experienced panel of judges evaluated the samples for different sensory attributes, viz., color and appearance, flavor, texture, juiciness, and overall acceptability, using an 8-point descriptive scale [11], where 8=excellent and 1=extremely poor. On each day of analysis, samples were cooked at 121°C for 15 min, cooled and then presented to the panelists for sensory evaluation along with a glass of water for rinsing of mouth.

Statistical analysis

Data were analyzed statistically on "SPSS-16.0" (SPSS Inc., Chicago, II USA) software package as per standard methods [12]. Duplicate samples were drawn for each parameter, and the whole experiment was repeated three times to have total number of observations, n=6 for all parameters. The entire data were subjected to two-way analysis of variance along with Duncan's multiple range test, and the significance was studied at 5% level ($p < 0.05$).

Results and Discussion

Physico-chemical quality

Cooking yields and cooking losses were estimated at day 0. Statistical analysis revealed that cooking yield was significantly higher ($p < 0.05$) for the T-4 (84.61 ± 0.02^{d0}%) followed by T-2 (82.63 ± 0.09^{c0}%), T-3 (82.50 ± 0.05^{b0}%), and T-1 (81.75 ± 0.05^{a0}%). It might be due to the extra uptake of salt and sugar, which were retained during processing, thus increasing water retention in T-4. The cooking loss was significantly higher ($p < 0.05$) for T-1 (18.25 ± 0.03^{d0}%) followed by T-3 (17.50 ± 0.15^{c0}%), T-2 (17.37 ± 0.03^{b0}%), and T-4 (15.39 ± 0.09^{a0}%). The heat treatment causes more moisture losses from the product, thereby resulting into more loss of meat fluid in T-1. Kanithaporn et al. [13] observed that the cooking loss in fully cooked RTE bacon heated for 30 s (20.91 ± 0.68) was lower than that of the RTE bacon heated for 60 s (24.23 ± 0.32).

The results for pH, texture analysis (hardness), TV, and TBA are presented in Table-2. The mean initial pH value of raw pork was 6.55. Initially, the pH values decreased up to 5th day of storage in all the treatment groups, but thereafter a rise in pH was observed gradually up to 15th day of storage, except in T-3, where progressive decrease in pH was recorded on 1st, 5th, and 10th days of storage followed by increased pH on 15th day of storage. CS samples, i.e., T-1 and T-3 for producing RTE Vawksa rep exhibited higher pH values compared to the ones who were directly smoked, i.e., T-2 and T-4. The pH of T-3 and T-4 samples was significantly higher ($p < 0.05$) on day 15 than day 1. Overall DS samples showed a faster fall in pH than CS samples of RTE Vawksa rep. Arnim and Marlida [14] also reported increase in pH values (at the end of storage) of meat balls treated with liquid smoke. Similar findings were observed by Kumar et al. [15] in pork nuggets during their refrigerated storage. The increase in pH of T-1, T-2, and T-4 on 10th and 15th day of storage, respectively, was in agreement with the findings of Karabagias et al. [16]. The variation in pH with curing ingredients, among the different treatments could be attributed to various factors such as the formation of bacterial metabolites, deamination of proteins, growth of facultative anaerobes, lactic acid bacteria, migration of antimicrobial substances, and formation of carbonic acid in vacuum packaging [17].

In texture profile, with the advancement of the storage period, there was continued and significant ($p < 0.05$) increase in hardness of all the Vawksa rep samples. In general, higher mean peak forces were required to cut CS as compared to DS RTE Vawksa rep samples. Between CS, i.e. T-1 and T-3; the T-3 (1775.50-2041.70 g) required low force than T-1 (2287.21-2869.17 g). In DS RTE Vawksa rep (T-2 and T-4), a relatively lower force was required in T-4 (1576.60-1712.50 g) as compared to T-2 (1890.41-2683.60 g). Garcia-Esteban et al. [18] also observed continued increase in hardness value of dry cured hams during storage under vacuum packaging conditions, with the highest hardness value (2669.00 g) observed in vacuum packed samples at the end of storage period. Cilla et al. [19] also observed a hardness value of 5220.99 g in vacuum packaged dry cured ham cuts stored at 4°C±2°C.

Table-2: Physico-chemical properties of Vawksa rep (smoked pork product) stored under vacuum packaging conditions at 4°C±1°C.

Treatments/Days	1	5	10	15
pH				
T-1	6.50 ± 0.01^{aA}	6.45 ± 0.01^{aA}	6.54 ± 0.13^{aA}	6.60 ± 0.01^{aA}
T-2	6.44 ± 0.01^{aAB}	6.25 ± 0.01^{cC}	6.37 ± 0.01^{bAB}	6.45 ± 0.01^{aB}
T-3	6.46 ± 0.02^{aB}	6.38 ± 0.01^{bcB}	6.36 ± 0.01^{cAB}	6.40 ± 0.01^{bC}
T-4	6.43 ± 0.01^{aB}	6.24 ± 0.01^{dC}	6.30 ± 0.01^{cB}	6.39 ± 0.01^{bC}
Hardness (g)				
T-1	2287.21 ± 0.06^{dA}	2687.80 ± 0.06^{cA}	2785.80 ± 0.10^{bA}	2869.17 ± 0.32^{aA}
T-2	1890.41 ± 0.06^{dB}	2412.90 ± 0.10^{cB}	2577.60 ± 0.06^{bB}	2683.60 ± 0.06^{aB}
T-3	1775.50 ± 0.06^{dC}	1832.90 ± 0.10^{cC}	1960.92 ± 0.11^{bC}	2041.70 ± 0.06^{aC}
T-4	1576.60 ± 0.10^{dD}	1650.30 ± 0.10^{cD}	1681.40 ± 0.10^{bD}	1712.50 ± 0.14^{aD}
TV (mg tyrosine/100 g)				
T-1	0.058 ± 0.05^{dB}	0.075 ± 0.05^{cB}	0.089 ± 0.01^{bB}	0.150 ± 0.01^{aB}
T-2	0.085 ± 0.08^{dA}	0.101 ± 0.01^{cA}	0.152 ± 0.06^{bA}	0.165 ± 0.09^{aA}
T-3	0.052 ± 0.06^{cC}	0.055 ± 0.06^{cD}	0.060 ± 0.01^{bC}	0.098 ± 0.09^{aD}
T-4	0.059 ± 0.06^{dB}	0.065 ± 0.09^{cC}	0.087 ± 0.05^{bB}	0.103 ± 0.01^{aC}
TBA (mg malondialdehyde/kg)				
T-1	0.28 ± 0.05^{dA}	0.34 ± 0.09^{cA}	0.65 ± 0.08^{bC}	1.21 ± 0.08^{aB}
T-2	0.25 ± 0.01^{dA}	0.32 ± 0.05^{cAB}	0.80 ± 0.09^{bA}	1.35 ± 0.01^{aA}
T-3	0.21 ± 0.08^{dB}	0.30 ± 0.05^{cB}	0.75 ± 0.01^{bB}	0.80 ± 0.09^{aD}
T-4	0.25 ± 0.01^{dA}	0.32 ± 0.05^{cAB}	0.78 ± 0.05^{bA}	0.90 ± 0.09^{aC}

n=6, mean±SE with different superscripts row wise (small alphabets) and column wise (capital alphabets) differ significantly ($p < 0.05$). SE=Standard error, TV=Tyrosine value, TBA=Thiobarbituric acid

The mean initial TV of raw pork was 0.220 mg tyrosine/100 g (0 day). Irrespective of the treatment groups, the TV increased in all the samples throughout the storage period (Table-2). The mean TV of all the samples increased significantly ($p < 0.05$) among the different days of analysis. At the end of the storage period, i.e., day 15, TV was significantly higher ($p < 0.05$) in T-2 followed by T-1, T-4, and T-3. Even though all the treatment groups showed a gradual increase in the TV from 1st to 15th day, the DS RTE *Vawksa rep* exhibited higher TV than the CS RTE *Vawksa rep* samples. Similar results were reported by Lalchamliani *et al.* [20] in *Vawksa rep* samples stored under different aerobic vacuum packaging conditions at 4°C±1°C. The findings are also in agreement with the statement of Pearson [8], who reported that TV of meat increases with storage period until deamination of amino acid limits the formation of free amino acid.

The TBA value of raw pork was 0.235 mg malondialdehyde/kg of meat. In general, TBA values of all the samples increased significantly ($p < 0.05$) throughout the storage period (Table-2). Compared to other treatments, T-3 sample maintained significantly ($p < 0.05$) lower values of TBA both at the beginning (day 1) and at the end (day 15) of storage period. At the end of the storage period, i.e., on day 15, the difference in TBA values of both CS and DS RTE *Vawksa rep* samples was significantly higher ($p < 0.05$) than day 1, 5 and 10 of storage periods. For TBA value, 0.5 mg malondialdehyde/kg is considered as the cut-off value for fat oxidation and 1 mg malondialdehyde/kg for rancidity in the products. From the Table-2, it is clear that all the treatments of RTE *Vawksa rep* experienced oxidation on the 10th day of storage. Overall, the combination of smoking and vacuum packaging resisted the lipid oxidation in RTE *Vawksa rep*. In this study, the increase in TBA values of all the samples was within the threshold limit of 1-2 mg malondialdehyde/kg meat. The increase in TBA value during storage might be attributed to the oxidation of meat lipid or both CS and DS RTE *Vawksa rep* at refrigeration temperature. Lalchamliani *et al.* [20] also observed increasing trends in TBA values of *Vawksa rep* samples during refrigerated storage. Kumar *et al.* [15] also reported that the TBARS values of pork nuggets significantly ($p < 0.01$) increased with the increase of storage period. Kumar and Sharma [21] also observed a linear increase in TBA value throughout the storage period while studying the quality characteristics of low-fat ground pork patties containing milk co-precipitate.

Microbiological quality

The data related to microbiological quality parameters of *Vawksa rep* are presented in Table-3. The TPC in raw pork was 5.50 $\log_{10}$ cfu/g. There was a continued and significant increase ($p < 0.05$) in TPC of all the samples from day 1 to 15, though the increase in the count was relatively less in T-3 and T-4 than T-1 and T-2. Moreover, it was evidenced that smoking caused decrease in the number of the viable aerobic micro-organisms from the initial mean value of raw meat. The increase in the TPC *Vawksa rep* during storage might be due to increasing in pH values of the sample, which favored the growth of bacteria. The reduction in the count of aerobic microbes could also be due to the antimicrobial effect of curing ingredients, smoking, and vacuum packaging. The findings are in agreement with the results of Lalchamliani *et al.* [20] in *Vawksa rep* meat samples stored at 4°C±1°C. Irkin *et al.* [22] also observed that minced beef samples treated with vacuum packaging showed lower viable counts than control. Kumar *et al.* [15] reported gradual but significant increase in total viable counts throughout the storage period in pork nuggets. Lawrie [23] reported that when smoking was combined with curing, the shelf-life of such products increases and the microbial load decreases especially on the meat surface.

The mean colititer value of raw pork was 780.00 MPN/g. The mean values of colititer counts

Table-3: Microbiological quality of *Vawksa rep* (smoked pork product) stored under vacuum packaging conditions at 4°C±1°C.

Treatments/Days	1	5	10	15
Total plate count ($\log_{10}$ cfu/g)				
T-1	3.60±0.06[dA]	3.90±0.06[cA]	4.80±0.04[bA]	5.30±0.06[aA]
T-2	3.80±0.10[dA]	4.10±0.06[cA]	4.90±0.06[bA]	5.40±0.10[aA]
T-3	2.51±0.12[bB]	2.60±0.10[bB]	3.50±0.14[aB]	3.80±0.06[aB]
T-4	2.60±0.10[bB]	2.70±0.06[bB]	3.70±0.13[aB]	3.90±0.06[aB]
Colititer (MPN/g)				
T-1	115.00±11.69[dB]	310.00±52.09[cB]	343.33±55.29[bB]	493.33±129.07[aB]
T-2	134.16±10.83[dA]	353.33±48.83[cA]	386.66±46.38[bA]	530.00±119.53[aA]
T-3	15.00±0.37[bC]	ND	ND	ND
T-4	18.00±1.71[bD]	ND	ND	ND
E. coli count ($\log_{10}$ cfu/g)				
T-1	1.57±0.05[cA]	1.73±0.05[bA]	1.82±0.09[abA]	1.93±0.05[aA]
T-2	1.62±0.05[dA]	1.75±0.05[cA]	1.85±0.05[bA]	1.98±0.03[aB]
T-3	ND	ND	ND	ND
T-4	ND	ND	ND	ND

n=6, mean±SE with different superscripts row wise (small alphabets) and column wise (capital alphabets) differ significantly ($p < 0.05$). ND=Not detected, SE=Standard error, *E. coli*=*Escherichia coli*

increased significantly (p<0.05) in T-1 and T-2. However, in T-3 and T-4 samples, colititer count was detected only on day 1 and was not detected subsequently. Among T-3 and T-4, colititer count was significantly lower (p<0.05) in T-3 sample. Hence, in terms of microbiological quality, T-3 sample of *Vawksa rep* was superior to other variants. Irkin *et al.* [22] reported that the number of coliforms increased slightly in all the minced beef samples until the end of storage and was below the accepted limit (3 $\log_{10}$ cfu/g) except in control samples stored at 4°C. Bacteriological isolation studies by Chaudhari *et al.* [6] in Mizoram involving 100 pork "*Sa-rep*" (smoked meat) samples revealed the presence of *E. coli* only in 9 isolates. The initial mean *E. coli* count was recorded to be 3.12 $\log_{10}$ cfu/g of meat. There was a significant increase (p<0.05) in *E. coli* counts in T-1 and T-2 from the mean value of 1.57 $\log_{10}$ cfu/g and 1.62 $\log_{10}$ cfu/g on the 1st day to 1.93 and 1.98 $\log_{10}$ cfu/g on the 15th day of storage, respectively. The *E. coli* count was negative for all the cured CS and DS (T-3 and T-4) products in all the storage periods. The absence of *E. coli* in T-3 and T-4 conforms to the national standard, i.e., nil presence of coliform organisms at 0.001g level the for entire storage period.

Organoleptic quality
Assessment of odor

The odor scores for different treatments decreased significantly with the advancement of the storage period (Table-4). In general, the scores were comparatively higher for T-3 and T-4 than T-1 and T-2. At the beginning of storage period, i.e., day 1, the odor scores for T-3 and T-4 were similar (9.60), but at the end of the storage period (day 15), the scores were slightly higher (p<0.05) for T-3 (7.80) than T-4 (7.60). The decrease in odor scores of samples might be due to continue and significant (p<0.05) increase in TBA value throughout the storage period. Many authors reported similar findings and observed that meat products were acceptable and did not show any perceivable rancidity or off odor/aroma up to 21 days of storage [24]. Nathappan *et al.* [25] also reported declining trends in odor scores of stored mutton (5°C±1°C) with the advancement of the storage period, and the scores also remained within the limit of acceptability up to 72 h of storage.

Sensory evaluation

The results of the sensory evaluation are presented in Table-5. The color and appearance scores were significantly higher (p<0.05) in T-3 and T-4, both at beginning (day 1) and at the end (day 15) of the storage period. However, in general, the scores for color decreased in all the samples as the storage advanced. At the end of storage, the scores for color and appearance were highest for T-3 (7.00) followed by T-4 (6.80), T-2 (5.70), and T-1 (5.50). The results were inconsistent with the findings of Lalchamliani *et al.* [20] in *Vawksa rep* meat samples stored at 4°C±1°C. Under vacuum packaging conditions, meat is protected from color fading due to the low level of oxygen [26]. Both the cured CS and DS (T-3 and T-4) RTE *Vawksa rep* showed superior flavor scores as compared to the uncured CS and DS (T-1 and T-2). The flavor scores also followed a declining trend starting from beginning till the end of the storage period, which might be due to increase in TBA, TPC, and coliform count. Overall the flavor scores were significantly higher (p<0.05) in T-3 and T-4 on all the storage days. Devatkal *et al.* [27] reported that there is deterioration of flavor due to microbial growth and oxidative rancidity in restructured pork rolls. As the storage period is advanced, the sharp decline in flavor scores might be due to oxidation of fat [28], liberation of fatty acids [29] and increased microbial load [30]. Both CS (T-1 and T-3) RTE *Vawksa rep* registered high texture scores as compared to the DS (T-2 and T-4) RTE *Vawksa rep*. Texture also followed declining trend throughout the storage in all the samples. Azad [31] also reported that during storage of smoked buffalo meat at 0°C and −4°C, it started losing color, texture, and odor. On all the storage days, juiciness was found to be significantly higher (p<0.05) in T-3 and T-4 batches than T-1 and T-2. Throughout the storage period, highest juiciness was observed in T-4 among the different samples. Overall, juiciness scores declined progressively from 1st to 15th day of storage, which might be due to significant (p<0.05) increase in hardness values in all the samples. Kumar *et al.* [15] also observed a significant decrease in flavor, texture, and juiciness of pork nuggets during storage. Decrease in texture and juiciness of samples might be due to loss of moisture during the storage. The overall acceptability was significantly higher (p<0.05) in T-3 on all the storage days. Both the cured CS and DS (T-3 and T-4) RTE *Vawksa rep* had registered higher overall acceptability as compared to their uncured counterparts, i.e. CS and DS (T-1 and T-2). In general, overall acceptability decreased in all the samples as the storage period advanced. These findings are in

Table-4: Odor scores of *Vawksa rep* (smoked pork product) stored under vacuum packaging conditions at 4°C±1°C.

Treatments/Days	1	5	10	15
T-1	9.20±0.05[aA]	8.50±0.05[bB]	6.70±0.05[cB]	6.20±0.05[dB]
T-2	9.40±0.05[aA]	8.40±0.05[bB]	6.50±0.05[cB]	6.10±0.09[dB]
T-3	9.60±0.05[aA]	9.50±0.05[abA]	8.30±0.05[cA]	7.80±0.05[dA]
T-4	9.60±0.05[aA]	9.40±0.05[abA]	8.20±0.05[cA]	7.60±0.05[dAB]

n=27, mean±SE with different superscripts row wise (small alphabets) and column wise (capital alphabets) differ significantly (p<0.05). SE=Standard error

Table-5: Sensory properties of *Vawksa* rep (smoked pork product) stored under vacuum packaging conditions at 4°C±1°C.

Treatments/Days	1	5	10	15
Color and appearance				
T-1	6.20±0.05[aB]	6.00±0.14[bA]	5.80±0.12[aB]	5.50±0.15[aB]
T-2	6.50±0.09[aB]	6.30±0.05[aB]	6.00±0.14[bB]	5.70±0.08[cB]
T-3	7.50±0.18[aA]	7.30±0.09[abA]	7.20±0.09[abA]	7.00±0.05[bA]
T-4	7.30±0.09[aA]	7.10±0.05[abA]	7.00±0.14[abA]	6.80±0.12[bA]
Flavor				
T-1	6.20±0.05[aB]	6.00±0.05[aB]	5.70±0.05[bB]	5.40±0.09[cB]
T-2	6.00±0.18[aB]	5.80±0.09[aB]	5.40±0.05[bC]	5.20±0.09[bB]
T-3	7.60±0.05[aA]	7.30±0.07[bA]	7.10±0.03[bcA]	7.00±0.14[cA]
T-4	7.40±0.12[aA]	7.20±0.09[abA]	7.00±0.14[bA]	6.90±0.03[bA]
Texture				
T-1	6.60±0.07[aB]	6.50±0.14[aB]	6.00±0.07[bB]	5.80±0.05[bBC]
T-2	6.40±0.05[aB]	6.20±0.07[bC]	5.90±0.05[cBC]	5.70±0.05[dC]
T-3	7.60±0.05[aA]	7.40±0.05[abA]	7.20±0.09[bcA]	7.00±0.13[cA]
T-4	7.40±0.07[aA]	7.30±0.05[aA]	7.10±0.05[bAB]	6.80±0.05[cAB]
Juiciness				
T-1	6.50±0.13[aB]	6.30±0.09[abB]	6.20±0.09[abB]	6.00±0.13[bB]
T-2	6.60±0.03[aB]	6.50±0.05[aB]	6.30±0.05[bB]	6.10±0.09[cB]
T-3	7.40±0.09[aA]	7.20±0.05[aA]	6.90±0.09[bA]	6.70±0.09[bA]
T-4	7.50±0.05[aA]	7.30±0.12[abA]	7.00±0.14[bcA]	6.80±0.13[cA]
Overall acceptability				
T-1	6.50±0.15[aB]	6.30±0.05[abC]	6.00±0.13[bB]	5.50±0.09[cB]
T-2	6.30±0.05[aB]	6.00±0.14[bD]	5.80±0.09[bB]	5.30±0.05[cB]
T-3	7.80±0.05[aA]	7.60±0.09[aA]	7.30±0.02[bA]	7.00±0.13[aA]
T-4	7.50±0.13[aA]	7.30±0.05[abB]	7.10±0.05[bA]	6.80±0.09[cA]

n=18, mean±SE with different superscripts row wise (small alphabets) and column wise (capital alphabets) differ significantly (p<0.05). SE=Standard error

Table-6: Economics of *Vawksa rep* (smoked pork product).

Commodities used	Cured (Rs.)	Uncured (Rs.)
Pork (25 kg)	6250.00	6250.00
Salt and sugar	26.25	-
Nitrate and nitrite	17.00	-
Spice mix	150.00	-
Yoghurt	100.00	-
STPP	93.00	-
Packaging	20.00	20.00
Sawdust/wood	20.00	20.00
Electricity	63.00	63.00
Total cost (25 kg)	6739.25	6353.00
Cost/kg	269.57	254.12

STPP=Sodium tripolyphosphate

agreement with the report of Iwanegbe *et al.* [32], who also observed significant differences (p<0.05) among the treatments groups (different cures, storage periods, and storage temperatures) in terms of color, flavor, juiciness, tenderness, and overall acceptability of smoked rabbit meat.

Production economics of cured versus uncured *Vawksa rep*

The comparative cost for the formulation of each of 25 kg CS (T-1 and T-3) and DS (T-2 and T-4) is presented in Table-6. It includes the cost of raw materials required, viz., cost of raw pork, curing ingredients (salt, sugar, nitrate, and nitrite), spice mix, yoghurt, STPP, packaging, saw dust/wood, and electricity. The cost of production of cured CS and DS RTE *Vawksa rep* was estimated to be Rs. 269.57/kg, whereas for uncured CS and DS RTE *Vawksa* rep, it

was Rs 254.12/kg. The expenditure incurred toward equipment and labor was not considered. The production cost of cured CS and DS RTE *Vawksa rep* was somewhat higher than the uncured CS and DS RTE *Vawksa rep,* but at the same time, it is much lower than the present market price of *Vawksa rep* in Aizawl city. Considering the above beneficial attributes superior in terms of sensory, physico-chemical, and most importantly the microbiological qualities of CS and DS RTE *Vawksa rep,* it would command higher market demand and price in comparison to the uncured CS and DS RTE *Vawksa rep,* because nowadays, consumers are more quality conscious and ready-to-pay more for the better quality products. Besides, production technology, up-gradation of traditional meat food products is the need of the hour as these products suit to the taste and flavor of local populates.

Conclusion

From the above study, it can be concluded that using combination of curing, cooking, and smoking, a new and quality assured RTE *Vawksa rep* could be developed. Compared to uncured CS and DS (T-1 and T-2), the cured CS and DS (T-3 and T-4) RTE *Vawksa rep* registered superior physico-chemical properties (higher cooking yield, favorable pH, lower TV, and lower TBA values), sensory properties (higher odor scores, higher color, flavor, texture, juiciness, and overall acceptability scores), and microbiological properties (lower TPC, absence of coltiter, and *E. coli* count) throughout the storage period of 15-day. Furthermore, cured CS and DS RTE *Vawksa rep* could be prepared easily with little technology up-gradation and with a negligible escalation of production cost.

Authors' Contributions

The present study was a part of DD's original research work during his M.V.Sc. thesis program. PH helped in designing of the work and gave the guidelines during experimental study. LC assisted in the processing of samples. TPS, PS, and ST assisted in statistical analysis, interpretation of the results and drafting of the manuscript. All the authors have read and approved the final manuscript.

Acknowledgments

The authors are thankful to the Dean, College of Veterinary Sciences and Animal Husbandry, CAU, Selesih, Aizawl, Mizoram, India, for providing the necessary infrastructure required for conducting this research work.

Competing Interests

The authors declare that they have no competing interests.

References

1. Singh, P., Sahoo, J., Chatli, M.K. and Biswas, A.K. (2014) Shelf life evaluation of raw chicken meat emulsion incorporated with clove powder, ginger and garlic paste as natural preservatives at refrigerated storage (4±1°C). *Int. Food Res. J.*, 21(4): 1363-1373.

2. Llave, Y., Suzuki, A., Fukuoka, M., Umiuchi, E. and Sakai, N. (2015) Migration of smoke components into pork loin ham during processing and storage. *J. Food Eng.*, 166: 221-229.

3. Gomez-Estaca, J., Gomez-Guillen, M.C., Montero, P., Sopelana, P. and Guillen, M.D. (2011) Oxidative stability, volatile components and polycyclic aromatic hydrocarbons of cold-smoked sardine (*Sardine pilchardus*) and dolphinfish (*Coryphaena hippurus*). *Food Sci. Technol.*, 44: 1517-1524.

4. Corzo, O., Bracho, N., Rodríguez, J. and Arias, J.M. (2015) Optimizing salting and smoking of Catfish (*Bagre Marinus*) using response surface methodology. *J. Aquat. Food Prod. Technol.*, DOI: 10.1080/10498850.2013.855286.

5. Sharma, B.D. and Kumar, R.R. (2013) Optimizing shelf life of meat and meat products using innovative packaging solutions. Proceedings of 5th Annual Conference and National Symposium of Indian Meat Science Association (IMSACON-V) on 'Emerging Technological Changes to Meet the Demands of Domestic and Export Meat Sector', 07-09 February, 2013. National Research Centre on Meat, Chengicherla, Hyderabad. p59-71.

6. Chaudhari, S.P., Tiwari, J.G. and Roychaudhury, P. (2007) Occurrence of *Escherichia coli* in smoked meat. *Indian J. Anim. Sci.*, 77(6): 442-445.

7. Bendall, J.R. (1973) Postmortem changes in muscle. In: Bourne, G.H., editor. The Structure and Function of Muscle. Academic Press, New York, NY. p244-306.

8. Pearson, D. (1968) Application of chemical methods for the assessment of beef quality and methods related to protein breakdown. *J. Sci. Food Agric.*, 19(2): 357-363.

9. Witte, V.C., Krause, G.F. and Bailey, M.E. (1970) A new extraction method for determining 2 Thiobarbituric acid

10. values of pork and beef during storage. *J. Food Sci.*, 35(5): 582-585.

10. APHA. (1992) Standard Methods for the Examination of Water and Wastewater. 18th ed. American Public Health Association Inc., Washington, DC.

11. Keeton, J.T. (1983) Effect of fat and NaCL/phosphate levels on the chemical and sensory properties of pork patties. *J. Food Sci.*, 48(3): 878-881.

12. Snedecor, G.W. and Cochran, W.G. (1995), Statistical Methods. 8th ed. Oxford and IBH Publishing, New Delhi.

13. Kanithaporn, P., Gadgil, P., Terry, A.H., Melvin, C.H. and Scott, S.J. (2011) Heterocyclic amine content in commercial ready to eat meat products. *J. Meat Sci.*, 88: 227-233.

14. Arnim, F. and Marlida, Y. (2012) The effect of liquid smoke utilization as preservative for meat balls quality. *Pak. J. Nutr.*, 11(11): 1078-1080.

15. Kumar, B.R., Kalaokannan, A. and Radhakrishnan, K.T. (2007) Studies on processing and shelf life of pork nuggets with liquid whey as replacer for added water. *Am. J. Food Technol.*, 2(1): 38-43.

16. Karabagias, I., Badeka, A. and Kontominas, M.G. (2011) Shelf life extension of lamb meat using thyme or oregano essential oils and modified atmosphere packaging. *Meat Sci.*, 88: 109-116.

17. Jay, J.M., Loessner, J.M. and Golden, D.A. (2005) Modern Food Microbiology. 7th ed. Springer Publications, New York, NY. p101-118.

18. Garcia-Esteban, M., Ansorena, D. and Astiasarán, I. (2004) Comparison of modified atmosphere packaging and vacuum packaging for long period storage of dry-cured ham: Effects on colour, texture and microbiological quality. *Meat Sci.*, 67(1): 57-63.

19. Cilla, I., Martínez, L., Beltrán, J.A. and Roncalés, P. (2006) Dry-cured ham quality and acceptability as affected by the preservation system used for retail sale. *Meat Sci.*, 73(4): 581-589.

20. Lalchamliani, L., Hazarika, P., Singh, T.P. and Talukder, S. (2015) Effects of curing ingredients and nisin on product characteristics of *Vawksa rep* (smoked pork product). *J. Nutr. Food Sci.*, 45(4): 634-645.

21. Kumar, M. and Sharma, B.D. (2003) Quality characteristics of low-fat ground pork patties containing milk co-precipitate. *Asian Aust. J. Anim.* Sci., 6(4): 588-595.

22. Irkin, R., Esmer, O.K., Degirmencioglu, N. and Degirmencioglu, A. (2011) Influence of packaging conditions on some microbial properties of minced beef meat at 4°C storage. *Bulg. J. Agric. Sci.*, 17(5): 655-663.

23. Lawrie, R.A. (1991) The eating quality of meat. In: Meat Science. 5th ed. Pergamon Press, New York, NY. p56-60.

24. Bullock, K.B., Huffman, D.L., Egbert, W.B., Mikel, W.B., Bradford, D.D. and Jones, W.R. (1994) Storage stability of low-fat ground beef made with lower value cuts of beef. *J. Food Sci.*, 59(1): 6-9.

25. Nathappan, M., Kolsalaraman, V.R. and Ramamurthi, R. (1985) A study of certain physic chemical changes in stored mutton in relation to odour score. *Cheiron*, 14: 2.

26. Parra, V., Viguera, J., Sánchez, J., Peinado, J., Espárrago, F., Gutierrez, J.I. and Andrésa, A.I. (2012) Effect of exposure to light on physico-chemical quality attributes of sliced dry-cured Iberian ham under different packaging systems. *Meat Sci.*, 90: 236-243.

27. Devatkal, S., Mendiratta, S.K. and Anjaneyulu, A.S.R. (2003) Effect of calcium lactate on the quality and shelf life of restructured pork rolls. *J. Meat Sci.*, 1: 1-6.

28. Santamaria, L., Lizarraga, T., Astiasaran, I. and Bello, J. (1992) Characterization of pamplona chorizo sausages, physico-chemical and sensory studies. *Rev. Esp. Cien. Tec. Ali.*, 32: 431-445.

29. Branen, A.L. (1979) Interaction of fat oxidation and microbial spoilage in muscle foods. Proceedings of the 31st Annual Reciprocal Meat Conference. p156-161.

30. Sahoo, J. and Anjaneyulu, A.S.R. (1997) Effect of natural antioxidants and vacuum packaging on the quality of buffalo meat nuggets during refrigerated storage. *Meat Sci.*, 47(3-4): 223-230.

31. Azad, Z.R.A. (2012) Role of smoking on the textural characteristics and shelf-life of buffalo meat. *J. Ind. Res.*

Technol., 2(2): 98-103.

32. Iwanegbe, I., Iwanegbi, A.I., Ebabhamiegbebho, P.A. and Bello, Y.O. (2011) Effect of cures and storage periods on the sensory and microbial evaluation of smoke - Dried vacuum packaged meat products. *Pak. J. Nutr.,* 10(11): 1032-1035.

29

Effect of incorporation of calcium lactate on physico-chemical, textural, and sensory properties of restructured buffalo meat loaves

A. Irshad[1], B. D. Sharma[2], S. R. Ahmed[2], S. Talukder[2], O. P. Malav[3] and Ashish Kumar[2]

1. Department of Livestock Products Technology, College of Veterinary and Animal Sciences, Kerala Veterinary and Animal Sciences University, Mannuthy, Thrissur - 680 651, Kerala, India; 2. Division of Livestock Products Technology, Indian Veterinary Research Institute, Izatnagar - 243 122, Uttar Pradesh, India; 3. Department of Livestock Products Technology, College of Veterinary Science, Guru Angad Dev Veterinary and Animal Sciences University, Ludhiana, Punjab, India.
Corresponding author: A. Irshad, e-mail: irshad2k6@gmail.com,
BDS: dr_bdsharma@yahoo.com, SRA: Sh.rafeh@gmail.com, ST: drttalukder@gmail.com,
OPM: drmalav_vet2007@rediffmail.com, AK: ashish07.vet@gmail.com

Abstract

Aim: The present study was conducted to develop a functional meat product by fortifying calcium (in the form of calcium lactate) with restructured buffalo meat loaf (RBML).

Materials and Methods: Deboned buffalo meat obtained from the carcass of adult female buffalo within 5-6 h of slaughter and stored under frozen condition. Calcium fortified RBML were prepared by replacing the lean buffalo meat with calcium lactate powder at 0%, 1%, 1.25%, and 1.5% level through the pre-standardized procedure. The developed products were evaluated for physico-chemical properties, proximate composition, calcium concentration (mg/100 g), water activity (a_w), Lovibond® tintometer color units, texture profile analysis (TPA), and sensory qualities as per-standard procedures.

Results: Of the various product quality parameters evaluated, cooking yield (%), product pH, moisture (%), protein (%), fat (%), and water activity (a_w) decreases significantly with increasing level of calcium lactate. Calcium content of fortified functional RBMLs was 135.02, 165.73, and 203.85 mg/100 g as compared to 6.48 mg/100 g in control. Most of the sensory scores at 1% and 1.25% levels of calcium lactate in treatment products remained comparable among themselves and control product, with a gradual decline.

Conclusions: The present study concluded that 1.25% calcium lactate was the optimum level for the fortification of calcium in RBML without affecting the textural and sensory properties which could meet out 15% of recommended dietary allowance for calcium.

Keywords: buffalo meat, calcium fortification, Lovibond® tintometer color units, meat loaves, restructured products, texture profile analysis and sensory attributes.

Introduction

Interest in the dietary calcium has intensified in the recent years as a result of increased awareness about the importance of higher calcium intake [1]. Calcium is one of the most important nutrients in the human diet. In addition to conferring structural integrity to mineralized tissue (where about 99% of total calcium is found), it plays a diverse role in maintaining cellular function such as cellular metabolism, blood clotting, enzyme activation, and so on [2,3]. Meat as such is relatively poor in calcium, containing only about 10 mg/100 g of meat [4]. So, there is a dire need to fortify meat products with calcium so that a sufficient amount of recommended dietary allowance (RDA) for calcium can be met through meat products

also [5]. The normal RDA for calcium in the age group of 19-50 is l000 mg/day [6,7].

The clinical implications of calcium deficiency include rickets, poor bone mass accrual as well as abnormal fetal programing during pregnancy, poor peak bone mass due to poor accrual in childhood and adolescence, postmenopausal osteoporosis, and osteoporosis of the elderly [1]. While the etiologies of all of these diseases are multi-factorial and poorly understood, there is some evidence to support the hypothesis that increased calcium intake will reduce the risk of each of the diseases [7-10]. A growing concern regarding bone health in people of all ages has prompted the food industry to respond by adding calcium to foods and beverages [11]. Various calcium containing beverages include fortified milk products, hot and cold drink mixes, orange juice, carbonated soft drinks, beer, and even water are available in the market [12]. So, there is a need to enrich meat products with calcium so that a sufficient amount of RDA for calcium can be met through meat products also [11]. Regarding meats, some work has been carried out on calcium enrichment in ground beef patties [13]; reduced fat beef emulsion [14]; pork sausage [15]; cooked meat sausage [2], and calcium enriched chicken meat rolls [11]. The ideal calcium source used to enrich foods should be highly absorbable, inexpensive, safe, and compatible with the food delivery vehicle [16]. Several salts of calcium are available, e.g. inorganic salts such as calcium carbonate, calcium chloride, calcium phosphate, and organic salts such as calcium citrate, calcium lactate, and calcium gluconate. In general, organic salts of calcium are more bioavailable than inorganic salts [17]. Many of the researchers recommended calcium lactate for the enrichment of the meat products due to its nutritional value with high calcium content (13%), bland taste, and neutral aroma [15,18-20].

India is endowed with the largest buffalo population in the world which is about 58% of the world's buffalo population. About 10.66 million buffaloes are slaughtered annually producing 1.53 million MT of buffalo meat which accounts 31% of total meat production of the country [21]. Buffalo meat has been the major one in Indian meat export accounting more than 85% of total meat export mostly in frozen form [22]. Buffalo meat is abundantly available in India and has enormous potential for development into valuable and highly palatable processed meat products. However, the production of processed buffalo meat is minimal at present. As per Agricultural and Processed Food Products Export Development Authority [23], only 2% of the total meat is processed in India. So, processing of buffalo meat is essential to exploit its undermined potential. The majority of buffaloes in India are slaughtered from aged/spent animals (about 10-15 years) after completion of their productive period resulting in tough meat with poor quality characteristics such as tough texture, less juiciness, and comparatively dark color [24,25]. This coarse textured meat needs to be subjected to special processing and cooking methods to improve tenderness [26]. Restructuring of meat enables the use of less valuable meat components to produce high-quality meat products at a reduced cost [27]. Therefore, the enhanced use of less demanded cuts and/or raw material from older maturity classes can be achieved using restructured meat technology. Meat processors and consumers can benefit from the development of efficient and economical technologies for processing buffalo meat into value-added convenience meat products with high acceptability at a reasonable cost.

Hence, the present study was carried out to develop a calcium fortified restructured buffalo meat loaves (RBMLs) by incorporating a suitable level of calcium lactate in spent buffalo meat readily available in the market.

Materials and Methods

Ethical approval

Since the study was conducted on the buffalo meat purchased from the local slaughter house, ethical approval from Animal Ethics Committee of the institute was not necessary.

Location

The study was undertaken at Indian Veterinary Research Institute (IVRI), Izatnagar, Bareilly, Uttar Pradesh located at 28°10' N, 78°23' E, and lies in the northern region of India. The place has a humid subtropical climate with an elevation of 268 m (879 ft) above mean sea level.

Buffalo meat and other ingredients

Deboned buffalo meat obtained from the carcass of adult female buffalo (>10 years of age) was procured from the local market of Bareilly within 5-6 h of slaughter. All visible fascia and external fat were trimmed off, and meat portions were made into cuts of approximately 0.5 kg. The cuts were then packaged separately in low-density polyethylene (LDPE) pouches and kept in the refrigerator (4±1°C) for conditioning for about 24 h. Thereafter, the samples were shifted to the deep freezer (Blue Star, FS345, Denmark) for storage at −18±2°C until further use.

To prepare condiment mix, onion, and garlic were peeled off, cut into small pieces and homogenized separately in a kitchen mixer to obtain a fine paste. For the preparation of RBMLs, onion and garlic were used in the ratio 2:1. The spice ingredients were purchased from local market, free from extraneous matter and dried in hot air oven at 50±2°C for 4 h. The ingredients were ground and sieved through a fine mesh. The powders were mixed in suitable proportion to obtain spice mixture. The spice mix was stored in a plastic container for subsequent use (Table-1). All the chemicals (analytical grade) were obtained from standard firms (Qualigen®, Hi-Media®, Sdefine®, etc.). Generally Recognized as Safe/Food Grade Chemicals were used for fortification were supplied by Qualigen® Fine Chemicals (A division of Glaxo India Limited), Mumbai. LDPE films (200 gauges) were procured from M/s Hitkari Industries Ltd., New Delhi - 14.

Table-1: Composition of spice mix for RBMLs.

Ingredients	Percentage (w/w)
Coriander powder (*Dhania*)	17
Cumin seed (*Jeera*)	10
Aniseed (*Soanf*)	10
Black pepper (*Kalimirch*)	10
Caraway seed (*Ajowan*)	10
Turmeric (*Haldi*)	10
Dried ginger (*Saundh*)	10
Capsicum (*Mirch powder*)	8
Cardamom (*Badi elaichi*)	5
Cinnamon (*Dal chini*)	5
Cloves (*Laung*)	3
Nutmeg (*Jaibhal*)	1
Lace (*Jaipatri*)	1
Total	100

RBMLs=Restructured buffalo meat loaves

Experimental design

Frozen meat was thawed (approximately 12 h at 4±1°C, reaching between −3 and −5°C). The partially thawed meat was carefully trimmed off adhering visible loose connective tissue and fascia was sliced across the grain into 1 cm thick slices. The sliced buffalo meat was then cut along and across to chunks of nearly 1 cm³. Temperature of the meat chunks was maintained below 2°C by keeping it immediately in a refrigerator at 0°C after chunking, so as to ensure temperature of meat chunks below 10°C throughout the processing. Meat chunks (77% of formulation) in semi-frozen state were placed in paddle mixture (HOBART, Model: N50G) and massaging was done initially at low speed with simultaneous addition of curing solution (15%) (Table-2) which facilitated the extraction of muscle proteins from meat and formed tacky exudates to bind meat pieces. After the initial 8 min of mixing at low speed, the refined wheat flour (3%), spices (2%), condiments (3%), and calcium lactate powder were added in order and concurrently mixed/blended for additional 4 min at medium speed for uniform mixing (Figure-1).

Four batters were prepared by replacing the lean buffalo meat with calcium lactate powder at 0, 1%, 1.25%, and 1.5% level. Once each mixing time was achieved, the meat batter was unloaded from the mixer, weighed and stuffed into stainless steel molds. Molds were squeezed with the wooden press to remove air pockets, closed tightly and placed in a pressure cooker filled with 1/3 boiling hot water and then cooked by steam without pressure. Slow heating rate was ensured by adjusting the flame regulating knob (Code: 637470, Regalia, Sun flame) to low so that the required internal temperature of 85°C of the product was achieved. The cooked meat block is cooled to room temperature, sliced into fillets, packaged into LDPE bags and analyzed for different parameters including sensory evaluation. The formulation of pre-standardized control RBMLs is shown in Table-3.

Table-2: Formulation of curing solution for RBMLs.

Ingredients	Quantity (g)
Sodium chloride (2%)	13.34
Cane sugar (0.76%)	5.07
STPP (0.32%)	2.13
Sodium nitrite (90 ppm)	0.06

Make the volume of each treatment to 100 ml with water. STTP=Sodium tripolyphosphate, RBMLs=Restructured buffalo meat loaves

Table-3: Formulation of pre-standardized control RBMLs.

Ingredients	Amount required for 100 g
Lean meat (g)	77.0
Curing solution (ml)	15.0
Refined wheat flour (g)	3
Spices (g)	2.0
Condiments (g)	3.0
Total	100

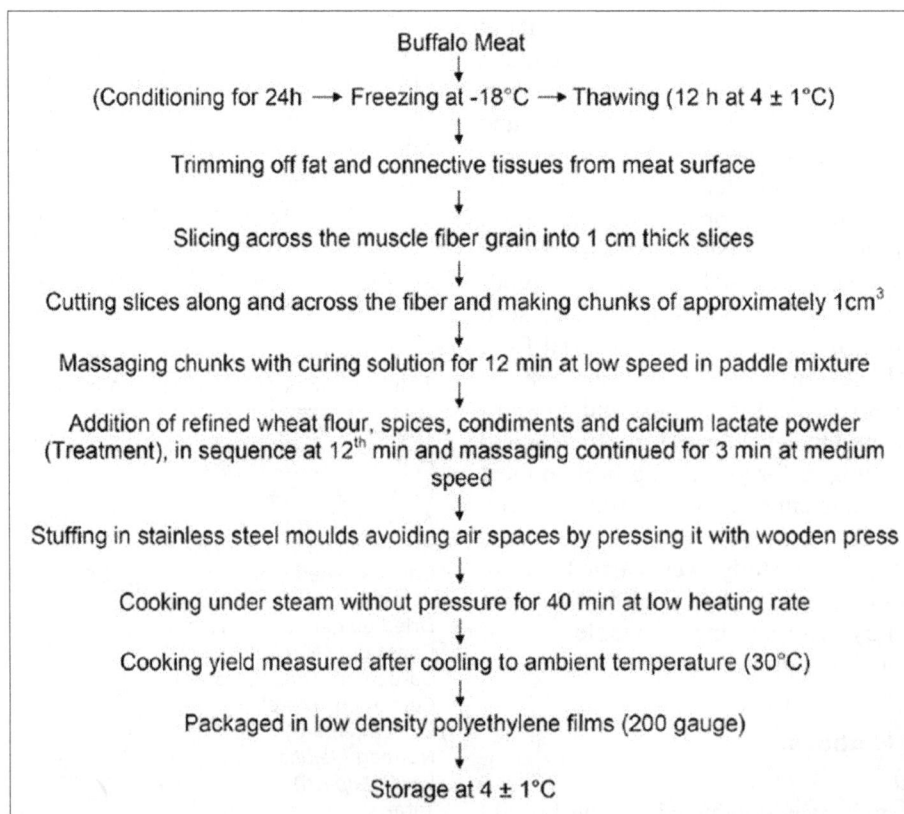

Buffalo Meat
↓
(Conditioning for 24h → Freezing at -18°C → Thawing (12 h at 4 ± 1°C)
↓
Trimming off fat and connective tissues from meat surface
↓
Slicing across the muscle fiber grain into 1 cm thick slices
↓
Cutting slices along and across the fiber and making chunks of approximately 1cm³
↓
Massaging chunks with curing solution for 12 min at low speed in paddle mixture
↓
Addition of refined wheat flour, spices, condiments and calcium lactate powder (Treatment), in sequence at 12th min and massaging continued for 3 min at medium speed
↓
Stuffing in stainless steel moulds avoiding air spaces by pressing it with wooden press
↓
Cooking under steam without pressure for 40 min at low heating rate
↓
Cooking yield measured after cooling to ambient temperature (30°C)
↓
Packaged in low density polyethylene films (200 gauge)
↓
Storage at 4 ± 1°C

Figure-1: Flow chart of processing protocol for the development of restructured buffalo meat loaves.

Analytical procedures

The pH of the cooked RBML was determined as per Trout et al. [28] method. 10 g of sample was homogenized with the help of ultra turrax tissue homogenizer (T-25 Germany) for about a minute in 50 ml of distilled water. The pH was recorded by immersing the electrode of a pH meter (model CP 901, Century Instrument Ltd., India) directly into the meat suspension. Cooking yield was determined by dividing cooked product weight by the raw uncooked weight and multiplying it by 100 to express as percent. The moisture, protein, fat, and ash content of the product were determined by standard methods using hot air oven, Kjeldahl assembly, Soxhlet extraction apparatus, and Muffle furnace, respectively, as per AOAC [29].

The calorific value of the sample was calculated using Gallenkamp and ballistic bomb calorimeter [30]. Approximately 1-2 pieces of meat sample were taken and weighed along with pre-weighed steel crucible. This crucible was placed on the support pillar in the base of the bomb. The firing wire and the sample were connected with the help of cotton thread. The bomb was fired under an oxygen pressure of 25 atm. The initial and final temperature readings on the galvanometer were noted. The deflection on the galvanometer was compared with 1 g standard benzoic acid of known calorific value (6.318 Kcal/g). The calorific value of the sample was calculated and expressed as Kcal/g.

Shear force value was determined as per the method described by Berry and Stiffler [31]. It is measured as the force required for shearing 1 cm^2 block on Warner-Bratzler Shear Press (81031307 GR Elec. MFG. Co., USA) and expressed in kg/cm^2. The calcium in the fortified RBMLs was estimated as per Talpatra et al. [32]. Water activity of functional RBMLs was measured by Aqua LAB dew point water activity meter 4TE (Decagon Devices Inc., United States). The samples were run in triplicate and the water activity meter was calibrated at regular intervals.

Lovibond® tintometer color units

The color of RBMLs was measured using a Lovibond® tintometer (Model F, Greenwich, UK). Samples were cut with the help of scissors to the inner diameter of the sample holder and secured against the viewing aperture. The sample color was matched by adjusting the red (a*) and yellow (b*) values while keeping the blue unit fixed at 0.1. The corresponding color units were recorded. The hue angle and chroma values were determined using the formulae, $\tan^{-1}(b/a)$ [33] and $(a^2+b^2)^{1/2}$ [34], respectively, where a = red unit, b = yellow unit.

Texture profile analysis (TPA)

The texture profile of RBMLs was measured with the help of instrumental TPA (TA.HDplus Texture Analyzer, Stable Micro Systems Ltd., UK).

The procedure used for instrumental TPA was similar to those described by Bourne [35]. Chilled samples were tempered to bring to room temperature and then cut into 1 cm^2. The samples were placed on a platform in a fixture and compressed twice to 85% of their original height by a compression probe (P75) at a crosshead speed of 10 mm/s through a two cycle sequence, using a 50 kg load cell. The calculation of TPA values was obtained by graphing a curve using force and time.

Sensory evaluation

Seven semi-trained experienced taste panel consisting of scientists and post-graduate students of the Division of LPT, IVRI, Izatnagar, India were involved in conducting the sensory evaluation of the product. Panelists were trained following the procedure of Means and Schmidt [36]. The sensory panel was organized around 3.30-4.00 PM every time. Loaves were cooked as described and served to panelists immediately after cooking. In every session, the products were evaluated for general appearance, saltiness, flavor, texture, binding, juiciness and overall acceptability using 8-point descriptive scale [37], where 8 is extremely desirable, and 1 is extremely undesirable. Each panelist was supplied with a plate, a knife, a fork, a glass of cold tap water, and a disposal cup. Panelists received = 30 g of products from each treatment. They were asked to rinse their mouths with cold tap water before evaluating each sample.

Statistical analysis

Three trials were conducted for each experiment in duplicate. The data generated from various trials under each experiment were pooled and analyzed by statistical method of one-way - analysis of variance and mean ± standard error using SPSS Statistics (version 20.0) software package developed as per the procedure of Snedecor and Cochran [38] and means were compared by using Dunkan's multiple range test [39].

Results and Discussion

Physico-chemical properties

The pH of the RBML with different levels of calcium lactate was found to be significantly lower (p<0.01) than that of control. There was a significant decline (p<0.01) in pH of the FRBML with each subsequent increase in the level of calcium lactate (Table-4). It may be attributed to acidic nature of the calcium lactate. The pH-reducing effect of calcium lactate in meat products was also documented by Alahakoon et al. [40], Devatkal and Mendiratta [19], and Caceres et al. [2].

Cooking yield of RBML fortified with calcium lactate was significantly low (p<0.01) at 1.5% treatment level as compared to the control. However, the values at 1% and 1.25% level of calcium lactate in treatment product remained comparable among themselves and control, with a gradual decline (Table-4). Similar kind of decrease in pH and cooking yield

Table-4: Effect of calcium lactate incorporation on the physico-chemical properties of calcium fortified RBMLs.

Parameters	Control	Level of calcium lactate incorporation		
		1%	1.25%	1.5%
Cooking yield (%)	93.07±0.30[a]	92.53±0.29[a]	91.96±0.33[a]	87.47±0.54[b]
Product pH	6.22±0.01[a]	6.10±0.01[b]	6.07±0.01[c]	5.90±0.02[d]
Moisture (%)	68.75±0.08[a]	68.23±0.11[b]	67.79±0.15[c]	65.99±0.46[d]
Protein (%)	19.57±0.10[a]	18.26±0.05[c]	18.08±0.09[c]	18.54±0.08[b]
Moisture protein ratio	3.19±0.02[c]	3.51±0.02[b]	3.73±0.01[a]	3.75±0.01[a]
Fat (%)	3.09±0.04[a]	2.77±0.03[bc]	2.74±0.03[c]	2.84±0.02[b]
Ash (%)	2.93±0.05[d]	3.11±0.03[c]	3.27±0.03[b]	3.42±0.02[a]
Calorific value (Kcal/100 g)	132.61±0.80[a]	130.97±0.52[b]	129.46±0.75[b]	127.99±0.82[b]
Shear force value (Kg/cm^2)	0.75±0.05[a]	0.66±0.05[ab]	0.68±0.05[ab]	0.57±0.05[b]
Calcium concentration (mg/100 g)	6.48±0.32[d]	135.02±2.35[c]	165.73±4.29[b]	203.85±2.95[a]

Mean±SE with different superscripts in a row differ significantly ($p<0.05$), n_1 (cooking yield and product pH)=3, n_2 (proximate analysis)=6, n_3 (shear force value)=30 for each treatment. SE=Standard error, RBMLs=Restructured buffalo meat loaves

was also reported by Sofos [41] in the meat product. In general, a decrease in moisture content was observed with the increase in the level of calcium lactate. The moisture percentage of control product was significantly higher ($p<0.01$) than treatment groups. Decrease in moisture percentage could be due to the property of calcium to compete with phosphates for protein binding sites and thus limiting protein-phosphate water interaction resulting in more water loss and less moisture in product [20]. However, Devatkal and Mendiratta [19] reported a significant improvement ($p<0.05$) in moisture content of restructured pork rolls due to the incorporation of different levels (0.4%, 0.7%, and 1.0%) of sodium alginate with 0.3% calcium lactate.

There was a significant increase ($p<0.05$) in the crude protein percentage with increase in the level of calcium lactate from 1% to 1.5% level. This might be due to decrease in the cooking yield of the product with increase of calcium lactate level. Some decrease ($p<0.05$) in protein percentage in the fortified products as compared to control may also be attributed to replacement of lean in the formulation (Table-4). Similar findings have been reported by Naveena et al. [42] in microwave cooked chicken patties incorporated with calcium lactate and in cooked meat sausage enriched with calcium lactate by Caceras et al. [2]. The significantly higher ($p<0.05$) moisture protein ratio for RBML prepared with calcium lactate as compared to control is self-explanatory, the value being dependent on the moisture and protein percentages of the product. The fat percentage of the RBML fortified with calcium lactate was significantly lower ($p<0.01$) than control. This could also be due to the replacement of lean meat and presence of calcium lactate in the formulation. Caceras et al. [2] also reported a decrease in fat content in meat sausage with an increase in the level of calcium lactate. The values of ash content in treatment products increased significantly ($p<0.01$) with increasing level of calcium lactate. This increase could probably be due to direct addition of calcium salt. Increase

in ash content in microwave cooked chicken patties and cooked sausages incorporated with calcium lactate were reported by Naveena et al. [42] and Caceras et al. [2], respectively.

The shear force values of the RBML fortified with calcium lactate were comparable ($p>0.05$) to the control up to 1.25% level. There was a significant decrease ($p<0.05$) in shear force value at 1.5% level in RBML as compared to control and other treatments (Table-4). Fortification with calcium lactate might interfere with protein-protein interactions or protein solubility, which could reduce shear force value. Similar findings have also been reported by Daengprok et al. [15] in Nhams (Thai-style fermented pork sausage). The calcium content in the fortified RBML was found to be significantly higher ($p<0.01$) than control. There was a significant increase ($p<0.01$) in the calcium concentration of treatment product with increase in calcium lactate level. Similar increase in the concentration of calcium had been reported by Daengpork et al. [15] and Caceres et al. [2] in Nhams and meat sausage fortified with calcium lactate, respectively. Water activity of the fortified RBML was found to be significantly lower ($p<0.05$) than control product, although both fortified and control product had high water activity due to high moisture content.

Lovibond® tintometer color units

The value of a* which denotes Lovibond® tintometer color score for redness in fortified RBML was significantly higher ($p<0.01$) than the control product. The increase in redness value in calcium lactate fortified products might be due to a reduction in myoglobin denaturation. Devatkal and Mendiratta [19] found that addition of calcium lactate along with phosphate decreased the metmyoglobin accumulation in restructured pork rolls (Table-5).

The value of Lovibond® tinometer color unit for yellowness denoted by b* was found to be significantly higher ($p<0.01$) in the RBML fortified with calcium as compared to control product. Although, the calcium lactate did not play a very important role in color development but a minor role of calcium lactate in enhancing the color stability of muscle could appear to be through the influx of lactate into the system. A similar result has also been reported by Devatkal and Mendiratta [19] in restructured pork rolls incorporated with calcium lactate. They found that enhancement with calcium resulted in less metmyoglobin discoloration and higher a* and b* values. Naveena et al. [42] also reported an increase in both a* and b* value in cooked chicken patties containing lactate as compared to control. Daengprok et al. [15] reported a non-significant increase ($p > 0.05$) in yellowness (b*) value with an increase in the level of commercial grade calcium lactate in calcium fortified Nhams.

Hue angle and chroma values were derived values and thus obtained according to their corresponding redness and yellowness values. The hue angle of the fortified RBML was found to be significantly higher than control product. Contrary findings were reported by Caceres et al. [2] with an increase in the hue value in control as compared to calcium lactate-treated cooked meat sausages. Naveena et al. [42] also reported a lower value for hue in the cooked chicken patties containing calcium lactate than control.

Chroma, which indicates the intensity of the color, was found to be significantly higher ($p < 0.01$) in the calcium fortified RBML than the control product. The increase in intensity could be due to the color stabilization by calcium lactate in the fortified product. Similar results were also observed by Naveena et al. [42] in cooked chicken patties containing calcium lactate.

TPA

The hardness value for calcium fortified RBML was found to be significantly higher ($p < 0.01$) as compared to control. The increase in hardness value with increased calcium lactate level could be due to forming bonds between meat proteins, in the presence of calcium, mainly myosin and favoring the formation of a stronger network that led to higher firmness [4]. An increase in hardness value with the incorporation of calcium lactate in both conventional and reduced fat cooked meat sausages was also reported by Caceres et al. [2]. Further, the hardness value could be higher ($p < 0.01$) in the fortified RBML than control because of the lower moisture content in the fortified product. Several workers had reported a decrease in product hardness with an increase in moisture content [43-45].

There was a significant increase ($p < 0.01$) in adhesiveness from control to fortified RBML with an increase in the level of calcium lactate, which might be attributed to better gelling by the salts of calcium present in the fortified product. Similar results were also reported by Caceres et al. [2] in reduced fat cooked meat sausages but in the case of conventional fat cooked meat sausages, they reported a decrease in the value of adhesiveness. Springiness, cohesiveness, and gumminess values did not show significant differences ($p > 0.05$) between control and the fortified RBML. Verma et al. [46] also observed no significant ($p > 0.05$) effect on cohesiveness in low-fat chicken nuggets due to the variation of contents. However, Ambadkar [47] and Caceres et al. [2] also reported an increase in values of both chewiness and gumminess in meat sausage and cooked buffalo meat salami respectively due to the incorporation of calcium lactate. Devatkal and Mendiratta [19] also reported an improvement in the texture profile of restructured pork rolls due to the addition of calcium lactate. Mehta [45] also found a similar result in fortified restructured chicken patties (Table-6).

Table-5: Lovibond® tintometer color units and water activity of RBMLs.

Parameters	Control	Level of calcium lactate incorporation		
		1%	1.25%	1.5%
Redness (a*) value	8.28±0.05[d]	9.57±0.13[c]	10.97±0.24[b]	11.68±0.09[a]
Yellowness (b*) value	6.28±0.05[c]	7.42±0.11[b]	8.98±0.04[a]	9.20±0.11[a]
Hue angle	37.18±0.35[b]	37.79±0.64[ab]	39.36±0.70[a]	38.21±0.19[ab]
Chroma	10.40±0.30[d]	12.11±0.10[c]	14.18±0.16[b]	14.87±0.14[a]
Water activity (a_w)	0.986±0.00[a]	0.976±0.00[b]	0.974±0.00[c]	0.971±0.00[d]

Mean±SE with different superscripts in a row differ significantly ($p < 0.05$), n=6 for each treatment. SE=Standard error, RBMLs=Restructured buffalo meat loaves

Table-6: Instrumental TPA of RBMLs.

Parameters	Control	Level of calcium lactate incorporation		
		1%	1.25%	1.5%
Hardness (N/cm^2)	46.62±1.07[c]	51.28±0.53[b]	55.04±1.30[a]	56.06±1.51[a]
Adhesiveness (Ns)	−0.17±0.00[c]	−0.16±0.00[bc]	−0.15±0.01[b]	−0.13±0.01[a]
Springiness (cm)	0.45±0.01	0.44±0.01	0.44±0.02	0.44±0.04
Cohesiveness (ratio)	0.31±0.01	0.26±0.05	0.31±0.01	0.281±0.01
Gumminess (N/cm^2)	14.47±0.41	13.09±2.24	16.88±0.55	15.57±0.85
Chewiness (N/cm)	6.41±0.14	5.75±1.05	7.37±0.53	6.57±0.77

Mean±SE with different superscripts in a row differ significantly ($p < 0.05$), n=6 for each treatment. SE=Standard error, RBMLs=Restructured buffalo meat loaves, TPA=Texture profile analysis

Table-7: Effect of calcium lactate incorporation on the sensory attributes of RBMLs.

Sensory attributes	Control	Level of calcium lactate incorporation		
		1%	1.25%	1.5%
General appearance	7.14±0.05[a]	7.05±0.04[a]	7.03±0.03[a]	6.85±0.05[b]
Flavor	7.10±0.06[a]	6.97±0.07[ab]	6.90±0.05[b]	6.71±0.05[c]
Juiciness	7.16±0.05[a]	7.03±0.06[a]	7.03±0.05[a]	6.67±0.07[b]
Texture	7.18±0.05[a]	7.03±0.05[a]	7.03±0.05[a]	6.76±0.07[b]
Binding	7.19±0.06[a]	7.06±0.05[ab]	7.10±0.03[b]	6.78±0.06[c]
Saltiness	7.12±0.05	7.00±0.05	7.02±0.04	6.98±0.06
Overall acceptability	7.16±0.06[a]	7.02±0.05[a]	7.01±0.05[a]	6.72±0.07[b]

Mean±SE with different superscripts in a row differ significantly (p<0.05), n=21 for each treatment. SE=Standard error, RBMLs=Restructured buffalo meat loaves

Sensory evaluation

Sensory scores for the general appearance of the RBML incorporated with 1.0% and 1.25% calcium lactate were compared to the control, in spite of marginally lower (p>0.05) scores. There was a significant reduction (p<0.05) in general appearance score of RBML fortified with 1.5% calcium lactate. Mehta [45] also reported the similar trend, in general, appearance scores of low-fat chicken meat patties. The flavor scores for the RBML gradually decreased with increased level of incorporation and were significantly low (p<0.05) at 1.25% and 1.5% (incorporation levels) as compared to control. The flavor scores of RBML were comparable (p>0.05) at 1% and 1.25% incorporation levels. The gradual decrease in flavor scores of RBML with an increase of calcium lactate incorporation could be due to poor solubility of calcium lactate, imparting its own flavor. Brewer *et al.* [48] reported an intense flavor in fresh pork sausage containing 2.0% and 3.0% lactate than in sausage containing 0% or 1.0% of the lactate. Got *et al.* [49] also reported that 0.3 M level of calcium lactate brought about flavor and taste defects. Contrary to this, Daengprok *et al.* [15] found that fortifying Nhams (Thai-style fermented pork sausage) with either commercial or egg shell calcium lactate did not change the perception of flavor compared to control (Table-7).

There was a gradual decrease (p>0.05) in juiciness score with increased level of calcium lactate but the scores remained comparable to control up to 1.25% incorporation. RBML prepared with 1.5% calcium lactate level had significantly lower (p<0.05) juiciness score as compared to control. This might be attributed to decrease in the moisture content in the RBML. This finding was in accordance with Ambadkar [47] who also reported a decrease in juiciness perception with an increase in the level of calcium lactate. However, Caceras *et al.* [2] reported an increase in juiciness perception for the meat sausage enriched with calcium using calcium lactate as a source of calcium. A decrease in juiciness score with increased the level of supplementation of calcium was also reported by Boyle *et al.* [14] and Mehta [45].

The texture scores for the RBML followed almost the same trend as that of flavor. The texture score of the product incorporated with 1.5% calcium

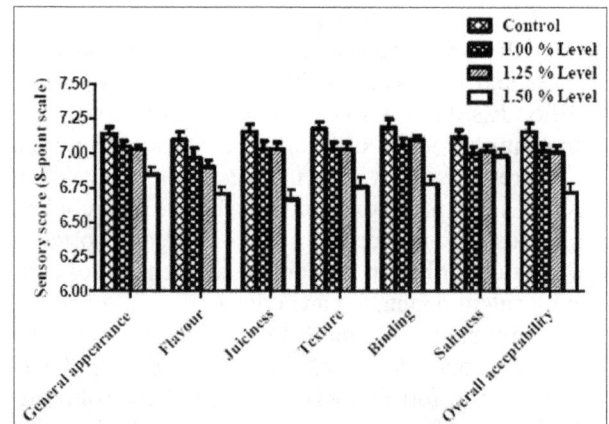

Figure-2: Effect of calcium lactate incorporation on the sensory attributes of restructured buffalo meat loaves.

lactate was significantly lower (p<0.05) than others, whereas up to 1.25% incorporation, the scores were comparable to control as well as 1.0% incorporation. A significant decrease (p<0.05) in texture score of low-fat meat sausage enriched with calcium was also reported by Caceras *et al.* [2]. Daengprok *et al.* [15] also reported that calcium fortified Nhams were less firm than control. Binding scores also showed a significant reduction (p<0.05) with increased incorporation level of calcium lactate. The sensory score for the saltiness of control was slightly higher (p>0.05) as compared to the fortified RBML. This was due to the taste of calcium lactate in the treatment products. The scores for the treatment products were marginally (p>0.05) different among themselves. The slightly sour taste of calcium lactate was masked by the addition of sucrose in the curing solution.

Overall acceptability scores of RBML declined gradually with increase in the incorporation level of calcium lactate. RBML with 1.5% calcium lactate had significantly lower (p<0.05) overall acceptability score as compared to control and fortified RBML with 1.25% calcium lactate incorporation, which remained comparable. The overall acceptability pattern reflected the related sensory rating for flavor, texture, juiciness, and saltiness of the products. Caceres *et al.* [2] also reported a lower overall acceptability score in cooked meat sausages enriched with calcium using calcium lactate as a source. Further, Mehta [45] also reported that the overall acceptability scores of fortified chicken patties gradually decreased with increase in incorporation level of calcium lactate (Figure-2).

Conclusion

Present study concluded that fortification of calcium in RBML is vital since buffalo meat is deficient in calcium. The addition of calcium lactate up to 1.25% (i.e., 15% recommended daily allowance), in RBML, improve the product color and textural properties besides maintaining sensory and physico-chemical attributes of the product.

Authors' Contributions

IA and BDS planned the study. IA carried out the study with assistance from BDS and SRA. ST and OPM revised the draft manuscript prepared by IA and AK. All authors read and approved the final manuscript.

Acknowledgments

The authors would like to acknowledge to Indian Council of Agricultural Research for providing financial assistance in the form of Junior Research fellowship to carry out the post-graduate research. The authors thank the Director, IVRI, Izatnagar - 243 122, Uttar Pradesh (India) for providing the necessary facilities for the current study.

Competing Interests

The authors declare that they have no competing interests.

References

1. Vavrusova, M. and Skibsted, L.H. (2014) Calcium nutrition, bioavailability and fortification. *Food Sci. Technol.*, 59(2): 1198-1204.
2. Caceres, E., Garcya, M.L. and Selgas, M.D. (2006) Design of a new cooked meat sausage enriched with calcium. *Meat Sci.*, 73: 368-377.
3. Adluri, R.S., Zhan, L., Bagchi, M., Maulik, N. and Maulik, G. (2010) Comparative effects of a novel plant-based calcium supplement with two common calcium salts on proliferation and mineralization in human osteoblast cells. *Mol. Cell. Biochem.*, 340(1-2): 73-80.
4. Jimenez-Colmenero, F., Herrero, A., Cofrades, S. and Capillas, C.R. (2012) Meat and functional foods. In: Hui, Y.H., editor. Handbook of Meat and Meat Processing. 2nd ed. CRC Press, Taylor & Francis Group, Boca Raton, London, New York. p225-242.
5. Jimenez-Colmenero, F., Sanchez-Muniz, F. and Olmedilla-Alonso, B. (2010) Design and development of meat-based functional foods with walnut: Technological, nutritional and health impact. *Food Chem.*, 123: 959-967.
6. Institute of Medicine (IOM). (2010) Dietary Reference Intakes: Recommended Intakes for Individuals. OIM, New York.
7. Soto, A.M., Morales, P., Haza, A.I., Garcia, M.L. and Selga, M.D. (2014) Bioavailability of calcium from enriched meat products using Caco-2 cells. *Food Res. Int.*, 55: 263-270.
8. Moseley, K. and de Beur, S. (2011) Principles of Gender-Specific Medicine. Elsevier Academic Press, London, UK. p716-736.
9. Neilson, A. and Ferruzi, M. (2013) Nutrition in the Prevention and Treatment of Disease. 3rd ed. Academic Press, London, UK.
10. Mesias, M., Seiquer, I. and Navarro, M.P. (2011) Calcium nutrition in adolescence. *Crit. Rev. Food Sci. Nutr.*, 51: 195-209.
11. Aggarwal, P., Ahlawat, S.S. and Sharma, D.P. (2009) Development of calcium enriched chicken meat rolls. *Indian J. Poultr. Sci.*, 44(2): 233-237.
12. Brant, L.A. (2003) Formulation challenge: Calcium the essential mineral, Issue December. Available from: http://www.preparedfoods.com/articles/103615-formulation-challenge-calcium-the-essential-mineral. Accessed on 03-06-2015.
13. Kilgore, L.T., Watson, K., Wren, N., Rogers, R.W. and Windham, F. (1977) Fortification of hamburger with calcium, vitamin A and ascorbic acid. *J. Am. Diet. Assoc.*, 71(2): 135-139.
14. Boyle, E.A.E., Addis, P.B. and Epley, R.J. (1994) Calcium fortified, reduced fat beef emulsion product. *J. Food Sci.*, 59(5): 928-932.
15. Daengprok, W., Garnjanagoonchorn, W. and Mine, Y. (2002) Fermented pork sausage fortified with commercial or hen egg shell calcium lactate. *Meat Sci.*, 62: 199-204.
16. Vavrusova, M. and Skibsted, L.H. (2014) Spontaneous super saturation of calcium D gluconate during isothermal dissolution of calcium L-lactate in aqueous sodium D-gluconate. *Food Funct.*, 5: 85-91.
17. Vavrusova, M., Raitio, R., Orlien, V. and Skibsted, L.H. (2013) Calcium hydroxy palmitate: Possible precursor phase in calcium precipitation by palmitate. *Food Chem.*, 138: 2415-2420.
18. Cilla, A., Lagarda, M.J., Alegría, A., Ancos, B., Cano, M.P., Sanchez-Moreno, C., Plaza, L. and Barberá, R. (2011) Effect of processing and food matrix on calcium and phosphorous bioavailability from milk-base fruit beverages in Caco-2 cells. *Food Res. Int.*, 44: 3030-3038.
19. Devatkal, S. and Mendiratta, S.K. (2001) Use of calcium lactate with salt-phosphate and alginate-calcium gels in restructured pork rolls. *Meat Sci.*, 58: 371-379.
20. Lawrence, T.E., Dikeman, M.E., Hunt, M.C., Kastner, C.L. and Johnson, D.E. (2004) Effects of enhancing beef longissimus with phosphate plus salt, or calcium lactate plus non-phosphate water binders plus rosemary extract. *Meat Sci.*, 67: 129-137.
21. FAO. (2012) Food and Agriculture Organization of the United Nations. FAOSTAT, Rome.
22. Suresh, A., Kavita, B. and Chaudhary, K.R. (2012) India's meat export: Structure, composition and future prospects. *J. Anim. Sci.*, 82(7): 749-756.
23. APEDA. (2014) Export of agro and processed food products including meat and meat products. Agricultural and Processed Food Products Export Development Authority. Ministry of Commerce, Government of India.
24. Kandeepan, G., Anjaneyulu, A.S.R., Kondaiah, N., Mendiratta, S.K. and Lakshmanan, V. (2009) Effect of age and gender on the processing characteristics of buffalo meat. *Meat Sci.*, 83: 10-14.
25. Naveena, B.M., Sen, A.R., Muthukumar, M., Babji, Y. and Kondaiah, N. (2011) Effects of salt and ammonium hydroxide on the quality of ground buffalo meat. *Meat Sci.*, 87: 315-320.
26. Aberle, E.D., Forrest, J.C., David, E.G. and Edward, W.M. (2012) Principles of Meat Science. 5rd ed. Kendall Hunt Publishing Company, Dubuque, Iowa, USA.
27. Gadekar, Y.P., Sharma, B.D., Shinde, A.K., Verma, A.K. and Mendiratta, S.K. (2014) Effect of natural antioxidants on the quality of cured, restructured goat meat product during refrigerated storage (4 ± 1°C). *Small Rumin. Res.*, 119(1-3): 72-80.
28. Trout, E.S., Hunt, M.C., Johnson, D.E., Claus, J.R., Kastner, C.L. and Kropt, D.H. (1992) Characteristics of low fat ground beef containing texture modifying ingredients. *J. Food Sci.*, 57(1): 19-24.

29. AOAC. (2012) Official Methods of Analysis of AOAC International. 19th ed. Association of Official Analytical Chemists, Washington, DC.

30. Haque, N. and Lai, M. (1999) Gross energy estimation In: Shastry, V.R.B., Kamra, D.N. and Pathak, N.N. editors. Laboratory Manual of Animal Nutrition. Indian Veterinary Research Institute, Izatnagar. p71.

31. Berry, B.W. and Stiffler, D.M. (1981) Effect of electric stimulator boiling temperature formulation and rate of freezing on sensory cooking chemical and physical properties of ground beef patties. *J. Food Sci.,* 46: 1103-1106.

32. Talpatra, S.K., Ray, S.C. and Sen, K.C. (1940) Estimation of phosphorus, choline, calcium, magnesium, sodium, potassium in feeding stuffs. *J. Vet. Sci. Anim. Husb.,* 10: 243-245.

33. Little, A.C. (1975) Off on a tangent. *J. Food Sci.,* 40: 410-412.

34. Froehlich, D.A., Gullet, E.A. and Usborne, W.R. (1983) Effect of nitrite and salt on the colour, flavour and overall acceptability of ham. *J. Food Sci.,* 48: 152-154.

35. Bourne, M.C. (1978) Texture profile analysis. *Food Technol.,* 32(7): 62-72.

36. Means, W.J. and Schmidt, G.R. (1986). Algin/calcium gel as a raw and cooked binder in restructured beef steaks. *J. Food Sci.,* 51: 60-65.

37. Keeton, J.T. (1983) Effect of fat and NaCl/phosphate levels on the chemical and sensory properties of pork patties. *J. Food Sci.,* 48: 878-881.

38. Snedecor, G.W. and Cochran, W.G. (1994) Statistical Methods. 1st ed. East West Press Pvt., Ltd., New Delhi.

39. Dunkan, D.B. (1995) Multiple range and multiple F-tests. *Biometrics,* 11: 1-42.

40. Alahakoon, A.U., Bae, Y.S., Kim, H.J., Jung, S., Jayasena, D.D., Yong, H.I., Kim, S.H. and Jo, C. (2013) The effect of citrus and onion peel extracts, calcium lactate, and phosvitin on microbial quality of seasoned chicken breast meat. *CNU J. Agric. Sci.,* 40(2): 131-137.

41. Sofos, J.N. (1983) Effects of reduced salt (NaCl) levels on sensory and instrumental evaluation of frankfurters. *J. Food Sci.,* 48: 1692-1695, 1699.

42. Naveena, B.M., Sen, A.R., Muthukumar, M., Vaithiyanathan, S. and Babji, Y. (2006) The effect of lactates on the quality of microwave-cooked chicken patties during storage. *J. Food Sci.,* 71: 603-608.

43. Talukder, S., Sharma, B.D., Mendiratta, S.K., Malav, O.P., Sharma, H. and Gokulakrishnan, P. (2013) Development and evaluation of extended restructured chicken meat block incorporated with Colocasia (*Colocasia esculenta*) flour. *J. Food Proc. Technol.,* 4: 207.

44. Sharma, H., Sharma, B.D., Mendiratta, S.K., Talukder, S. and Ramasamy, G. (2013) Efficacy of flaxseed flour as bind enhancing agent on the quality of extended restructured mutton chops. *Asian-Aust. J. Anim. Sci.,* 27(2): 247-255.

45. Mehta, N. (2008) Studies on fortification of low fat chicken meat patties with calcium, vitamin E and vitamin C. Thesis, M.V.Sc. Deemed University, Indian Veterinary Research Institute, Izatnagar, India.

46. Verma, A.K., Sharma, B.D. and Banerjee, R. (2010) Effect of sodium chloride replacement and apple pulp inclusion on the physico-chemical, textural and sensory properties of low fat chicken nuggets. *Food Sci. Technol.,* 43: 715-719.

47. Ambadkar, R.K. (2002) Studies on the effect of lactates on the quality of cooked salami from buffalo meat. Thesis, Ph.D. Deemed University, Indian Veterinary Research Institute, Izatnagar, India.

48. Brewer, M.S., Mckeith, F., Martin, S.E., Dallnier, A.W. and Meyer, J. (1991) Sodium lactate effects on shelf life, sensory and physical characteristics of fresh pork sausage. *J. Food Sci.,* 56(5): 1176-1178.

49. Got, F., Rouseel-Akrim, S., Bayle, M.C. and Culioli, J. (1995) Effects of calcium lactate on tenderness and flavour of beef. *Viandes-et-Produits-Cames,* 17(6): 328-330.

30

Impact of heat stress on health and performance of dairy animals

Ramendra Das[1], Lalrengpuii Sailo[2], Nishant Verma[1], Pranay Bharti[3], Jnyanashree Saikia[4], Imtiwati[5] and Rakesh Kumar[1]

1. Department of Animal Genetics & Breeding, Indian Council of Agricultural Research - National Dairy Research Institute, Karnal - 132 001, Haryana, India; 2. Division of Animal Genetics, Indian Council of Agricultural Research - Indian Veterinary Research Institute, Izatnagar - 243 122, Uttar Pradesh, India; 3. Department of Livestock Production & Management, Indian Council of Agricultural Research - National Dairy Research Institute, Karnal - 132 001, Haryana, India; 4. Department of Animal Genetics & Breeding, College of Veterinary Sciences & Animal Husbandry, Agartala - 799 008, Tripura, India; 5. Department of Livestock Production & Management, College of Veterinary Sciences & Animal Husbandry, Agartala - 799 008, Tripura, India.
Corresponding author: Ramendra Das, e-mail: ramenvets@gmail.com,
LS: lrp.sailo@gmail.com, NV: nish99verma@gmail.com, PB: dr12pranay@gmail.com, JS: gsaikia123@gmail.com,
IM: imtiba777@gmail.com, RK: rakesh05vet@gmail.com

Abstract

Sustainability in livestock production system is largely affected by climate change. An imbalance between metabolic heat production inside the animal body and its dissipation to the surroundings results to heat stress (HS) under high air temperature and humid climates. The foremost reaction of animals under thermal weather is increases in respiration rate, rectal temperature and heart rate. It directly affect feed intake thereby, reduces growth rate, milk yield, reproductive performance, and even death in extreme cases. Dairy breeds are typically more sensitive to HS than meat breeds, and higher producing animals are, furthermore, susceptible since they generates more metabolic heat. HS suppresses the immune and endocrine system thereby enhances susceptibility of an animal to various diseases. Hence, sustainable dairy farming remains a vast challenge in these changing climatic conditions globally.

Keywords: amelioration, health, heat stress, production, reproduction.

Introduction

Stress is a reflex reaction of animals in harsh environments and causes unfavorable consequences ranges from discomfort to death. Climate change is one of the major threats for survival of various species, ecosystems and the sustainability of livestock production systems across the world, especially in tropical and temperate countries. Intergovernmental Panel on Climate Change [1] reported that temperature of the earth has been increased by 0.2°C per decade and also predicted that the global average surface temperature would be increased to 1.4-5.8°C by 2100. It was also indicated that mainly developing countries tend to be more vulnerable to extreme climatic events as they largely depend on climate sensitive sectors like agriculture and forestry [1]. Recently, Silanikove and Koluman [2] also forecasted the severity of heat stress (HS) issue as an increasing problem in near future because of global warming progression.

The thermoneutral zone (TNZ) of dairy animals ranges from 16°C to 25°C, within which they maintained a physiological body temperature of 38.4-39.1°C [3].

However, air temperatures above 20-25°C in temperate climate and 25-37°C in a tropical climate like in India, it enhance heat gain beyond that lost from the body and induces HS [4,5]. As a results body surface temperature, respiration rate (RR), heart rate and rectal temperature (RT) increases which in turn affects feed intake, production and reproductive efficiency of animals. RT >39.0°C and RR >60/min indicated cows were undergoing HS sufficient to affect milk yield and fertility [6]. However, the animal being homeotherms can resist to HS up to some extents depending on species, breed and productivity [7,8]. Among dairy animals, goats were the most adapted species to imposed HS in terms of production, reproduction and also to disease resistance [2]. Studies stipulated that the native breeds survive and perform better as compared to exotic breeds and their crosses under tropical environmental conditions may be due to inability of the exotic genes to express/adapt under tropical conditions [8-10]. Further, the sensitivity of dairy cattle to HS increases with increase in milk production [5], which might be due increase in metabolic heat output with increase production levels in dairy animals. The present review is targeted to collate and synthesize information pertaining HS and its impacts on health, production and reproduction in dairy animals.

Effects of HS on Health of Dairy Animals

HS effects health of dairy animals by imposing direct or indirect affects in normal physiology, metabolism, hormonal, and immunity system.

Feed intake and rumen physiology

Increase in environmental temperature has a direct negative effect on appetite center of the hypothalamus to decreases feed intake [11]. Feed intake begins to decline at air temperatures of 25-26°C in lactating cows and reduces more rapidly above 30°C in temperate climatic condition and at 40°C it may decline by as much as 40% [12], 22-35% in dairy goats [13] or 8-10% in buffalo heifers [14]. Reducing feed intake is a way to decrease heat production in warm environments as the heat increment of feeding is an important source of heat production in ruminants [15]. As results, animals experience a stage of negative energy balance (NEB), consequently body weight and body condition score goes down [16].

Increase environmental temperature alters the basic physiological mechanisms of rumen which negatively affects the ruminants with increased risk of metabolic disorders and health problems [17,18]. Nonaka *et al.* [19] reported animal under HS has reduced acetate production whereas propionate and butyrate production increased as rumen function altered. As a response animal consumed less roughages, changes rumen microbial population and pH from 5.82 to 6.03 [20], decreasing rumen motility and rumination [17,18]. Subsequently, affects health by lowering saliva production, variation in digestion patterns and decrease dry matter intake (DMI) [17,18]. Moreover, HS also results into hypofunction of the thyroid gland and effects on metabolism patterns of the animal to reduce metabolic heat production [21].

Acid-base balance

Animal under HS has increased RR and sweating which results increased body fluid loss that lift up maintenance requirements to control dehydration and blood homeostasis. As RR increases, expiration of CO_2 via the lungs increases. This results to respiratory alkalosis, as blood carbonic acid concentration decreases [22]. Therefore, animal needs to compensate for higher blood pH by excreting bicarbonate in the urine to maintain the carbonic acid: bicarbonate ratio [23]. Compensation results in urinary bicarbonate loss in an attempt to balance the ratio of carbonic acid to bicarbonate in the blood [21]. Chronic hyperthermia also causes severe or prolonged inappetence which further aggravates the increased supply of total carbonic acid in the rumen and decrease ruminal pH thereby, resulting into subclinical and acute rumen acidosis [15].

Oxidative stress

Oxidative stress results to increase in reactive oxygen species (ROS) in different cells and tissues of HS animals that have negative impacts on normal physiology and body metabolism. However, body has antioxidants in the form of enzymatic (superoxide dismutase [SOD], glutathione (GSH) peroxidase and catalase), non-enzymatic (albumin, L-cysteine, homocysteine, melatonin and protein sulfhydryl groups), and non-enzymatic low molecular weight antioxidants (ascorbic acid, GSH, uric acid, α-tocopherol, β-carotene, pyruvate and retinol), which increases as a results of HS to provide protection against negative effects of ROS. Significantly ($p<0.05$) higher levels of stress indices catalase, SOD, GSH reductase, and malondialdehyde was observed in lactating and non-lactating buffaloes [24] and cattle [25] during summer compared to spring seasons. Significantly higher levels of stress indices were believed due to lactation stress since increased milk production predispose to HS-induced oxidative damages in the body [25].

Immune system

The immune system is the major body defense systems to protect and cope against environmental stressors. Primary indicators of immunity response include white blood cells (WBCs), red blood cells (RBCs), hemoglobin (Hb), packed cell volume (PCV), glucose and protein concentration in blood get altered on thermal stress. WBC (leukocytes) count increase by 21-26% [26] and RBC count decrease by 12-20% [27] in thermally stressed cattle that could be due to thyromolymphatic involution or destruction of erythrocytes. Sejian *et al.* [28] reported highly significant variation of Hb, PCV, plasma glucose, total protein and albumin for the different temperature exposure in malpura ewes. This higher PCV value was an adaptive mechanism to provide water necessary for evaporative cooling process [29]. However, in contrast to these findings reduction of Hb and PCV levels were observed as results of RBC lysis either by increased attack of free radicals on its membrane or inadequate nutrient availability for Hb synthesis as the animal consumes less feed or decreases voluntary intake upon HS [30]. The blood glucose significantly decreased in HS dairy cows in accordance to greater blood insulin activity [9,31]. Release of plasma cortisol increases in stressed animals which causes down-regulation or suppression of L-selectin expression on the neutrophils surface [32]. Further, this poor L-selectin expression responsible for weak neutrophils function by failing to move into the tissue being invaded by pathogens and resulted clinical outcome of disease following exposure to an infective organism [33]. Increase circulating cortisol also causes increase cellular levels heat shock proteins (HSPs) that function as a danger signal to the immune system to encourage increased killing of pathogenic bacteria by neutrophils and macrophages against invading bacteria [34]. Hence, regular assessment of blood constituents is useful in appraisal of the health status of animals in hot-humid regions.

Health problem like subclinical or clinical ketosis [16] and higher risk of liver lipidosis and impairs liver function [35] were encountered. Sanders *et al.* [36] observed that lameness incidence increases with an increase in air temperature that could be due to increase in standing time [37]. Further, lameness causes thin soles, white line disease, ulcers, and sole punctures [36] and increases the likelihood for early culling from the herd. Climate change may bring about substantial shifts in disease distribution and outbreaks of disease prevalence in previously unexposed animal populations possibly with the breakdown of endemic stability [38]. Changes in rainfall and temperature regimes may affect both the distribution and the abundance of disease-causing vectors was also reported by Thornton et al. [38]. In accordance, Dhakal et al. [39] also observed incidence of external parasite as the first ranked (43.3%) problems in the warm temperate. The increase in THI resulted in increased incidence of mastitis in cows ($p < 0.01$) while Murrah buffaloes were less affected [40]. Further incidence was more in Sahiwal and Tharparkar cows ($p < 0.01$) than the crossbred Karan Swiss and Karan Fries cows [40]. Higher incidence of mastitis in dairy cows could be due to high temperatures facilitating survival and multiplication of pathogens carrier fly population associated with hot-humid conditions. Excess heat load in extreme cases not only compromises animal welfare but also results into death of the animals [2,41].

Effect of HS on Production and Reproduction Performance of Dairy Animals

Milk production and composition

HS adversely affects milk production and its composition in dairy animals, especially animals of high genetic merit [42-46]. Berman [7] estimated that effective environmental heat loads above 35°C activate the stress response systems in lactating dairy cows. In response dairy cows reduce feed intake which is directly associated with NEB, which largely responsible for the decline in milk synthesis [46]. Moreover, maintenance requirements of energy also increased by 30% in HS dairy animal [47]. Therefore, energy intake would not be enough to cover the daily requirements for milk production. West [43] reported a reduction in DMI by 0.85 kg with every 1°C rise in air temperature above a cow's TNZ, this decrease in intake accounts approximately 36% of the decrease in milk production [31]. According to Bouraoui et al. [42] daily THI negatively correlated to milk yield, as increase of THI value from 68 to 78 decreases DMI by 9.6% and milk production by 21%. Spiers et al. [44] reported that milk yield decreases by 0.41 kg/cow/day for each THI unit increase of above 69, feed intake decreased within a day after initiation of HS, while milk yield decreased after 2 days of HS. Gaafar et al. [48] reported that with increases in THI from 59.82 in the winter season to 78.53 in the summer season, HS reduced total (305 days) and daily milk yield by 39.00%, 31.40% and 29.84%, respectively. Total average milk production/cow was significantly ($p < 0.05$) higher in spring period (42.74±4.98 L) compared to summer (39.60±5.091 L) [49]. Drop in milk

production up to 50% in dairy animals might be due to reduced feed intake [9], whereas, rest could be reasons of metabolic adaptations to HS as HS response markedly alters post-absorptive carbohydrate, lipid, and protein metabolism a part of reduced feed intake [9]. Increased in basal insulin levels with improved insulin response in heat-stressed cows [9,12,46] and in ewes [50] were observed that explains the shift in glucose utilization in non-mammary gland tissue affecting milk synthesis [12]. HS during the dry period (i.e., last 2 months of gestation) reduced mammary cell proliferation and so, decreases milk yield in the following lactation [51]. Moreover, HS during the dry period negatively affects the function of the immune cell in dairy cows facing calving and also extended to the following lactation [51]. Singh et al. [52] also reported negative impacts of HS on lactation length, dry period, calving interval, milk constituents and milk yield in Murrah buffaloes. Upadhyay et al. [45] reported that the annual total milk loss due to thermal stress at the all-India level was 1.8 million tonnes or approximately 2% of the total milk production of the country amounting to a whopping Rs. 2661.62 crores per year. The negative impact of global warming on total milk production in India is also estimated to about 3.2 million tons by 2020 and more than 15 million tons by 2050.

The stage of lactation is an important factor for severity of imposed HS and animals which were in mid-lactation is mostly heat sensitive compared to early and late lactating counterparts [35,53]. The decline in milk production due to HS was 14% in early lactation and 35% in mid-lactation [35,53]. Average milk production in Holstein-Friesian during early lactation period (first 60 days of lactation) was significantly ($p < 0.05$) higher in spring (42.74±4.98 L) than in summer (39.60±5.09 L) seasons [49]. Similar results were also observed [13] in early lactating dairy goats under HS with greater milk yield losses (9%) compared to late lactating animals (3%) and also reported greater reductions in milk fat at early lactation (12%) compared to late lactation (1%). Kumar et al. [10] also observed that high temperature with high humidity during calving had a detrimental effect on lactation yield and lactation length of Holdeo crossbred (Holstein Friesian × Deoni) cattle.

Hot and humid environment not only affects milk yield but also effects milk quality. Kadzere et al. [15] reported that milk fat, solids-not-fat (SNF) and milk protein percentage decreased by 39.7, 18.9 and 16.9%, respectively. Bouraoui et al. [42] observed lower milk fat and milk protein in the summer season. When THI value goes beyond 72, milk fat and protein content declines. In addition, the analysis of protein fractions also showed a reduction in percentages of casein, lactalbumin, immunoglobulin G (IgG) and IgA. 80% of these were associated with loss of productivity and 20% with health issues which might be due to disruption of internal homeostasis mechanism [54]. Zheng *et al.* [55] observed that HS significantly reduces the production of milk, the percentage of milk fat and percentage of proteins, but that it has no effect on the content of lactose in milk. Milk protein contents decline, whereas the response of milk fat content seems delayed and results are contradictory when THI is above 72 [53]. The content of proteins and fats was significantly (p<0.01) higher in spring period than in summer. However, values for percentage of lactose varied slightly (4.45±0.54% in spring vs. 4.03±0.24% in summer period; p>0.05) in these two seasons [49]. HS significantly reduced milk fat, protein, lactose, SNF and ash contents from 3.79%, 3.20%, 4.78%, 8.69%, 12.48% and 0.71% during the winter season to 3.49%, 3.07%, 4.59%, 8.34%, 11.83% and 0.67% during summer season [48]. A reduction in casein percentage and casein index (casein/total proteins ratio) was also decreased in summer (2.18% vs. 2.58% and 72.4% vs. 77.7%, respectively) compared to spring season [35,53]. Hamzaoui *et al.* [13] also reported milk with lower protein (6-13%) and lactose (1-5%) contents in HS goats. Continual genetic selection for greater performance results to increased HS sensitivity and decreasing trend in lactation curve as well as poor milk quality in of dairy animals during summer seasons.

Effects on reproductive performance

High air temperature and humidity affects cellular functions by direct alteration and impairment of various tissues or organs of the reproductive system in both the sexes of the animal.

Effects on female reproductive performance

Estrous period and follicular growth

HS reduces the length and intensity of estrus besides increases incidence of anestrous and silent heat in farm animals [6,52,56]. It increases ACTH and cortisol secretion [52], and blocks estradiol-induced sexual behavior [57]. Roth *et al.* [58] reported that developed follicles suffer damage and become non-viable when the body temperature exceeds 40°C. When female goats exposed to 36.8°C and 70% relative humidity for 48 h follicular growth to ovulation suppresses, accompanied by decreased LH receptor level and follicular estradiol synthesis activity [59]. Reduced granulosa cells aromatase activity and viability also contributed to poor estradiol secretion [59,60]. Low estradiol secretion suppresses signs of estrus, gonadotropin surge, ovulation, transport of gametes and ultimately reduced fertilization [60]. A temperature rise of more than 2°C in unabated buffaloes may cause negative impacts due to low or desynchronized endocrine activities particularly pineal-hypothalamo-hypophyseal-gonadal axis altering respective hormone functions [45]. They also reported that low estradiol level on the day of estrus during summer period may be the likely factor for poor expression of heat in Indian buffaloes [45].

Fertility

Multifactorial mechanisms involved in reducing fertility of dairy animals depending on the magnitude of HS. HS reduces oocyte development by affecting its growth and maturation [52]. It increases circulating prolactin level in animal's results to acyclicity and infertility [52,61]. Moreover, 80% of estrus may be unnoticeable during summer [62] which further reduces fertility. A period of high-temperature results to increase secretion of endometrial PGF-2α, thereby threatening pregnancy maintenance leads to infertility [63]. Plasma follicle-stimulating hormone (FSH) surge increases and inhibin concentrations decrease during HS leading to variation in follicular dynamics and depression of follicular dominance that could be associated with low fertility of cattle during the summer and autumn [58]. However, FSH secretion is elevated under HS condition probably due to reduced inhibition of negative feedback from smaller follicles which ultimately affect the reproductive efficiency of dairy animals [64]. Conception rates were drop from about 40% to 60% in cooler months to 10-20% or lower in summer, depending on the severity of the thermal stress [65]. About 20-27% drop in conception rates [66] or decrease in 90-day non-return rate to the first service in lactating dairy cows were recorded in summer [67]. Amundson *et al.* [68] reported a reduction (p<0.01) in pregnancy rate in summer (62%) and decreasing in spring (44%) when the average daily minimum temperature and average daily THI were equal to or above 16.7°C and 72.9 respectively. Moreover, severe HS, only 10-20% of inseminations were resulted, in normal pregnancies, were also reported [58]. Oocytes of cows exposed to thermal stress lose their competence for fertilization [69] and development to the blastocyst stage [70]. Recently, Lacerda and Loureiro [71] also reported HS decreases fertility by diminishing quality of oocytes and embryos through direct and indirect effects.

Embryonic growth and development

Embryonic growth and survival also affected during thermal stress in dairy animals. HS causes embryonic death by interfering with protein synthesis [72], oxidative cell damage [60], reducing interferon-tau production for signaling pregnancy recognition [63] and expression of stress-related genes associated with apoptosis [73]. Low progesterone secretion limits endometrial function and embryo development [60,64]. Exposure of lactating cows to HS on the 1st day after estrus reduced the proportion of embryos that developed to the blastocyst stage on the day 8th after estrus [74]. Further, exposure of post-implantation embryos (early organogenesis) and fetus to HS also leads to various teratologies [60]. The deleterious effects of HS in the embryo are most evident in early stages of its development [75]. However, embryos subjected to high temperatures *in vitro* or *in vivo* until day 7 of development (blastocyst) showed lower pregnancy rates at day 30 [75] and higher rates of embryonic loss on day 42 of gestation [75] and lactation yield as well as postpartum ovarian activity. Fetal malnutrition and eventually fetal growth retardation under thermal stress were also reported [6,51].

Effects on male reproductive performance

Bull is recognizing as more than half of the herd and hence, bull's fertility is equally or more important for fertilization of oocyte to produce a good, viable and genetically potential conceptus. It is well known that bull testes must be 2-6°C cooler than core body temperature for fertile sperm to be produced. Therefore, increased testicular temperature results from thermal stress could changes in seminal and biochemical parameters leads to infertility problems in bulls. The significant seasonal difference in semen characteristics was reported by several studies [76-80]. Cardozo *et al.* [76] reported seasonal effects on changes in testicular volume, hormonal profiles, sexual behavior and semen quality that affect the reproductive performance of males. Balic *et al.* [77] studied seasonal influence on 19 *Bos taurus* (simmental) bulls and found summer HS declined semen quality parameters. They also reported that younger bulls are more sensitive to elevated air temperatures during the summer seasons. Mishra *et al.* [78] in a study observed that membrane integrity status of fresh spermatozoa in four different breeds of bulls (crossbred, Red Sindhi, Haryana and Jersey) were affected significantly (p<0.01) with increases in air temperature from 10 to 18°C to more than 35°C. Rahman *et al.* [79] also reported that HS spermatozoa showed a highly reduced (p<0.01) fertilization rate in comparison to non-HS or normal control spermatozoa (53.7% vs. 70.2% or 81.5%, respectively). Bhakat *et al.* [80] observed optimal semen qualities during winter, poor during summer and intermediate during rainy season and conclude that hot-dry or summer season adversely affect the various bio-physical characteristics of semen in Karan Fries bulls. Hence, HS significantly lowers conception as well as fertility rates per insemination of male and subsequently reduces male's fitness.

Strategies for Ameliorating HS

Physical modifications of the environment, nutritional management and genetic development of thermotolerance breeds are key components for sustainable livestock production in tropical hot climates [81].

Physical modifications of environment

The most common approach to ameliorate HS is to alter the cow's environment through provision of house or shade (along with feed and drinking water), evaporative cooling system with water in the form of fog, mist or sprinkling with natural or forced air movement, and possibly cooling ponds [81]. Modification of microenvironment to enhance heat dissipation mechanism to relieve HS is one of the most important measures to be considered in hot environment.

Cooling ponds and sprinklers can also be used to cool the environment. Cooling can also improve reproductive performance in cows and heifers, and probably, the most effective cooling systems currently in use are those that couple evaporative cooling with tunnel ventilation or cross ventilation [6]. Dairy cattle allowed access to sprinklers (with and without forced ventilation) have increased milk production, improved reproduction and improved conversion of feed to milk [82]. Shading is one of the cheapest ways to modify an animal's environment during hot weather. For outdoors animals, provision of shade (natural or artificial) is one of the simplest and cost-effective methods to minimize heat from solar radiations. Trees are very effective and natural shading materials providing shade to the animals combined with beneficial cooling as moisture evaporates from the leaves. Artificial shades can be used to protect from the effects of solar radiation in absence of natural shade. Various types of roofing materials can be used from metal to synthetic materials for shade structures among which a white galvanized or aluminum roof is considered best.

Nutritional management

Nutritional modifications could help animals to maintain homeostasis or prevent nutrient deficiencies that result from HS. Lower DMI during hot weather reduces nutrients available for absorption, and absorbed nutrients are used less efficiently [83]. Rations should be >18% protein on a dry basis as overfeeding requires more energy to excrete excess nitrogen as urea. Optimizing ruminally undegraded protein improves milk yield in hot climates [83]. DMI and milk yield increased for cows fed with diets containing 14% versus 17 or 21% acid detergent fiber (ADF). However, milk yield was less sensitive to change in dairy temperature for cows fed with 14% ADF diet [43]. Increasing dietary fat content enhanced milk production efficiency and yield in the warm season [84]. Feed containing low fiber rations during hot weather is logical since heat production is highly associated with metabolism of acetate compared with propionate [81]. HS causes oxidative damage which could be minimized through supplementation of vitamins C, E and A and also mineral such as zinc [85]. Vitamin E acts as an inhibitor −"chain blocker"- of lipid peroxidation and ascorbic acid prevents lipid peroxidation due to peroxyl radicals. It also recycles vitamin E, vitamin C and zinc are known to scavenge ROS during oxidative stress. Further, vitamin C assist in the absorption of folic acid by reducing it to tetrahydrofolate, the latter again acts as an antioxidant. Use of vitamin C along with electrolyte supplementation was found to relieve the animals of oxidative stress and boosts cell-mediated immunity in buffaloes [86]. West [83] reported that Na^+ and K^+ status of the body stayed normal during HS when supplemented with electrolytes could be due to better regulation of acid-base balance in the blood. Yeast product supplementation plays an important role in digestibility of nutrient by altering the volatile fatty acids production in the rumen, decrease the production of ruminal ammonia and increase in ruminal microorganism population. Live yeast was also reported as beneficial to small ruminant nutrition and production [87].

Genetic selection

Advances in environmental modifications and nutritional management in part alleviate the impact of thermal stress on animal performance during the hotter seasons. However, long-term strategies have to be evolved for adaptation to climate change. Differences in thermal tolerance exist between livestock species provide clues or tools to select thermotolerant animals using genetic tools. The identification of heat-tolerant animals within high-producing breeds will be useful only if these animals are able to maintain high productivity and survivability when exposed to HS conditions. Cattle with shorter hair, hair of greater diameter and lighter coat color are more adapted to hot environments than those with longer hair coats and darker colors [53]. This phenotype has been characterized in *B. taurus* tropical cattle (senepol and carona), and this dominant gene is associated with an increased sweating rate, lower RT and lower RR in homozygous cattle under hot conditions [88]. There is heat shock gene related to thermotolerance that was identified and being used as marker in marker assisted selection and genome-wide selection to developed thermotolerant bull that are used in breeding program. Major families of Hsps are Hsp100, Hsp90, Hsp70, Hsp60, Hsp40 and the small Hsps (so-called Hsps of sizes below 30 kDa). HSPs have a critical role in the recovery of cells from stress and in cytoprotection as well as guarding cells from subsequent insults. Hsp gene expression under thermal stress changes include: (i) Activation of heat shock transcription factor 1 (HSF1); (ii) increased expression of Hsp genes and decreased expression and synthesis of other proteins; (iii) increased glucose and amino acid oxidation and reduced fatty acid metabolism; (iv) endocrine system activation of the stress response; and (v) immune system activation via extracellular secretion of Hsp. If the stress persists, these gene expression changes lead to an altered physiological state referred to as "acclimation," a process largely controlled by the endocrine system [8]. Several reports showed associations of SNP in the Hsp genes with thermal stress response and tolerance in farm animals. Association of polymorphisms in Hsp90AB1 with heat tolerance has also been reported in Thai native cattle [89], Sahiwal and Frieswal cattle [90], HSF1 gene [91], HSP70A1A gene [92], HSBP1 [93] in Chinese Holstein cattle. There are non-Hsps genes also revealed to undergo changes in expression in response to HS. For example ATP1B2 gene in Chinese Holstein cows [94] and ATP1A1 gene in jersey crossbred cows [95] was observed to have associated with thermotolerance.

These SNPs could be used as markers in marker assisted selection to developed thermotolerant animal in early ages. Further, thermotolerant bull can be used in breeding policy to have thermal adapted offspring.

Conclusion

Extended periods of high air temperature coupled with high relative humidity compromise the ability of dairy animal to dissipate excess body heat which affects feed intake, milk production, and reproductive efficiency and ultimately reducing profitability for dairy farmers. However, by minimizing body temperature, greater feed intake could be encouraged. Moreover, the gross efficiency with which dietary nutrients are used by the cow for performance could also be improved. The loss of electrolytes via skin secretions has to be minimized by improvement of housing and cooling of the animals. Standardization of mineral supplement to control acid-base balance should be considered in animal under different level of thermal stress. Increase pregnancy rate of HS cows could be achieved by improving various managemental conditions. Identification of genes associated with thermotolerance and using these genes as markers in the breeding program or marker assisted selection should be applied to identify animals adapted to thermal stress considering genotype-environment interactions (G × E) in addition to higher productivity. Further research on climate resilient animal agriculture is the need of the hour for sustainability in dairy farming system, especially in hot humid climatic regions.

Authors' Contributions

RD prepared the initial version of the manuscript. LS, NV, PB, JS and RK assisted in literature collection. RD and IM drafted and revised the manuscript for critical scientific corrections. All authors read and approved the final manuscript.

Acknowledgments

The authors are thankful to National Library in Dairying, NDRI, Karnal, India for providing scientific literature.

Competing Interests

The authors declare that they have no competing interests.

References

1. Intergovernmental Panel on Climate Change (IPCC). (2007) Climate Change: Synthesis Report. Available from: http://www.ipcc.ch/pdf/assessment report/ar4/syr/ar4_syr_sym.pdt. Accessed on 28-11-2015.

2. Silanikove, N. and Koluman, N.D. (2015) Impact of climate change on the dairy industry in temperate zones: Predications on the overall negative impact and on the positive role of dairy goats in adaptation to earth warming. *Small Rumin. Res.*, 123: 27-34.

3. Yousef, M.K. (1985) Stress Physiology in Livestock. Vol. 1. CRC Press, Boca Raton. p67-73.

4. Vale, W.G. (2007) Effects of environment on buffalo

reproduction. *Ital. J. Anim. Sci.,* 6(2): 130-142.

5. Sunil Kumar, B.V., Kumar, A. and Kataria, M. (2011) Effect of heat stress in tropical livestock and different strategies for its amelioration. *J. Stress Physiol. Biochem.,* 7(1): 45-54.

6. Kadokawa, H., Sakatani, M. and Hansen, P.J. (2012) Perspectives on improvement of reproduction in cattle during heat stress in a future Japan. *Anim. Sci. J.,* 83(6): 439-445.

7. Berman, A.J. (2005) Estimates of heat stress relief needs for Holstein dairy cows. *J. Anim. Sci.,* 83(6): 1377-1384.

8. Collier, R.J., Collier, J.L., Rhoads, R.P. and Baumgard, L.H. (2008) Invited review: Genes involved in the bovine heat stress response. *J. Dairy Sci.,* 91(2): 445-454.

9. Baumgard, L.H. and Rhoads, R.P. (2013) Effects of heat stress on postabsorptive metabolism and energetics. *Annu. Rev. Anim. Biosci.,* 1: 311-337.

10. Kumar, S., Mote, S., Singh, D., Chauhan, S.S. and Ghosh, N. (2014) Effects of environmental factors on lactation yield and lactation length of Holdeo crossbred cattle. *Indian J. Appl. Res.,* 4(10): 4-7.

11. Baile, C.A. and Forbes, J.M. (1974) Control of feed intake and regulation of energy balance in ruminants. *Physiol. Rev.,* 54(1): 160.

12. Rhoads, R.P., Baumgard, L.H., Suagee, J.K. and Sanders, S.R. (2013) Nutritional interventions to alleviate the negative consequences of heat stress. *Adv. Nutr.,* 4(3): 267-276.

13. Hamzaoui, S., Salama, A.A.K., Caja, G., Albanell, E., Flores, C. and Such, X. (2012) Milk production losses in early lactating dairy goats under heat stress. *J. Dairy Sci.,* 95(2): 672-673.

14. Hooda, O.K. and Singh, S. (2010) Effect of thermal stress on feed intake, plasma enzymes and blood bio-chemicals in buffalo heifers. *Indian J. Anim. Nutr.,* 27(2): 122-127.

15. Kadzere, C.T., Murphy, M.R., Silanikove, N. and Maltz, E. (2002) Heat stress in lactating dairy cows: A review. *Livest. Prod. Sci.,* 77(1): 59-91.

16. Lacetera, N., Bernabucci, U., Ronchi, B. and Nardone, A. (1996) Body condition score, metabolic status and milk production of early lactating dairy cows exposed to warm environment. *Riv. Agric. Subtrop. Trop.,* 90(1): 43-55.

17. Nardone, A., Ronchi, B., Lacetera, N., Ranieri, M.S. and Bernabucci, U. (2010) Effect of climate changes on animal production and sustainability of livestock systems. *Livest. Sci.,* 130(1-3): 57-69.

18. Soriani, N., Panella, G. and Calamari, L. (2013) Rumination time during the summer season and its relationships with metabolic conditions and milk production. *J. Dairy Sci.,* 96(8): 5082-5094.

19. Nonaka, I., Takusari, N., Tajima, K., Suzuki, T., Higuchi, K. and Kurihara, M. (2008) Effects of high environmental temperatures on physiological and nutritional status of prepubertal Holstein heifers. *Livest. Sci.,* 113(1): 14-23.

20. Hall, M.B. (2009) Heat stress alters ruminal fermentation and digesta characteristics, and behavior in lactating dairy cattle. In: Chilliard, Y., Glasser, F., Faulconnier, Y., Bocquier, F., Veissier, I. and Doreau, M., editors. Proceeding of 11ᵗʰ International Symposium on Ruminant Physiology. Wageningen Academic Publication, Wageningen, The Netherlands. p204.

21. Helal, A., Hashem, A.L.S., Abdel-Fattah, M.S. and El-Shaer, H.M. (2010) Effect of heat stress on coat characteristics and physiological responses of Balady and Damascus goats in Sinai, Egypt. *Am. Euresian J. Agric. Environ. Sci.,* 7(1): 60-69.

22. Benjamin, M.M. (1978) Fluid and electrolytes. In: Outline of Veterinary Clinical Pathology. Iowa State Univ. Press, Ames. p213.

23. Schneider, P.L., Beede, D.K., Wilcox, C.J. and Collier, R.J. (1984) Influence of dietary sodium and potassium bicarbonate and total potassium on heat-stressed lactating dairy cows. *J. Dairy Sci.,* 67(11): 2546-2553.

24. Lallawmkimi, M.C., Singh, S.V., Upadhyay, R.C. and De, S. (2013) Impact of vitamin supplementation on heat shock protein 72 and antioxidant enzymes in different stages of Murrah buffaloes during seasonal stress. *Indian J. Anim. Sci.,* 83(9): 909-915.

25. Yatoo, M.I., Dimri, M. and Sharma, M.C. (2014) Seasonal changes in certain blood antioxidants in cattle and buffaloes. *Indian J. Anim. Sci.,* 84(2): 173-176.

26. Abdel-Samee, A.M. (1987) The role of cortisol in improving productivity of heat-stressed farm animals with different techniques. Ph.D. Thesis, Faculty of Agriculture, Zagazig University, Zagazig, Egypt.

27. Habeeb, A.A.M. (1987) The role of insulin in improving productivity of heat stressed farm animals with different techniques. Ph.D. Thesis, Faculty of Agriculture, Zagazig University, Zagazig, Egypt.

28. Sejian, V., Indu, S. and Naqvi, S.M.K. (2013) Impact of short term exposure to different environmental temperature on the blood biochemical and endocrine responses of Malpura ewes under semi-arid tropical environment. *Indian J. Anim. Sci.,* 83(11): 1155-1160.

29. Al-Haidary, A.A. (2004) Physiological responses of Naimey sheep to heat stress challenge under semi-arid environments. *Int. J. Agric. Biol.,* 6(2): 307-309.

30. Srikandakumar, A. and Johnson, E.H. (2004) Effect of heat stress on milk production, rectal temperature, respiratory rate and blood chemistry in Holstein, Jersey and Australian Milking Zebu cows. *Trop. Anim. Health Prod.,* 36(7): 685-692.

31. Rhoads, M.L., Rhoads, R.P., Baale, M.J., Collier, R.J., Sanders, S.R., Weber, W.J., Croocker, B.A. and Baumgard, L.H. (2009) Effects of heat stress and plane of nutrition on lactating Holstein cows: I. Production, metabolism, and aspects of circulating somatotropin. *J. Dairy Sci.,* 92(5): 1986-1997.

32. Burton, J.L. and Ronald, J.E. (2003) Immunity and mastitis: Some new ideas for an old disease. *Vet. Clin. Food Anim.,* 19(1): 1-45.

33. Kansas, G.S. (1996) Selectins and their ligands: Current concepts and controversies. *Blood,* 88(9): 3259-87.

34. Do Amaral, B.C., Connor, E.E., Tao, S., Hayen, M.J., Bubolz, J.W. and Dahl, G.E. (2011) Heat stress abatement during the dry period influences metabolic gene expression and improves immune status in the transition period of dairy cows. *J. Dairy Sci.,* 94(1): 86-96.

35. Basirico, L., Bernabucci, U., Morera, P., Lacetera, N. and Nardone, A. (2009) Gene expression and protein secretion of apolipoprotein B100 (ApoB100) in transition dairy cows under hot or thermoneutral environments. *Ital. J. Anim. Sci.,* 8(2): 592-594.

36. Sanders, A.H., Shearer, J.K. and De Vries, A. (2009) Seasonal incidence of lameness and risk factors associated with thin soles, white line disease, ulcers, and sole punctures in dairy cattle. *J. Dairy Sci.,* 92(7): 3165-3174.

37. Privolo, G. and Riva, E. (2009) One year study of lying and standing behaviour of dairy cows in a freestall barn in Italy. *J. Agric. Eng.,* 2: 27-33.

38. Thornton, P., van de Steeg, J., Notenbaert, M.H. and Herrero, M. (2009) The impacts of climate change on livestock and livestock systems in developing countries: A review of what we know and what we need to know. *Agric. Syst.,* 101(3): 113-127.

39. Dhakal, C.K., Regmi, P.P., Dhakal, I.P., Khanal, B., Bhatta, U.K., Barsila, S.R. and Acharya, B. (2013) Perception, impact and adaptation to climate change: An analysis of livestock system in Nepal. *J. Anim. Sci. Adv.,* 3(9): 462-471.

40. Jingar, S.C., Mehla, R.K. and Singh, M. (2014) Climatic effects on occurrence of clinical mastitis in different breeds of cows and buffaloes. *Arch. Zootec.,* 63(243): 473-482.

41. Vitali, A., Segnalini, M., Bertocchi, L., Bernabucci, U., Nardone, A. and Lacetera, N. (2009) Seasonal pattern of mortality and relationships between mortality and

temperature humidity index in dairy cows. *J. Dairy Sci.,* 92(8): 3781-3790.

42. Bouraoui, R., Lahmar, M., Majdoub, A., Djemali, M. and Belyea, R. (2002) The relationship of temperature-humidity index with milk production of dairy cows in a Mediterranean climate. *Anim. Res.,* 51(6): 479-491.

43. West, J.W. (2003) Effects of heat-stress on production in dairy cattle. *J. Dairy Sci.,* 86(6): 2131-2144.

44. Spiers, D.E., Spain, J.N., Sampson, J.D. and Rhoads, R.P. (2004) Use of physiological parameters to predict milk yield and feed intake in heat-stressed dairy cows. *J. Therm. Biol.,* 29(7-8): 759-764.

45. Upadhyay, R.C., Ashutosh and Singh, S.V. (2009) Impact of climate change on reproductive functions of cattle and buffalo. In: Aggarwal, P.K., editor. Global Climate Change and Indian Agriculture. ICAR, New Delhi. p107-110.

46. Wheelock, J.B., Rhoads, R.P., Van Baale, M.J., Sanders, S.R. and Baumgard, L.H. (2010) Effect of heat stress on energetic metabolism in lactating Holstein cows. *J. Dairy Sci.,* 93(2): 644-655.

47. NRC. (2007) Nutrient Requirements of Small Ruminants, Sheep, Goats, Cervids, and New World Camelids. National Academy Press, Washington, DC.

48. Gaafar, H.M.A., Gendy, M.E., Bassiouni, M.I., Shamiah, S.M., Halawa, A.A. and Hamd, M.A. (2011) Effect of heat stress on performance of dairy Friesian cow's milk production and composition. *Researcher,* 3(5): 85-93.

49. Joksimović-Todorović, V.M., Hristov Davidović, S. and Stanković, B. (2011) Effect of heat stress on milk production in dairy cows. *Biotechnol. Anim. Husb.,* 27(3): 1017-1023.

50. Sejian, V., Maurya, V.P. and Naqvi, S.M.K. (2010c) Adaptive capability as indicated by endocrine and biochemical responses of Malpura ewes subjected to combined stresses (thermal and nutritional) in a semi-arid tropical environment. *Int. J. Biometeorol.,* 54(6): 653-661.

51. Tao, S. and Dahl, G.E. (2013) Heat stress effects during late gestation on dry cows and their calves. *J. Dairy Sci.,* 96(7): 4079-4093.

52. Singh, M., Chaudhari, B.K., Singh, J.K., Singh, A.K. and Maurya, P.K. (2013) Effects of thermal load on buffalo reproductive performance during summer season. *J. Biol. Sci.,* 1(1): 1-8.

53. Bernabucci, U., Lacetera, N., Baumgard, L.H., Rhoads, R.P., Ronchi, B. and Nardone, A. (2010) Metabolic and hormonal acclimation to heat stress in domesticated ruminants. *J. Anim. Sci.,* 4(7): 1167-1183.

54. Nardone, A., Ronchi, B., Lacetera, N. and Bernabucci, U. (2006) Climatic effects on productive traits in livestock. *Vet. Res. Commun.,* 30(1): 75-81.

55. Zheng, L., Chenh, M., and Zhi-Cheng, G. (2009) Effects of heat stress on milk performance and fatty acids in milk fat of Holstein dairy cows. *J. Chin. Dairy Ind.,* 37(9): 17-19.

56. Singhal, S.P., Dhanda, O.P. and Razdan, M.N. (1984) Some managemental and therapeutic approaches in the treatment of physiological infertility of water buffaloes (*Bubalus bubalis*). In: Proceedings of 10th International Congress Animal Reproduction and Artificial Insemination. Vol. 3. p471.

57. Hein, K.G. and Allrich, R.D. (1992) Influence of exogenous adrenocorticotropic hormone on estrous behavior in cattle. *J. Anim. Sci.,* 70(1): 243-247.

58. Roth, Z., Meidan, R., Braw-Tal, R. and Wolfenson, D. (2000) Immediate and delayed effects of heat stress on follicular development and its association with plasma FSH and inhibin concentration in cows. *J. Reprod. Infertil.,* 120(1): 83-90.

59. Ozawa, M., Tabayashi, D., Latief, T.A., Shimizu, T., Oshima, I. and Kanai, Y. (2005) Alterations in follicular dynamics and steroidogenic abilities induced by heat stress during follicular recruitment in goats. *Reproduction,* 129(5): 621-630.

60. Wolfenson, D., Roth, Z. and Meidan, R. (2000) Impaired

reproduction in heat stressed cattle: Basic and applied aspects. *Anim. Rep. Sci.,* 60-61: 535-547.

61. Alamer, M. (2011) The role of prolactin in thermoregulation and water balance during heat stress in domestic animals. *Asian J. Anim. Vet. Adv.,* 6(12): 1153-1169.

62. Rutledge, J.J. (2001) Use of embryo transfer and IVF to bypass effects of heat stress. *Theriogenology,* 55(1): 105-111.

63. Bilby, T.R., Baumgard, L.H., Collier, R.J., Zimbelman, R.B. and Rhoads, M.L. (2008) Heat stress effects on fertility: Consequences and possible solutions. In: The Proceedings of the 2008 South Western Nutritional Conference.

64. Khodaei-Motlagh, M.M., Zare, Shahneh, A., Masoumi, R. and Fabio, D. (2011) Alterations in reproductive hormones during heat stress in dairy cattle. *Afr. J. Biotechnol.,* 10(29): 5552-5558.

65. Cavestany, D., El-Whishy, A.B. and Foot, R.H. (1985) Effect of season and high environmental temperature on fertility of Holstein cattle. *J. Dairy Sci.,* 68(6): 1471-1478.

66. Chebel, R.C., Santos, J.E.P., Reynolds, J.P., Cerri, R.L.A., Juchem, S.O. and Overton, M. (2004) Factor affecting conception rate after artificial insemination and pregnancy loss in lactating dairy cows. *Anim. Rep. Sci.,* 84(3-4): 239-255.

67. Al-Katanani, Y.M., Webb, D.W. and Hansen, P.J. (1999) Factors affecting seasonal variation in 90-day non return rate to first service in lactating Holstein cows in a hot climate. *J. Dairy Sci.,* 82(12): 2611-2616.

68. Amundson, J.L., Mader, T.L., Rasby, R.J. and Hu, Q.S. (2006) Environmental effects on pregnancy rate in beef cattle. *J. Anim. Sci.,* 84(12): 3415-3420.

69. Gendelman, M., and Roth, Z. (2012a) Seasonal effect on germinal vesicle-stage bovine oocytes is further expressed by alterations in transcript levels in the developing embryos associated with reduced developmental competence. *Biol. Reprod.,* 86(1): 1-9.

70. Gendelman, M. and Roth, Z. (2012b) *In vivo* vs. *In vitro* models for studying the effects of elevated temperature on the GV-stage oocyte, subsequent developmental competence and gene expression. *Anim. Reprod. Sci.,* 134(3-4): 125-134.

71. Lacerda, T.F. and Loureiro, B. (2015) Selecting thermotolerant animals as a strategy to improve fertility in Holstein cows. *Glob. J. Anim. Sci. Res.,* 3(1): 119-127.

72. Edwards, J.L. and Hansen, P.J. (1996) Elevated temperature increases heat shock protein 70 synthesis in bovine two-cell embryos and compromises function of maturing oocytes. *Biol. Reprod.,* 55(2): 340-346.

73. Fear, J.M. and Hansen, P.J. (2011) Developmental changes in expression of genes involved in regulation of apoptosis in the bovine preimplantation embryo. *Biol. Reprod.,* 84(1): 43-51.

74. Ealy, A.D., Drost, M. and Hansen, P.J. (1993) Developmental changes in embryonic resistance to adverse effects of maternal heat stress in cows. *J. Dairy Sci.,* 76: 2899-2905.

75. Demetrio, D.G.B., Santos, R.M., Demetrio, C.G.B. and Vasconcelos, J.L.M. (2007) Factors affecting conception rates following artificial insemination or embryo transfer in lactating Holstein cows. *J. Dairy Sci.,* 90(11): 5073-5082.

76. Cardozo, J., Fernández-Juan, M., Forcada, F., Abecia, A., Muiño-Blanco, T. and Cebrián-Pérez, J.A. (2006) Monthly variations in ovine seminal plasma proteins analyzed by two-dimensional polyacrylamide gel electrophoresis. *Theriogenology,* 66(4): 841-850.

77. Balic, I.M., Milinkovic-Tur, S., Samardzija, M. and Vince, S. (2012) Effect of age and environmental factors on semen quality, glutathione peroxidase activity and oxidative parameters in Simmental bulls. *Theriogenology,* 78(2): 423-431.

78. Mishra, S.R., Kundu, A.K. and Mahapatra, A.P.K. (2013) Effect of ambient temperature on membrane integrity of spermatozoa in different breeds of bulls. *The Bioscan,* 8(1): 181-183.

79. Rahman, M.B., Kamal, M.M., Rijsselaere, T., Vandaele, L., Shamsuddin, M. and Soom, A.V. (2013) Altered chromatin condensation of heat stressed spermatozoa perturbs the dynamics of DNA methylation reprogramming in the paternal genome after *in vitro* fertilisation in cattle. *Reprod. Fertil. Dev.,* 26(8): 1107-1116.

80. Bhakat, M., Mohanty, T.K., Gupta, A.K. and Abdullah, M. (2014) Effect of season on semen quality of crossbred (Karan Fries) bulls. *Adv. Anim. Vet. Sci.,* 2(11): 632-637.

81. Atrian, P. and Shahryar, H.A. (2012) Heat stress in dairy cows. *Res. Zool.,* 2(4): 31-37.

82. Wolfenson, D. (2009) Impact of heat stress on production and fertility of dairy cattle. In: Proceedings of the 18th Annual Tri-State Dairy Nutrition Conference. Fort Wayne, IN, USA. 21-22 April 2009. p55-59.

83. West, J.W. (1999) Nutritional strategies for managing the heat stressed dairy cows. *J. Anim. Sci.,* 77(2): 21-35.

84. Linn, J., Reath-Knight, M. and Larson, R. (2004) Managing heat stressed lactating dairy cows. *Hubbard Feeds Inc.,* 26: 9-10.

85. McDowell, L.R., editor. (1989) Vitamins in Animal Nutrition: Comparative Aspects to Human Nutrition. Academic Press, London. p10-52, 93-131.

86. Sunil Kumar, B.V., Singh, G. and Meur, S.K. (2010) Effects of Addition of electrolyte and ascorbic acid in feed during heat stress in buffaloes. *Asian-Aust. J. Anim. Sci.,* 23(7): 880-888.

87. Stella, A.V., Paratte, R., Valnegri, L., Cigalino, G., Soncini, G., Chevaux, E., Dell'Orto, V. and Savoini, G. (2007) Effect of administration of live *Saccharomyces cerevisiae* on milk production, milk composition, blood metabolites, and faecal flora in early lactating dairy goats. *Small Rumin. Res.,* 67: 7-13.

88. Mariasegaram, R., Chase, C.C., Jr Chaparro, J.X., Olson, T.A., Brenneman, R.A. and Niedz, R.P. (2007) The slick air coat locus maps to chromosome 20 in Senepol-derived cattle. *Anim. Genet.,* 38: 54-59.

89. Charoensook, R., Gatphayak, K., Sharifi, A.R., Chaisongkram, C., Brenig, B. and Knorr, C. (2012) Polymorphisms in the bovine HSP90AB1 gene are associated with heat tolerance in Thai indigenous cattle. *Trop. Anim. Health Prod.,* 44: 921-928.

90. Deb, R., Sajjanar, B., Singh, U., Kumar, S., Singh, R., Sengar, G., Sharma, A. (2014) Effect of heat stress on the expression profile of Hsp90 among Sahiwal (*Bos indicus*) and Frieswal (*Bos indicus* × *Bos taurus*) breed of cattle: A comparative study. *Gene,* 536: 435-440.

91. Li, Q.L., Ju, Z.H., Huang, J.M., Li, J.B., Li, R.L., Hou, M.H., Wang, C.F. and Zhong, J.F. (2011a) Two novel SNPs in HSF1 gene are associated with thermal tolerance traits in Chinese Holstein cattle. *DNA Cell Biol.,* 30: 247-254.

92. Li, Q., Han, J., Du, F., Ju, Z., Huang, J., Wang, J., Li, R., Wang, C. and Zhong, J. (2011b) Novel SNPs in HSP70A1A gene and the association of polymorphisms with thermo tolerance traits and tissue specific expression in Chinese Holstein cattle. *Mol. Biol. Rep.,* 38: 2657-2663.

93. Wang, Y., Huang, J., Xia, P., He, J., Wang, C., Ju, Z., Li, J., Li, R., Zhong, J. and Li, Q. (2013) Genetic variations of HSBP1 gene and its effect on thermal performance traits in Chinese Holstein cattle. *Mol. Biol. Rep.,* 40: 3877-3882.

94. Wang, Z., Wang, G., Huang, J., Li, Q., Wang, C. and Zhong, J. (2011) Novel SNPs in the ATP1B2 gene and their associations with milk yield, milk composition and heat-resistance traits in Chinese Holstein cows. *Mol. Biol. Rep.,* 38: 1749-1755.

95. Das, R., Gupta, I.D., Verma, A., Singh, A., Chaudhari, M.V., Sailo, L., Upadhyay, R.C. and Goswami, J. (2015) Genetic polymorphisms of ATP1A1 gene and their association with heat tolerance in Jersey crossbred cows. *Indian J. Dairy Sci.,* 68(1): 50-54.

31

Neonatal mortality in dogs: Prognostic value of Doppler ductus venosus waveform evaluation - Preliminary results

Gabriele Barella, Stefano Faverzani, Massimo Faustini, Debora Groppetti and Alessandro Pecile

Department of Veterinary Medicine, State University of Milan, Via Celoria 10; 20133; Milan, Italy.
Corresponding author: Gabriele Barella, e-mail: gabriele.barella@gmail.com,
SF: stefano.faverzani@unimi.it, MF: massimo.faustini@unimi.it, DG: debora.groppetti@unimi.it,
AP: alessandro.pecile@unimi.it

Abstract

Aim: To define the prognostic value of Doppler ultrasonographic morphology of ductus venosus (DV) waveform on canine neonatal mortality.

Materials and Methods: Fifty-four healthy pregnant bitches underwent fetal ultrasonographic assessment. The DV waveforms were classified as diphasic (dDVw) or triphasic (tDVw) and compared with neonatal mortality.

Results: Ninety-three fetuses were evaluated. Twenty fetuses belonged to litters with neonatal mortality, in which tDVw was observed. Seven fetuses belonged to litters without neonatal mortality, in which tDVw was observed. Fifty-eight fetuses belonged to litters without neonatal mortality, in which only dDVw was observed. Eight fetuses belonged to litters with neonatal mortality, in which only dDVw was observed. The correlation between tDVw and neonatal mortality was statistically significant (odds ratio [OR], 20.7; $p<0.0001$). Considering only pregnancies with one or two fetuses with the same DV waveform: Two fetuses with tDVw belonged to litters with neonatal mortality; 1 foetus with tDVw belonged to litter without neonatal mortality and 26 fetuses showed dDVw without neonatal mortality. The correlation between tDVw and neonatal mortality even in litters up to two pups was statistically significant (OR, 88.3; $p=0.01$).

Conclusion: Echo-Doppler assessment of DV is feasible in canine fetuses, and the presence tDVw seems to be related to neonatal mortality.

Keywords: dog, Doppler, ductus venosus, neonatal mortality, ultrasound.

Introduction

The ultrasonographic evaluation of ductus venosus (DV) hemodynamic plays an important role in human medicine since it is considered a relevant indicator of fetal well-being [1,2]. The DV is a small trumpet-shaped vessel of a few millimeters length and width, originating from the umbilical vein and reaching the caudal vena cava near the confluence of the hepatic veins, gradually reducing its diameter. Several studies reported ultrasonographic evaluation of DV blood flow in fetal lambs [3,4] and in dogs [5]. According to human literature the ultrasonographic Doppler waveforms of DV are classified as monophasic, diphasic or triphasic (dDVw or tDVw) [6], while only two different types of waveforms have been described in canine fetuses (diphasic or triphasic) [5].

In humans, the presence of a triphasic waveform in the DV (reverse a-wave which corresponds to a deflection during atrial contraction) is considered a strong predictor of neonatal mortality independently of gestational age [7].

This preliminary study aims to evaluate the Doppler ultrasonographic waveforms of the DV and to verify the predictive ability of the tDVw in neonatal mortality in dogs.

Materials and Methods

Ethical approval

The present study has been carried out on privately owned dogs and include no any clinical trials. The present study was performed in accordance with the ethical guidelines of animal welfare committee and informed consent was obtained from each owner.

Data collection

Fifty-four clinically healthy private owned pregnant bitches (primiparous or multiparous) were recruited. The population was composed by mixed and purebred dogs such as American Staffordshire, Bernese Mountain Dog, Boston Terrier, Chihuahua, Dogo Argentino, Dogue de Bordeaux, English Bulldog, French Bulldog, Golden Retriever, Great Dane, Jack Russel Terrier, Labrador Retriever, Pinscher, Rhodesian Ridgeback, Shetland Sheepdog, and Yorkshire Terrier. All dogs were considered healthy based on physical examination, blood cell count, serum chemistry, and urinalysis results. No clinical pathological evidence of disease was recorded through any pregnancy. Neonatal mortality defined stillborn pups and those died within 6 h of life. The present study was performed in accordance with the ethical guidelines of animal welfare committee and informed consent was obtained from each owner.

To deduce the LH peak and the optimal time for mating, all bitches underwent an accurate reproductive cycle monitoring by vaginal cytology and plasma progesterone measurement [8,9].

Plasma progesterone concentration was determined using a quantitative test based on ELFA technique (Enzyme Linked Fluorescent Assay; MiniVidas, Biomerieux). Assay principle combines an enzyme immunoassay competition method with a final fluorescent detection [10]. Bitches were included in the study if the initial progesterone sample at proestrus was <2 ng/mL. The first day on which the serum progesterone was ≥2 ng/mL was regarded as the LH peak [8,9]. Gestational age was calculated from the estimated LH peak (Day 0). The number of born puppies, the date and type of delivery were recorded.

All dogs underwent ultrasonographic evaluation once during pregnancy. The bitches were evaluated in dorsal or lateral recumbency (without any pharmacological restraint), clipping the hair from the costal arch to the inguinal region, and applying a conductive gel to the skin. Ultrasonographic diagnosis of pregnancy and fetal monitoring were performed using two-dimensional and Doppler ultrasound (Esaote MyLab 70, Genua, Italy) with a high multi-frequency linear probe (7.5-13 MHz). Waveform in the DV was measured in only two fetuses [11,12] during each examination, except in cases of singleton pregnancy). The fetuses selected for measurements were the ones that were located most cranially and caudally within the uterus, but all recognizable fetuses were evaluated for viability based on ultrasonographic evaluations of the fetal movements [13] and heartbeat [13,14]. The DV was identified following the intra-abdominal course of the umbilical vein until a trumpet-shaped vessel was seen entering the caudal vena cava, as previously described by Kiresud et al. [1]. The color aliasing artifact was used for correctly identify the DV (this color phenomenon is responsible for the "mosaic" appearance of the DV).

Pulsed-wave Doppler was then applied to acquire the waveforms. The angle of the pulsed Doppler sample volume was set for angle-dependent measurements between 20° and 60°. To avoid the signal from nearby vessels, the sample volume was set to 1-2 mm. The Doppler and color filters were set at 40-100 Hz, and the velocity was set at 8-12 waveforms in one screen image. A sequence of at least three successive and symmetric waves was required to classify them as monophasic, diphasic or triphasic. The DV waveform was considered monophasic (Figure-1) if there were no modulations other than those attributable to breathing; diphasic (Figure-2) if all the modulations were in the same direction and none of them reached the baseline; triphasic (Figure-3) if two modulations

were seen on one side of the baseline and one was seen on the opposite side of the baseline. Images were collected and downloaded to a computer.

Statistical analysis

Odds ratios (OR) were calculated, with 95% confidence intervals (CI), to compare the chance of neonatal mortality between litters with one or more tDVw and litters without tDVw. The test sensibility (Se) and specificity (Sp) were also calculated as the relative positive predicting value (PPV) and negative predicting value (NPV).

Results

Fifty-four bitches were included in the study. The bitches ranged in age from 1 to 7 years (2.8±1.2 years), and weighed from 4 to 50 kg (16.6±12.3 kg). Ninety-three fetuses out of the 213 born pups were evaluated (43.7%).

Sixty puppies were born by elective cesarean section from 25 bitches, and 153 puppies were born by vaginal parturition from 29 bitches. All bitches with vaginal delivery were monitored during labor. No fetal ingestion occurred. During gestational period, the pups number was not determined. However, all bitches were evaluated again after labor with ultrasound to confirm that each bitch delivered every pups that were in uterus. Litter sizes ranged from 1 to 10

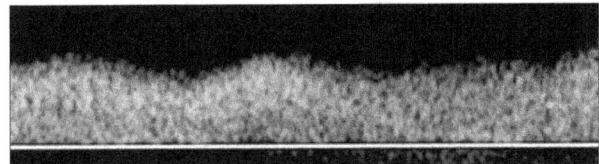

Figure-1: Pulsed-wave Doppler image of monophasic waveform of a portal vein as an example.

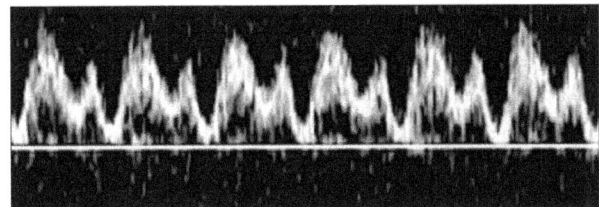

Figure-2: Pulsed-wave Doppler image of a diphasic waveform of a ductus venosus.

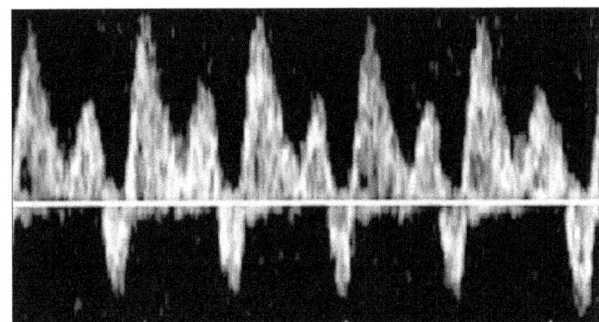

Figure-3: Pulsed-wave Doppler image of a triphasic waveform of a ductus venosus.

(mean value of 4±3 puppies). Neonatal mortality (within 6 h of birth) was 9.8% (21 out of 213) with nine dead necropsied pups affected by: One pup had severe chest wall deformation; one pup was anasarca; three pups had bilateral renal agenesis; four pups had a premature appearance. The remaining 192 pups (90.1%) were healthy. All bitches underwent ultrasonographic evaluation once from 36 to 66 days of pregnancy (mean 53.5±8 days). No bitch had an abortion. Considering that the earlier Doppler measurement was performed at day 36 of gestation, we can assume that no measured foetus was reabsorbed. The DV was identified in all the 93 fetuses considered and the waveform was classified as diphasic (66 waveforms out of 93; 71%) or triphasic (27 waveforms out of 93; 29%). No monophasic DV waveform was detected.

Distribution of dDVw and tDVw respect to neonatal mortality is showed in Table-1. The OR showed a statistically significant correlation between the presence of a tDVw and neonatal mortality (OR, 20.7; 95% CI, 6.7-64.4; p<0.0001). Se and Sp were 71.4% and 89.2% with PPV 74.1% and NPV 87.9%, respectively. If we consider the pregnancies with only one or two fetuses, 35 fetuses were evaluated (15 singleton from 15 bitches and 20 fetuses from 10 bitches). Among the 10 pregnancies with two fetuses, only in seven the fetuses presented the same DV waveform (either tDVw or dDVw). The distribution of dDVw and tDVw respect to neonatal mortality in pregnancies with one foetus (n=15) and in pregnancies (n=7) with two fetuses with the same DV waveform (n=29 fetuses) is represented in Table-1. The OR showed a statistically significant correlation between the presence of a tDVw and neonatal mortality (OR, 88.3; 95% CI, 2.8-2791.9; p=0.01). The Se and Sp were 100% and 96.3% with PPV 66.67% and NPV 100%, respectively.

Discussion

The bloodflow waveform of DV is commonly used in hemodynamic evaluation of human fetuses [15]. It reflects the cardiac cycle: the S-wave corresponds to the ventricular systole, the v-wave corresponds to the atrial diastole, the D-wave corresponds to the ventricular diastole and the a-wave corresponds to the atrial systole (Figure-4). The abnormalities of DV waveform such as reverse flow during the atrial systole, that is triphasic waveform, are considered strong predictors of stillbirth [7]. The a-wave reflects the capacity of the heart to accommodate venous return that depends on venous volume, cardiac function (relaxation, compliance and contractility) and downstream arterial bloodflow resistance. The presence of a maintained dDVw in fetuses predicts an intact survival [7].

Our study shows the feasibility to access the hemodynamic of canine fetal DV during pregnancy. However, Doppler recording requires some training

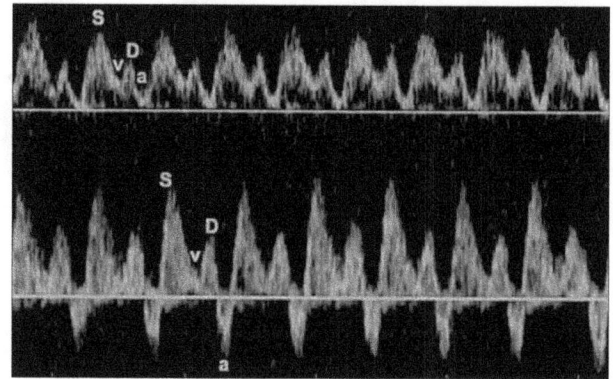

Figure-4: At the top a diphasic ductus venosus waveform of a canine fetus; at the bottom a triphasic ductus venosus waveform of another fetus. S=Ventricular systole, v=Atrial diastole, D=Ventricular diastole, a=Atrial systole.

and patience to reach a reliable level of skill [16]. The DV was identified in all the 93 fetuses considered; the waveform was diphasic in 71% of subjects while the remaining 29% of fetuses presented a tDVw. As expected a monophasic DV waveform was not observed in this study; indeed, this wave depends on breathing movements that cannot be present in the foetus.

Neonatal mortality was significantly associated with reverse DV a-wave (tDVw): Litters in which tDVw was recorded had more chance (almost 21 times more) to present neonatal mortality (one or more dead pups per litter) than those with only dDVw.

The inability to identify the single foetus among other littermates (both in subsequent ultrasonographic evaluations through pregnancy) is a common limit occurring in fetal evaluation of polytocous species. The evaluation of only 2 fetuses in our work is obviously a biasing factor of our results; however in every obstetric study concerning the ultrasonographic evaluation of canine fetuses only 2 pups are normally evaluated [11,12] and in many studies even just one [17-19]. In our study, we evaluated two fetuses to be sure to evaluate 2 different subjects. To our knowledge the only way we can evaluate every subjects would be during cesarean section, using an intraoperative ultrasound technique. Statistical correlation between tDVw and neonatal mortality resulted in an acceptable Sp (89.2%) and a poor Se (71.4%). This finding could depend on decision to evaluate only two fetuses per litter. Regarding the eight fetuses belonged to litters with neonatal mortality in which only dDVw was recorded (Table-1), we hypothesized that there might be other puppies not valued in the same litter presenting tDVw.

Further, seven fetuses belonged to litters without neonatal mortality in which at least a tDVw was observed (Table-1). We cannot explain this finding, but we noticed that all these fetuses belonged to bitches that underwent cesarean section. However, our study does not describe, in any way, the influence of Cesarean section on neonatal mortality.

Table-1: Table summarizing population data.

ID	Breed	Weight (kg)	Age (year)	GA (day)	Waveform	Type of parturition	Neonatal mortality	Number of pups
1	Dogo Argentino	33	3	50	dDV	C	No	2
2	Labrador retriever	25	2.5	43	dDV	C	No	2
3	Bouledogue	8	3	63	tDV	C	Yes	6
4	Staffordshire bull t.	18	4	52	dDV	N	No	6
5	Shetland	9	4.5	56	dDV/tDV	N	Yes	5
6	Dogo Argentino	35.5	2	57	dDV	C	No	2
7	Am. Staffordshire t.	34.5	3	49	dDV	N	No	7
8	Great Dane	50	5	58	dDV/tDV	N	No	10
9	Chihuahua	4	2	57	dDV	N	No	3
10	Yorkshire	5.5	3	51	tDV	N	Yes	4
11	Bulldog	21	1.5	49	dDV	C	No	1
12	Bulldog	19	2	60	dDV	C	No	1
13	Boston t.	12.5	4	64	dDV	C	No	2
14	Chihuahua	3.5	2.5	58	dDV/tDV	C	Yes	2
15	Pinscher	9	2	46	dDV	N	No	1
16	Pug	9.5	2.5	40	dDV	N	Yes	3
17	Jack russel t.	8.5	2.5	64	tDV	N	Yes	1
18	Bulldog	8	2	55	dDV	N	Yes	5
19	Rhodesian Ridgeback	33	2	38	dDV	N	No	10
20	Chihuahua	6	2	47	dDV/tDV	C	No	4
21	Bulldog	21.5	3	58	dDV	C	No	1
22	Bouledogue	8	3	60	dDV	C	No	5
23	Boston t.	9	5	66	dDV	C	No	1
24	Am. Pit bull t.	28	2	36	dDV	N	No	10
25	Cross breed	9	3	53	tDV	N	Yes	4
26	Bouledogue	7.5	1	39	dDV	N	No	1
27	Staffordshire bull t.	17	3	59	dDV	N	No	6
28	Pinscher	9.5	2	43	tDV	C	No	1
29	Bouledogue	9	2.5	61	tDV	C	Yes	5
30	Pug	8	5	63	dDV	C	No	2
31	Chihuahua	5	2.5	38	dDV	C	No	4
32	Dogo Argentino	31.5	2	54	dDV	N	No	9
33	Bouledogue	9.5	4	60	dDV/tDV	N	No	7
34	Am. Staffordshire t.	28.5	2	45	dDV	N	No	7
35	Benese Mountain dog	30.5	3.5	39	dDV	N	No	9
36	Yorkshire	5	4.5	60	tDV	N	Yes	4
37	Golden r.	30	2	52	dDV	N	No	9
38	Chihuahua	4	2	55	dDV/tDV	N	Yes	2
39	Bouledogue	10.5	5	47	tDV	C	Yes	7
40	Pinscher	9.5	1	60	dDV	N	No	2
41	Shetland	7	5	49	tDV	N	Yes	4
42	Rhodesian Ridgeback	38	2	53	dDV	N	No	8
43	Pug	13	2	62	dDV	C	No	1
44	Bulldog	20	1	56	dDV	C	No	1
45	Dogo Argentino	30.5	2.5	50	dDV	C	No	2
46	Jack russel t.	6	3	60	tDV	N	Yes	1
47	Boston t.	8	2	66	dDV	C	No	1
48	Dogue de Bordeaux	38	3	50	dDV	N	No	9
49	Great dane	47.5	4	60	dDV	N	No	5
50	Chihuahua	4,5	2	52	dDV/tDV	C	Yes	2
51	Boston t.	7	6,5	64	tDV	C	No	3
52	Yorkshire	8.5	2	51	dDV	C	No	1
53	Boston t.	10	1	48	dDV	N	No	1
54	Bulldog	17.5	2	63	dDV	C	No	1

dDV=Diphasic ductus venosus waveform, tDV=Triphasic ductus venosus waveform, C=Cesarean section, N=Natural vaginal delivery, GA=Gestational age

It is known that pregnancies with one or two fetuses are predisposed to higher neonatal mortality, and so we decided to analyze data referring only to these subjects. The OR calculated in singleton or twin concordant fetuses showed 88 times higher risk of death in fetuses with tDVw compared to those with dDVw, and Se and Sp were very high (respectively 100% and 96.3%).

We remark that tDVw is not the cause of death of these pups, it can be considered as a parameter of fetal disvitality as an expression of a circulatory distress.

In humans, the abnormalities of DV bloodflow have been associated to some pathological conditions such as aneuploidy, congenital heart diseases, fetal acidosis, hypoxemia, intrauterine growth restriction, oligohydramnios, and fetal anemia [20,21]. As mentioned above, it was not possible to correlate DV bloodflow characteristics to specific diseases we found in our sample. Further, four pups died within 6 h after birth (two French bouledouge, one Boston terrier) had bilateral renal agenesis. A relationship between renal agenesis and tDVw has never been postulated. However, in human fetuses with severe urinary tract malformations, a cardiorenal syndrome characterized by a bilateral ventricular hypertrophy (caused by an increased afterload) was described by Merz et al. [22] and it is known that a reverse DV a-wave (tDVw) can be a consequence of an increase afterload [7].

Conclusions

Our study does not correlate at all the presence of tDVw and a specific cause of death, but rather the presence of tDVw seems to be predicting the risk of neonatal mortality in the litter. When reverse DV a-wave is found, an accurate pregnancy monitoring and perinatal assistance should be scheduled. Although these preliminary results are encouraging, further studies are needed to deepen the relationship between fetal DV abnormalities and specific pathologies in dogs.

Authors' Contributions

GB, SF, and DG designed the study project and retrieved all data during the study period. GB, SF, DG and AP performed the clinical procedures. MF, GB, SF, and DG analyzed the data. The paper was written by GB, SF and DG. All authors read and approved the final manuscript.

Acknowledgments

The authors are thankful to the Faculty of Veterinary Medicine of University of Milan for providing facilities.

Competing Interests

The authors declare that they have no competing interests.

References

1. Kiresud, T., Eik-Nes, S.H., Blaas, H.G. and Hellevik, L.R. (1992a) Foramen ovale: An ultrasonographic study of its relation to the inferior vena cava, ductus venosus and hepatic veins. *Ultrasound Obstet. Gynecol.*, 2: 389-396.
2. Kiresud, T., Eik-Nes, S.H., Blaas, H.G., Hellevik, L.R. and Simensen, B. (1992b) Ductus venosus. A longitudinal Doppler velocimetric study of the human fetus. *J. Mater. Fetal Invest.*, 11: 2-5.
3. Panarace, M., Garnil, C., Cané, L., Rodriguez, E. and Medina, M. (2008) Echo-Doppler assessment of resistance and velocity of blood flow in the ductus venosus throughout gestation in fetal lambs. *Theriogenology*, 70: 648-654.
4. Tchirikov, M., Eisermann, K., Rybakowski, C. and Schroder, H.J. (1998) Doppler ultrasound evaluation of ductus venosus blood flow during acute hypoxemia in fetal lambs. *Ultrasound Obstet. Gynecol.*, 11: 426-431.
5. Barella, G., Faverzani, S., Faustini, M., Groppetti, D. and Pecile, A. (2014) Doppler ultrasonographic evaluation of ductus venosus blood flow in 55 canine fetuses. *J. Ultrasound*, 17: 287-292.
6. Vade, A., Lim-Dunham, J. and Iqbal, N. (2001) Imaging of the ductus venosus in neonates. *J. Ultrasound Med.*, 20: 681-687.
7. Turan, O.M., Turan, S., Berg, C., Gembruch, U., Nicolaides, K.H., Harman, C.R. and Baschat, A.A. (2011) Duration of persistent abnormal ductus venosus flow and its impact of perinatal outcome in fetal growth restriction. *Ultrasound Obstet. Gynecol.*, 8: 295-302.
8. Concannon, P., Hansel, W. and McEntee, K. (1977) Changes in LH, progesterone and sexual behavior associated with preovulatory luteinisation in the bitch. *Biol. Reprod.*, 7: 604-613.
9. Michel, E., Spörri, M., Ohlerth, S. and Reichler, I. (2011) Prediction of parturition date in the bitch and queen. *Reprod. Domest. Anim.*, 46: 926-939.
10. Brugger, N., Otzdorff, C., Walter, B., Hoffmann, B. and Braun, J. (2011) Quantitative determination of progesterone (P4) in canine blood serum using an enzyme-lined fluorescence assay. *Reprod. Domest. Anim.*, 46: 870-873.
11. Groppetti, D., Vegetti, F., Bronzo, V. and Pecile, A. (2015) Breed-specific fetal biometry and factors affecting the prediction of whelping date in the German shepherd dog. *Anim. Reprod. Sci.*, 152: 117-122.
12. Kutzler, M.A., Yeager, A.E., Mohammed, H.O. and Meyers-Wallen, V.N. (2003) Accuracy of canine parturition date prediction using fetal measurements obtained by ultrasonography. *Theriogenology*, 60: 1309-1317.
13. Zone, M.A. and Wanke, M.M. (2011) Diagnosis of canine fetal health by ultrasonography. *Reproduction*, 57: 215-219.
14. Yeager, A.E. and Concannon, P.W. (1990) Association between the preovulatory luteinizing hormone surge and the early ultrasonographic detection of pregnancy and fetal heartbeats in beagle dogs. *Theriogenology*, 34: 655-665.
15. Martins, W.P. and Kiresud, T. (2013) How to record ductus venosus blood velocity in the second half of pregnancy. *Ultrasound Obstet. Gynecol.*, 42: 245-245.
16. Maiz, N., Kagan, K.O., Milovanovic, Z., Celik, E. and Nicolaides, K.H. (2008) Learning curve for Doppler assessment of ductus venosus flow at 11 + 0 to 13 + 6 weeks' gestation. *Ultrasound Obstet. Gynecol.*, 31: 503-506.
17. Blanco, P.G., Rodriguez, R., Olguin, S., Rubea, A., Tortora, M. and Gobello, C. (2014) Doppler ultrasonographic assessment of maternal and fetal arteries during normal feline gestation. *Anim. Reprod. Sci.*, 146: 63-69.
18. Di Salvo, P., Bocci, F., Zelli, R. and Polisca, A. (2006) Doppler evaluation of maternal and fetal vessels during normal gestation in the bitch. *Res. Vet. Sci.*, 81: 382-388.
19. Scotti, L., Di Salvo, P., Bocci, F., Pieramati, C. and Polisca, A. (2008) Doppler evaluation of maternal and foetal vessels during normal gestation in queen. *Theriogenology*, 69: 1111-1119.
20. Gallarreta, F.M.P., Martins, W.P., Nastri, C.O., Filho, F.M., Nicolau, L.G.C., Barra, D.A., Morais, E.N. and Crott, G.C. (2011) Evaluation of ductus venosus and inferior vena cava by using multiple Doppler ultrasound parameters in healthy fetuses. *Arch. Gynecol. Obstet.*, 283: 959-963.
21. Gilani, S.A., Javaid, A. and Bala, A.A. (2010) Fetal Doppler ultrasound assessment of ductus venosus in a 20-40 weeks gestation normal fetus in the Pakistani population. *Med. Ultrasound*, 12: 110-113.
22. Merz, W.M., Kubler, K., Fimmers, R., Willruth, A., Stoffel-Wagner, B. and Gembruch, U. (2013) Cardiorenal syndrome is present in human fetuses with severe, isolated urinary tract malformations. *PLoS One*, 8(5): 63664.

32

Clinical and ultrasonographic observations of functional and mechanical intestinal obstruction in buffaloes (*Bubalus bubalis*)

Arafat Khalphallah[1], Nasr-Eldin M. Aref[1], Enas Elmeligy[2] and Sayed F. El-Hawari[3]

1. Department of Animal Medicine, Faculty of Veterinary Medicine, Assiut University, Assiut, Egypt; 2. Veterinary Teaching Hospital, Faculty of Veterinary Medicine, Assiut University, Assiut, Egypt; 3. Department of Surgery, Anesthesiology and Radiology, Faculty of Veterinary Medicine, Sohag University, Sohag, Egypt.
Corresponding author: Nasr-Eldin M. Aref, e-mail: nasreldeen.aref@vet.au.edu.eg,
AK: arafatvet2003@yahoo.com, EE: enaselmeligy@yahoo.com, SFE: newvet911@yahoo.com

Abstract

Aim: This study was designed for clinical and laboratory evaluation of intestinal obstruction (IO) in buffaloes *(Bubalus bubalis)* with special emphasis on the diagnostic value of ultrasonographic findings.

Materials and Methods: A total number of 30 buffaloes were included in the study and divided into 2 groups: Healthy (n=10) and diseased group (n=20). Diseased buffaloes were admitted to the Veterinary Teaching Hospital at Assiut University, Egypt, with a history of anorexia, abdominal pain, various degrees of abdominal distention, and absence or presence of scanty mucoid faces. These animals were subjected to clinical and ultrasonographic as well as laboratory examinations.

Results: Based on ultrasonographic findings, various forms of IO were diagnosed. Functional obstruction, paralytic ileus, was diagnosed in 17 cases (85%) while mechanical IO was diagnosed only in 3 cases (15%). Out of 17 cases of paralytic ileus, both proximal and distal ileuses were successfully imaged in 8 and 9 cases, respectively. Proximal ileus was imaged from the right dorsal flank region as a single dilated loop of diameter >6 cm, while distal ileus was imaged as multiple dilated loops of diameter <6 cm. Mechanical obstruction due to duodenal intussusception was visualized as two concentric rings with outer echogenic wall and hypoechoic lumen. All cases of IO showed leukocytosis, hypoproteinemia, and increased activity of alkaline phosphatase and aspartate aminotransferase.

Conclusion: Ultrasonography proved to be an essential tool for diagnosis and differential diagnosis of various forms of IO in buffaloes.

Keywords: buffalo, ileus, intestine, intussusception, ultrasonography.

Introduction

Intestinal obstruction (IO) represents an abdominal emergency that is potentially life-threatening to the affected animals. It is seen in all large animal species but is most common in horses [1]. Cattle are the most commonly affected ruminants and diagnosis in sheep and goats is rare (except for intestinal volvulus in lambs) [1]. According to our best knowledge, few available data about IO in buffaloes with no exact monitoring figure for its incidence or prevalence in Egypt.

Two common types of IO that interrupt the flow of ingesta have been recognized in large ruminants: Mechanical and functional [1,2]. Mechanical IO occurs due to a wide variety of causes and is characterized as being luminal or extraluminal. Luminal obstructions include hemorrhagic jejunitis (jejunal occlusion with blood clots); phytobezoars; cecocolic

volvulus; impacted ingesta and atresia coli, recti, and ani. Extraluminal obstructions include intussusceptions, strangulation, and volvulus of the gastrointestinal tract as well as intestinal compression with an expanding abdominal mass such as lymphosarcoma or fat necrosis [3-5].

Unlike mechanical obstruction; functional obstruction, called ileus or paralytic ileus, occurs because of cessation of peristalsis movement of the intestinal tract. The inciting cause of functional obstruction is not well determined; however, they are often associated with dietary or management factors, phytobezoars, parasite infection, enteritis, peritonitis, or electrolyte abnormalities [1]. Paralytic ileus has no gross abnormality but is characterized by generalized intestinal hypomotility or atony. This condition occurs more frequently than mechanical obstruction and is common in pregnant and recently parturient cows [1]. Recently, this syndrome has been reported in camels [6] and buffalos [7]. Animals with paralytic ileus show unspecific clinical signs and rectal findings [2].

IO may compose a large proportion of abdominal emergency situations for the bovine specialists, and may occur under different management conditions that put challenges in making a definitive diagnosis. Although the case history, signalment, and physical examination are important to formulate a tentative diagnosis, other diagnostic tools such as radiography and ultrasonography should be included to reach an accurate diagnosis and an effective therapeutic plan in a timely and orderly manner.

Therefore, this study was designed to clinical and laboratory evaluate the syndrome of IO in buffaloes *(Bubalus bubalis)* with special emphasis on the diagnostic value of ultrasonographic findings.

Materials and Methods

Ethical approval

The present study was approved by the Institutional Animal Ethics Committee of The Faculty of Veterinary Medicine at Assiut University.

Animals

The study was carried out on 30 buffaloes of different ages and sex. They were divided into two groups: Control group (n=10) and diseased group (n=20). The control group was selected from healthy non-pregnant female buffaloes belonged to a herd at the Veterinary Teaching Hospital (VTH), Faculty of Veterinary Medicine, Assiut University, Egypt. The diseased buffaloes were admitted to the VTH with a history of anorexia, decrease fecal output, and abdominal pain. Various degrees of abdominal distention, mucoid scanty faces, and reduction of milk production separately or collectively were also reported in some cases. All Institutional and National Guidelines for the care and use of animals were followed.

Clinical examination

All buffaloes underwent a thorough clinical examination according to Cockcroft [8]. The general condition and demeanor, rectal temperature, heart rate, respiratory rate, and lung sounds were determined. Swinging and/or percussion auscultation on both sides of the abdomen and tests for a reticular foreign body and rectal palpation were also carried out. Animals were treated in accordance with guidelines established by the Faculty of Veterinary Medicine atAssiut University.

Ultrasonographic examination

Ultrasonographic examination was performed according to Braun and Marmier [9]. Briefly, The small intestine (SI) of was examined ultrasonographically with a 3.5 MHz sector transducer (FF Sonic, Model UF-4000, Tokyo, Japan). Buffaloes were examined on the right side, from the tuber coxae to the eighth intercostal space (ICS) and from the transverse processes of the vertebrae to the linea alba. The appearance of loops of SI and their contents and motility were assessed.

Blood sampling

Whole blood and serum samples were collected, and all precautions of sample collections and preparation for accurate evaluation of hematological and biochemical indices were taken into consideration according to Otter [10].

Complete blood count assessment

A fully automated blood cell counter machine, Medonic CA620 Vet hematology analyzer–Sweden, was used to determine various hematological parameters. The differential leukocyte count was determined using four field meander method.

Biochemical assays

A spectrophotometric method was adopted to determine serum concentrations of liver enzymes: Aspartate aminotransferase (AST), gamma-glutamyl transferase (γGT), alkaline phosphatase (ALP), and serum total protein. All kits and reagents were obtained from Spectrum Reagents (Egyptian Company for Biotechnology, Egypt).

Statistical analysis

Data were analyzed using SPSS statistical software packaged program for windows version 10.0.1 (SPSS Inc., Chicago, IL, USA). All data were presented as mean±standard deviation. Analysis of variance of (one-way ANOVA) was performed and the significance level was set at $p \leq 0.05$.

Results

Clinical signs

The clinical signs varied according to nature of IO. Two conditions have been identified in this study (Table-1): Mechanical obstruction due to intussusceptions and paralytic ileus.

All admitted cases showed some degree of depression, anorexia, and cessation of ruminal motility. Rectal examination revealed empty rectum and the presence of mucus and dilated loop(s) of the intestine. Buffaloes with intestinal intussusception showed signs of abdominal pain, lack of defecation, and lethargy but no abdominal distention. Rectal findings could not detect intussusception; however, distended loops of the SI were palpable. Slight systemic changes, including elevated heart rate (90±5 beats/min), respiratory rate (32±7/min), and congested mucous membranes, were observed. Buffaloes with paralytic ileus showed slight abdominal distension, absent peristalsis, and marked reduction of defecation. Ballottement with simultaneous auscultation and percussion of the right abdominal cavity revealed ping sound in four cases. Rectal palpation was unspecific; however, distended intestinal loop was palpable.

Table-1: Classification of intestinal obstruction in buffaloes based on ultrasonography findings.

Group	Number
I. Control	10
II. Disease	20
A. Mechanical obstruction	
Intussusception of duodenum	3
B. Paralytic ileus alone	
Distal ileus of the SI with partial obstruction	4
Distal ileus of the SI with complete obstruction	5
Proximal ileus with complete obstruction of SI	3
Proximal ileus with partial obstruction of SI	5

SI=Small intestine

Ultrasonographic findings

Ultrasonographic examination of the intestinal tract of the control group was conducted to setup a reference image on comparing with the diseased ones. Intestinal tract was imaged from the right flank region at different points of the last ICSs. The duodenum appeared as echogenic envelope with a diameter of 1.5-4 cm (Figure-1a) while the jejunum and ileum were imaged as loops with two echogenic wall in cross section with echoic or hypoechoic contents with a diameter of 2.5-4.2 cm (Figure-1b). The two walls (closest and furthest ones) of the SI were imaged as an echogenic wall. The cecum, proximal loop of the colon, and the spiral colon could be clearly imaged from the right flank region. The closest wall of the proximal loop of colon and cecum was imaged as a continuous or slightly curved echogenic line while the furthest wall of cecum and colon could not be imaged (Figure-1c).

In diseased animals, two types of IO were identified based on ultrasound findings: Functional and mechanical. Cases of functional obstruction, ileus of the SI (n=17), could be distal at the area of the jejunum and ileum (distal ileus, n=9) or proximal at the area of the duodenum (proximal ileus, n=8) (Table-1). Ultrasonogram in distal ileus revealed the presence of multiple dilated loops of the jejunum and ileum with a diameter (Ø) of < 6 cm (4.5-6 cm), two hyperechoic walls and echoic contents (Figure-2a and b). The peristaltic movement was either reduced (partial obstruction, n=4) or cessated (complete obstruction, n=5) with empty post-stenotic loops of the ileum and jejunum with anechoic contents (Figure-2c).

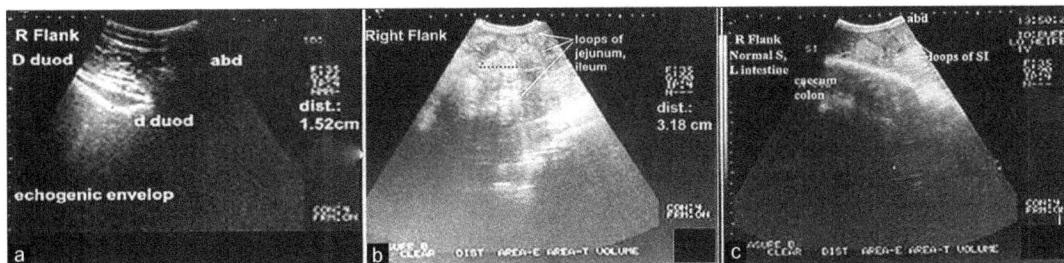

Figure-1: Ultrasonogram in 3-year-old healthy female buffalo imaged from right flank showed the descending part of duodenum of 1.5-4 cm Ø (echogenic wall and envelope) (a); loops of jejunum and ileum (two echogenic wall with echoic or hypoechoic contents and of 2.5-4.2 cm Ø) (b), and proximal loop of cecum and colon (c).

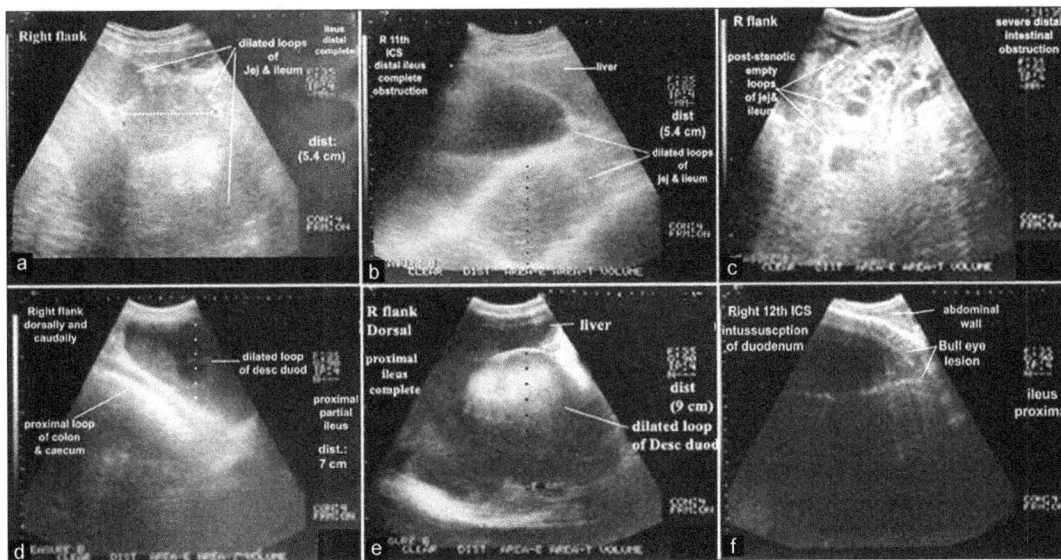

Figure-2: Ultrasonogram in a buffalo-heifer imaged from the right 11th intercostal spaces (ICSs) and the right flank (RF) region suffered from distal ileus with complete obstruction. Small intestine showed multiple dilated loops of <6 cm Ø, two hyperechoic walls, echoic contents (a and b) and empty post-stenotic loops of ileum and jejunum with anechoic contents (c). Ultrasonogram in 5-year-old female buffalo imaged from the dorsal RF suffered from proximal ileus and partial obstruction (d) showed cross section (CS) in a dilated loop of the duodenum of >6 cm Ø (echogenic wall and envelope) with hypoechoic contents and anechoic lumen. Ultrasonogram in buffalo-bull suffered from proximal ileus with complete obstruction imaged from the ventral RF, middle 10th and 11th ICSs and caudodorsal RF showed CS in dilated loop of descending duodenum with cessation of the peristaltic movement (e). Ultrasonogram in 4-year-old buffalo-bull imaged from the RF showed CS dilated loop of the duodenal intussusception. Intussusception was visualized as two concentric rings with outer echogenic wall and hypoechoic lumen then inner highly reflective rings with anechoic center (f).

On the other hand, ultrasonogram of proximal ileus showed the presence of one dilated loop of the duodenum with a diameter of >6 cm (Figure-2d and e). In proximal ileus with partial obstruction, the dilated loop of the descending part of the duodenum was clearly visualized as echogenic wall and envelop with hypoechoic contents and anechoic lumen (Figure-2d) along with the observation of normal loops of the jejunum and ileum as well as the proximal loop of the colon. The peristaltic movement was reduced. The dilated loop of the descending duodenum did not interfere with the liver or obscure the right kidney. In proximal ileus with complete obstruction (Figure-2e) dilated loop of the duodenum was imaged from the right with visualization of empty loops of the SI and complete reduction of the peristaltic movement of the SI.

Table-2: Mean values±standard deviation of blood picture and serum biochemical indices in control and diseased buffaloes.

Parameter	Control	IO
T. WBCs (G/L)	6.71±1.63	17.35±3.6*
Neutrophils (%)	26.4±9.13	28.09±4.49
Lymphocytes (%)	60.80±7.73	48.42±6.69*
Monocytes (%)	7.80±4.63	19.04±2.6*
Eosinophils (%)	3.60±2.07	3.25±1.5
Band cells (%)	1.40±0.52	1.2±0.42
Total proteins (g/L)	94.7±10.7	68.9±5.9*
γGT (U/L)	14.95±5.23	18.14±3.03
ALP (U/L)	36.11±8.40	71.46±7.54*
AST (U/L)	32.92±4.77	84.34±8.92*

IO=Intestinal obstruction, T. WBC=Total white blood cell, γGT=Gamma-glutamyl transferase, ALP=Alkaline phosphatase, AST=Aspartate aminotransferase. *Significant ($p < 0.05$)

Buffaloes with mechanical IO (n=3) due to intussusception were imaged from the right flank region in cross section as bull's eyes lesion or bowel within bowel lesion (Figure-2f). The bull's eyes lesion was visualized as two concentric rings with outer echogenic wall and hypoechoic lumen then inner highly reflective rings with the anechoic center.

Blood picture and serum biochemical analysis (Table-2)

The hematological profiles in IO showed a significant increase ($p < 0.05$) in the total leukocyte count. The population of individual WBC showed a significant decrease ($p < 0.05$) in the percentage of lymphocytes and significant increase ($p < 0.05$) in the percentage of monocytes. On the other hand, blood serum biochemical levels showed significant decrease $p < 0.05$) in serum total protein and significant increase $p < 0.05$) in blood serum activities of AST and ALP.

Discussion

IO represents an abdominal emergency that is potentially life-threatening to the affected animals. IO could be tentatively diagnosed based on the results of the clinical examination. The first alarming sign associated with all admitted cases was no or significant reduction of fecal output, and the presence of mucus covering the figured fecal matter. Laboratory findings showed leukocytosis and hypoproteinemia, which could be attributed to prolonged anorexia, stress, and pain associated with IO [11]. The significant increase in the serum activities of AST and ALP could be attributed tissue destruction associated with intussusception [12]. These

Table-3: Differential diagnosis of various forms of intestinal obstruction in buffaloes based on ultrasonography findings.

Parameters	Intussusception	Proximal ileus obstruction		Distal ileus obstruction	
		Partial	Complete	Partial	Complete
Sites of the probe					
	Right abdominal side, from the tuber coxae to the 8th ICS and from the transverse processes of the vertebrae to the linea alba				
Ultrasonogram					
Duodenum	Multiple concentric rings (Bull eye's lesion), One loop >6 cm Ø	One dilated loop>6 cm Ø (9-15 cm)	One dilated loop> 6 cm Ø (9-15 cm)	Imaged normal	Nonvisualized
Jejunum and ileum	Imaged normal	Imaged normal	Nonvisualized	Multiple dilated loops<6 cm Ø (4.5-<6 cm)	Multiple dilated loops <6 cm Ø (4.5-<6 cm) Empty post-stenotic loops
Large intestine	Not imaged	Imaged normal	Not imaged	Imaged normal	Not imaged
Right kidney	Not imaged	Imaged normal	Not imaged	Imaged normal	Not imaged
Liver	Affection was intertangled with liver dorsally and occupied the ventral part of the last R-3 ICSs	Imaged Normal	Affection was intertangled with liver dorsally and occupied the ventral part of the last R-3 ICSs	Imaged normal	Affection was intertangled with liver dorsally and occupied the ventral part of the last R-3 ICSs
Peristaltic movement of SI	Reduced	Reduced	Ceased	Reduced	Ceased

ICSs=Intercostal spaces, SI=Small intestine

findings may have limited value in IO, and they do not reflect the exact diagnosis. Ultrasonography is an essential tool for diagnosis of several abdominal disorders [13]. In this study, ultrasonography was applied to diagnose IO and evaluate its forms in buffaloes. Differential diagnosis of various forms of IO in buffaloes based on ultrasonography findings was presented in Table-3. Imaging of the intestinal tract could be successfully performed from the right flank over the last 3 ICS. The descending part of the duodenum in healthy animal had a diameter of 1.7-4 cm, and the loops of jejunum and ileum had diameters of 2.5-4.2 cm. The normal peristaltic movement of the SI was clearly demonstrated. These findings agreed with that reported by Braun [13] in cattle. The closest wall of the proximal loop of the colon and cecum was also clearly imaged from right flank over the last 3 ICS as a continuous or slightly curved echogenic line while the furthest wall could not be imaged. Similar findings were reported by Braun and Amrein [14] in healthy cows.

In comparison with healthy animals, ultrasound examination of IO due to ileus revealed different diameters and number of dilated loops of the duodenum, jejunum, and ileum according to the site of ileus. Proximal ileus showed the presence of one to five dilated loops of diameter >6 cm (9-15 cm) while distal ileus showed the presence of more than 5 dilated loops of diameter <6 cm (4.5-6 cm). These findings were in agreement with several studies conducted on cattle [15]. The authors reported that the larger diameter of dilated loops of SI; the more ileus of the proximal part of SI was indicated. In cows with proximal ileus, distal ileus at the jejunum and distal ileus at the ileum, the diameter of the intestine measured from the last right ICS varied from 6.5-9.9, 3.5-9.8, and 4.4-5.5 cm, respectively.

Mechanical obstruction due to intussusception of SI was also imaged just caudal to the last rib or last ICS at the level of the dorsal right flank region in a cross section as bull's eye lesions. The bull's eye lesions were visualized as two concentric rings with outer echogenic wall and hypoechoic lumen then inner highly reflective rings with the anechoic center. This ultrasonographic description agreed with that described in cattle [7,16]. The number of the dilated loops was only one loop at the site of intussusceptions suggests that the intussusception is in the duodenum.

Partial versus complete obstruction of the SI refers to the reduction or absence of peristaltic movement, respectively. In both proximal and distal partial obstruction, large intestine and right kidney could be visualized while they could not be imaged in the case of complete obstruction because dilated loops of the SI fully occupied the right flank region and the ventral part of the last right three ICS, and intertangled with liver lobes dorsally.

Conclusion

It could be concluded that ultrasonography is a necessary tool for diagnosis of IO and to describe the nature and site of obstruction in buffaloes. The obtained results also suggested that functional obstruction (paralytic ileus) is a common form of IO in buffaloes.

Authors' Contributions

Authors have formulated the research plan. AK and NMA conducted clinical and ultrasonography examination, samples collection and analysis, and recorded the information. EE provided help in the analysis of data. SE helped in ultrasonography examination. AK drafted the manuscript and NMA revised it. All authors read and approved the final manuscript.

Acknowledgments

The authors are grateful to the Director of Veterinary Teaching Hospital and Head Department of Animal Medicine at Assiut University for their kind support during conducting this study.

Competing Interests

The authors declare that they have no competing interests.

References

1. Kahn, C.M. and Line, S. (2010) Overview of acute intestinal obstructions in large animals. In: eBook Merck Veterinary Medicine Manual. 10th ed. Merck & Co., Whitehouse Station, NJ.
2. Radostits, O.M., Gay, C.C., Hinchcliff, K.W. and Constable, P.D., editors. (2007) Diseases of the alimentary tract. Veterinary Medicine: A Textbook of the Diseases of Cattle, Horses, Sheep, Pigs and Goats. 10th ed. Saunders, Elsevier, Philadelphia, PA. p189-382.
3. Smith, B.P. (2014) Large Animal Internal Medicine. 5th ed. Mosby, St. Louis. p820.
4. Dharmaceelan, S., Rajendran, N., Nanjappan, K., Subramanian, M. and Balasubramaniam, G.A. (2012) Incidence of bovine gastrointestinlal obstruction in a teaching veterinary hospital of Tamilnadu, India. *Int. J. Vet. Sci.*, 1(3): 112-114.
5. Hussain, S.A., Uppal, S.K., Randhawa, C.S. and Sood, N.K. (2015) Bovine intestinal obstruction: Blood gas analysis, serum C-reactive protein and clinical, haematological and biochemical alterations. *J. Appl. Anim. Res.*, 43(2): 224-230.
6. Tharwat, M., Al-Sobayil, F. and Ali, A. (2012) Ultrasonographic evaluation of abdominal distension in 52 camels *(Camelus dromedarius)*. *Res. Vet. Sci.*, 93: 448-456.
7. Tharwat, M. (2011) Diagnostic ultrasonography in cattle and buffaloes with intestinal obstruction. *J. Agric. Vet. Sci.*, 4(1): 67-80.
8. Cockcroft, P. (2015) Diagnosis and clinical reasoning in cattle practice. In: Bovine Medicine. 3rd ed. John Wiley & Sons, Ltd., New Jersey. p124-132.
9. Braun, U. and Marmier, O. (1995) Ultrasonographic examination of the small intestine of cows. *Vet. Rec.*, 36: 239-244.
10. Otter, A. (2013) Diagnostic blood biochemistry and haematology in cattle. *Practice*, 35(1): 7-16.
11. Weiss, D.G. and Wardrop, J.K. (2010) Interpretation of

ruminant leukocyte responses. In: Schalm's Veterinary Hematology. 6th ed. Blackwell Publishing Ltd., Oxford. p307-313.

12. Davoudi, S.M. (2013) Study of hepatic problems in livestock. *Eur. J. Zool. Res.,* 2(4): 124-132.

13. Braun, U. (2003) Ultrasonography in gastrointestinal disease in cattle. *Vet. J.,* 166(2): 112-124.

14. Braun, U. and Amrein, E. (2001) Ultrasonographic examination of the caecum and proximal and spiral loop of the colon of cattle. *Vet. Rec.,* 149: 45-48.

15. Braun, U., Marmier, O. and Pusterla, N. (1995) Ultrasonographic examination of the small intestine of cows with ileus of the duodenum, jejunum or ileum. *Vet. Rec.,* 137: 209-215.

16. Imran, S., Tyagi, S.P., Kumar, A., Kumar, V., Sharma, A. and Sharma, S. (2011) Usefulness and limitation of ultrasonography in the diagnosis of intestinal intussusception in cows. *Vet Med Int.,* 2011: 1-6.

PERMISSIONS

LIST OF CONTRIBUTORS

Yusuf Hüseyinoğlu
Department of Biology, Faculty of Science and Letters, Mersin University, Mersin, Turkey

Musa Ibrahim Waziri
Department of Veterinary Medicine Ahmadu Bello University, Zaria, Nigeria

Kaltungo Bilkisu Yunusa
Veterinary Teaching Hospital Ahmadu Bello University, Zaria, Nigeria

James. Higenyi and John. David. Kabasa
College of Veterinary Medicine, Animal Resources and Bio-security, Makerere University, Kampala, Uganda

Charles. Muyanja
College of Agriculture and Environmental Sciences, Makerere University, Kampala, Uganda

Hala Ali Abdel-Salam
Department of Zoology, Faculty of Science, Cairo University, Egypt

Anton Lazarinov Antonov and Plamen Ivanchev Georgiev
Department of Obstetrics, Reproduction and Reproductive Disorders, Faculty of Veterinary Medicine, Trakia University, 6000, Stara Zagora, Bulgaria

Department of Immunobiology of Reproduction, Institute of Biology and Immunology of Reproduction "Acad. K. Bratanov", Tzarigradsko shose 73, 1113 Sofia, Bulgaria

Julieta Dineva Dineva
Department of Immunobiology of Reproduction, Institute of Biology and Immunology of Reproduction "Acad. K. Bratanov", Tzarigradsko shose 73, 1113 Sofia, Bulgaria

Sunanda Sharma
Department of Veterinary Gynaecology and Obstetrics, College of Veterinary and Animal Science, Rajasthan University of Veterinary & Animal Sciences, Bikaner-334001, Rajasthan, India

Narendra K. Sharma
Divisional Mobile Veterinary Surgery and Infertility Unit, Animal husbandry Department, Government of Rajasthan, Bikaner, India

N. K. Sinha
Former Principal Scientist (Animal Reproduction), Central Institute for Research on Goats, Makhdoom, Mathura, Uttar Pradesh, India

S. S. Sharma
Former Professor and Head, Department of Veterinary Gynaecology and Obstetrics, College of Veterinary and Animal Science, Rajasthan University of Veterinary & Animal Sciences, Bikaner-334001, Rajasthan, India

Taghi Madadzadeh
Graduated from the Faculty of Veterinary Medicine, University of Islamic Azad, Urmia, Iran

Mohsen Nouri
Mehregan Veterinary Group, Tehran, Iran

Iradj Nowrouzian
Department of Clinical Sciences, Faculty of Veterinary Medicine, University of Tehran, Tehran, Iran

Gebremedhin Romha
Dilla University, College of Agriculture and Natural Resource, Department of Animal and Range Science, P.O. Box 419, Dilla, Ethiopia

Gebremedhin Gebre egziabher
Samera University, College of Veterinary Medicine, P.O. Box 132, Samera, Ethiopia

Gobena Ameni
Aklilu Lemma Institute of Pathobiology, Addis Ababa University, P.O. Box 1176, Addis Ababa, Ethiopia

Jaime Parejo Garcia
Researcher in Animal Behaviour and Specialized Instructor for Search and Rescue Dogs, Firefighter in Seville Town Hall, Spain

Philip Cheriose Nzien Alikwe
Animal Science Department, Niger Delta University, Yenagoa, Nigeria

Elijah Ige Ohimain
Biological Sciences Department, Niger Delta University, Yenagoa, Nigeria

Soladoye Mohammed Omotosho
SMO Laboratory Consult, 5 Joyce B Shopping Complex, Ibadan, Nigeria

Amira A. Goma
Dept. of Animal Husbandry and wealth development, Faculty of Veterinary Medicine, Alexandria University, Egypt

Usama E. Mahrous
Dept. of Animal Husbandry and wealth development, Faculty of Veterinary Medicine, Damanhour University, Egypt

Mohsen Nouri
Mehregan Veterinary Group, Tehran, Iran

Javad Ashrafi-Helan
Department of Pathology, Faculty of Veterinary Medicine, the University of Tabriz, Tabriz, Iran

James Higenyi
College of Medicine and Veterinary Medicine, University of Edinburgh, Scotland, England

John David Kabasa
Department of Biosecurity, Makerere University, Kampala, Uganda

U. M. Garba, A. Audu and E. U. Onwuhafua
Veterinary Clinic, Equitation Wing, Nigerian Defence Academy, Kaduna, Nigeria

M. Bisalla
Department of Veterinary Pathology, Faculty of Veterinary Medicine, Ahmadu Bello University Zaria, Nigeria

Luana Araújo Saraiva, Patrick Elvis Paraguaio, Morgana Santos Araújo, Sheila Vilarindo de Sousa and Luciana Pereira Machado1
University Federal of Piauí, Campus Professora Cinobelina Elvas, Bom Jesus, Piauí, Brazil

Tairon Pannunzio Dias e Silva
Center for Nuclear Energy in Agriculture, Animal Nutrition Laboratory, University of São Paulo, Piracicaba, São Paulo, Brazil

Ban-bo Bebanto Antipas and Nadjilem Digamtar
Faculty of Exact and Applied Sciences - University of N'Djamena

Bidjeh Kebkiba
Research Institute of Livestock Development

Alhaji Mahamat Souleymane
Office of Veterinary Services - Epidemiosupervision Network – OVS

Andarawous Ballah Tina
Institute of Agro-sylvo pastorals sciences

Mohsen Nouri, Alireza Vajhi, Iradj Nowrouzian and Davoud Faskhoudi
Department of Clinical Sciences, Faculty of Veterinary Medicine, the University of Tehran, Tehran, Iran

Seyyed Hossein Marjanmehr
Department of Pathology, Faculty of Veterinary Medicine, the University of Tehran, Tehran, Iran

Adane Haile
Department of Animal Science, Faculty of Agricultural Sciences, Wachemo University, P.O.Box: 667, SNNP, Ethiopia

Yisehak Tsegaye and Niguse Tesfaye
College of Veterinary Medicine, Mekelle University, Tigray, Ethiopia

Getahun Kebede Yadete
Department of Livestock Research, Debre Zeit Agricultural Research Center, Debre Zeit, Ethiopia

Hala Ali Abdel-Salam
Department of Zoology, Faculty of Science, Cairo University, Egypt

Meseret Gebreselama
Elfora Agro-industries export abattoir, Bishoftu, P. O. Box 2500, Bishoftu, Ethiopia

Fikre Zeru
College of Veterinary Medicine, Samara University, P.O. Box 132, Samara, Ethiopia

Gebremedhin Romha
Dilla University, College of Agriculture and Natural Resource, Department of Animal and Range Science, P.O. Box 419, Dilla, Ethiopia

Stanimir Angelov Yotov and Anatoli Stefanov Atanasov
Dept. of Obstetrics, Reproduction and Reproductive Disorders, Faculty of Veterinary Medicine, Trakia University, Stara Zagora, Bulgaria

Sibel YavruOguzhan Avci
Department of Virology, Faculty of Veterinary Medicine, University of Selcuk, 42075 Konya, Turkey

Mehmet Kale
Department of Virology, Faculty of Veterinary Medicine, University of Mehmet Akif Ersoy, Burdur, 15100, Turkey

Thyagarajan Desikan
Distance Education, Tamilnadu Veterinary and Animal Sciences University, Chennai, India

Barathi Megarajan
SRF, Directorate of Distance Education, Tamilnadu Veterinary and Animal Sciences University, Chennai, India

Oguzhan Avci and Sibel Yavru
Department of Virology, Faculty of Veterinary Medicine, University of Selcuk, 42075, Konya, Turkey

Mehmet Ekik
Virology Laboratory, Veterinary Control Institute, 42080, Konya, Turkey

James. Higenyi and John. David. Kabasa
College of Veterinary Medicine, Animal Resources and Bio-security, Makerere University, Kampala, Uganda

Charles. Muyanja
College of Agriculture and Environmental Sciences, Makerere University, Kampala, Uganda

Mohsen Nouri, Iradj Nowrouzian and Seyed Mohamad Karbalaee Seyed Javad
Department of Clinical Sciences, Faculty of Veterinary Medicine, the University of Tehran, Tehran, Iran

Fateme Katouli and Fahime Zibaee
Iranian Arad Pajouh Veterinary University Center, Tehran, Iran

Oguzhan Avci
Department of Virology, Faculty of Veterinary Medicine, University of Selcuk, Konya, Turkey

Burak Dik
Department of Pharmacology and Toxicology, Faculty of Veterinary Medicine, University of Selcuk, Konya, Turkey

Hala A. Abdel- Salam and Salwa A. H. Hamdi
Department of Zoology, Faculty of Science, Cairo University, Egypt

Vijay Kumar
Veterinary Officer, Monkey Sterilization centre, Gopalpur - Zoo, Palampur, Distt – Kangra, H.P, India

Vipin Kumar
Veterinary Officer, Monkey Sterilization centre, Saster Distt- Hamirpur, Himachal Pradesh, India

Hamid Karimi
Department of Basic science, Faculty of Veterinary Medicine, University of Tabriz, Tabriz, Iran

Hossein Daghigh Kia and Ali Hosseinkhani
Faculty of Agriculture, University of Tabriz, Tabriz, Iran

Gharari Kia
Department of Animal Science, Islamic Azad University, Germi, Iran

Ghasemi Mehdi and Radjabalizade Keyvan
Department of Biology, Islamic Azad University, Ardabil, Iran

Teppei Hirata, Yoshihito Yonahara, Faramarz Asharif and Shiro Tamaki
Department of Information Engineering, Faculty of Engineering, University of the Ryukyus, Nishihara town, Japan

Takeshi Miyagi, Tsutomu Omatsu and Tetsuya Mizutani
Research and Education Center for Prevention of Global Infectious Disease of Animals, Faculty of Agriculture, Tokyo University of Agriculture and Technology, Tokyo, Japan

Yasushi Shiroma and Yasunori Nagata
Department of Electrical and Electronic Engineering, Faculty of Engineering, University of the Ryukyus, Nishihara town, Japan

Safa Mohamed A/Wahab El-Tazi
Faculty of Agriculture, Omdurman Islamic University P.O. Box 382, Sudan

Talha ELsadig Abbas
Department of Animal Production, University of ALneelain, Khartoum, Sudan

Dejene Takele Gebissa
Oromia Agricultural Research Institute, Yabello Pastoral and Dryland Agriculture Research Center, Yabello, Ethiopia

Aaron Ross Flakemore and Peter David McEvoy
Animal Science and Genetics, Tasmanian Institute of Agriculture, School of Land and Food, Faculty of Science, Engineering and Technology, University of Tasmania, Private Bag 54 Sandy Bay, Hobart, Tasmania 7001, Australia

Razaq Oladimeji Balogun
Coprice Feeds, PO Box 104 Cobden, Victoria 3266, Australia

Bunmi Sherifat Malau-Aduli
School of Medicine and Dentistry, Faculty of Medicine, Health and Molecular Sciences, James Cook University, Townsville, Queensland 4811, Australia

Peter Nichols
Commonwealth Scientific and Industrial Research Organisation Food Futures Flagship, Division of Marine and Atmospheric Research, G.P.O. Box 1538, Hobart, Tasmania 7001, Australia

Aduli Enoch Othniel Malau-Aduli
Animal Science and Genetics, Tasmanian Institute of Agriculture, School of Land and Food, Faculty of Science, Engineering and Technology, University of Tasmania, Private Bag 54 Sandy Bay, Hobart, Tasmania 7001, Australia
School of Veterinary and Biomedical Sciences, Faculty of Medicine, Health and Molecular Sciences, James Cook University, Townsville, Queensland 4811, Australia

Index